AFFECTIVE DISORDERS AND THE FAMILY

THE GUILFORD FAMILY THERAPY SERIES
ALAN S. GURMAN, EDITOR

Affective Disorders and the Family: Assessment and Treatment
John F. Clarkin, Gretchen L. Haas, and Ira D. Glick, *Editors*

Families and Larger Systems: A Family Therapist's Guide through the Labyrinth
Evan Imber-Black

Family Transitions: Continuity and Change over the Life Cycle
Celia Jaes Falicov, *Editor*

Handbook of Family Therapy Training and Supervision
Howard A. Liddle, Douglas C. Breunlin, and Richard C. Schwartz, *Editors*

Marital Therapy: An Integrative Approach
William C. Nichols

Family Therapy Sourcebook
Fred P. Piercy, Douglas H. Sprenkle, and Associates

Systemic Family Therapy: An Integrative Approach
William C. Nichols and Craig A. Everett

Family Resources: The Hidden Partner in Family Therapy
Mark A. Karpel, *Editor*

Family Paradigms: The Practice of Theory in Family Therapy
Larry L. Constantine

Systems Consultation: A New Perspective for Family Therapy
Lyman C. Wynne, Susan H. McDaniel, and Timothy T. Weber, *Editors*

Clinical Handbook of Marital Therapy
Neil S. Jacobson and Alan S. Gurman, *Editors*

Marriage and Mental Illness: A Sex-Roles Perspective
R. Julian Hafner

Living through Divorce: A Developmental Approach to Divorce Therapy
Joy K. Rice and David G. Rice

Generation to Generation: Family Process in Church and Synagogue
Edwin H. Friedman

Failures in Family Therapy
Sandra B. Coleman, *Editor*

Casebook of Marital Therapy
Alan S. Gurman, *Editor*

Families and Other Systems: The Macrosystemic Context of Family Therapy
John Schwartzman, *Editor*

The Military Family: Dynamics and Treatment
Florence W. Kaslow and Richard I. Ridenour, *Editors*

Marriage and Divorce: A Contemporary Perspective
Carol C. Nadelson and Derek C. Polonsky, *Editors*

Family Care of Schizophrenia: A Problem-Solving Approach to the Treatment of Mental Illness
Ian R. H. Falloon, Jeffrey L. Boyd, and Christine W. McGill

The Process of Change
Peggy Papp

Family Therapy: Principles of Strategic Practice
Allon Bross, *Editor*

Aesthetics of Change
Bradford P. Keeney

Family Therapy in Schizophrenia
William R. McFarlane, *Editor*

Mastering Resistance: A Practical Guide to Family Therapy
Carol M. Anderson and Susan Stewart

Family Therapy and Family Medicine: Toward the Primary Care of Families
William J. Doherty and Macaran A. Baird

Ethnicity and Family Therapy
Monica McGoldrick, John K. Pearce, and Joseph Giordano, *Editors*

Patterns of Brief Family Therapy: An Ecosystemic Approach
Steve de Shazer

The Family Therapy of Drug Abuse and Addiction
M. Duncan Stanton, Thomas C. Todd, and Associates

From Psyche to System: The Evolving Therapy of Carl Whitaker
John R. Neill and David P. Kniskern, *Editors*

Normal Family Processes
Froma Walsh, *Editor*

Helping Couples Change: A Social Learning Approach to Marital Therapy
Richard B. Stuart

Affective Disorders and the Family

Assessment and Treatment

Edited by
JOHN F. CLARKIN, PhD
GRETCHEN L. HAAS, PhD
IRA D. GLICK, MD

Foreword by Gerald L. Klerman, MD

THE GUILFORD PRESS
New York   London

© 1988 The Guilford Press
A Division of Guilford Publications, Inc.
72 Spring Street, New York, NY 10012

Printed in the United States of America

Last digit is print number: 9 8 7 6 5 4 3 2 1

Library of Congress Cataloging in Publication Data

Affective disorders and the family : assessment and treatment / edited
    by John F. Clarkin, Gretchen L. Haas, Ira D. Glick.
        p. cm. — (The Guilford family therapy series)
    Includes bibliographies and index.
    ISBN 0-89862-101-1
    1. Affective disorders. 2. Affective disorders—Patients—Family
relationships. 3. Family psychotherapy. I. Clarkin, John F.
II. Haas, Gretchen, L. III. Glick, Ira D., 1935-   . IV. Series.
    [DNLM: 1. Affective Disorders—diagnosis. 2. Affective Disorders
—therapy. 3. Family Therapy. WM 207 A2563]
    RC537.A316 1988
    616.85′2—dc 19   87-28175
                                                              CIP

Contributors

MARVIN L. ADLAND, MD. Washington Psychoanalytic Institute, Washington, DC; and Department of Psychiatry, Georgetown University School of Medicine, Chevy Chase, Maryland

DUANE S. BISHOP, MD. Department of Psychiatry and Human Behavior, Brown University, Providence, Rhode Island; and Butler Hospital, Providence, Rhode Island

JOHN F. CLARKIN, PhD. Department of Psychiatry, Cornell University Medical College, New York, New York; and The New York Hospital—Cornell Medical Center, Westchester Division, White Plains, New York

JAMES C. COYNE, PhD. Department of Psychiatry and Family Practice, University of Michigan Medical School, Ann Arbor, Michigan

YOLANDE B. DAVENPORT, MSW. Chestnut Lodge Hospital, Rockville, Maryland

KEITH S. DOBSON, PhD. Department of Psychology, University of British Columbia, Vancouver, British Columbia, Canada

JOHN DOCHERTY, MD. Nashua Brookside Hospital, Nashua, New Hampshire

NATHAN B. EPSTEIN, MD. Department of Psychiatry and Human Behavior, Brown University, Providence, Rhode Island; and Parkwood Hospital, New Bedford, Massachusetts

IAN R. H. FALLOON, MD. Buckingham Mental Health Service, Buckingham, England

IRA D. GLICK, MD. Department of Psychiatry, Cornell University Medical College, New York, New York; and The New York Hospital—Payne Whitney Clinic, New York, New York

GRETCHEN L. HAAS, PhD. Department of Psychiatry, Cornell University Medical College, New York, New York; and The New York Hospital—Payne Whitney Clinic, New York, New York

VICTOR HOLE, RMN. Buckingham Mental Health Service, Buckingham, England

NEIL S. JACOBSON, PhD. Department of Psychology, University of Washington, Seattle, Washington

GABOR I. KEITNER, MD. Department of Psychiatry and Human Behavior, Brown University, Providence, Rhode Island; and Butler Hospital, Providence, Rhode Island

MELVIN R. LANSKY, MD. Department of Psychiatry, University of California at Los Angeles Medical School, Los Angeles, California; and Brentwood VA Medical Center, Los Angeles, California

IVAN W. MILLER, MD. Department of Psychiatry and Human Behavior, Brown University, Providence, Rhode Island; and Butler Hospital, Providence, Rhode Island

LESLEY MULROY, RMN. Buckingham Mental Health Service, Buckingham, England

LYNNE J. NORRIS, RMN. Buckingham Mental Health Service, Buckingham, England

TERENCE PEMBLETON, RMN. Buckingham Mental Health Service, Buckingham, England

STEVEN D. TARGUM, MD. Department of Psychiatry, University of South Florida School of Medicine, Tampa, Florida; and Sarasota Palms Hospital, Sarasota, Florida

JOYCE VICTOR, MSW, ACSW. Department of Psychology, University of Washington, Seattle, Washington

Foreword

This volume represents the confluence of three important trends in contemporary mental health research and practice: (1) the focus on individual illness or groups of disorders—in this case, affective disorders; (2) the maturation of family therapy as a therapeutic intervention; and (3) the "new wave" of psychotherapy research.

AFFECTIVE ILLNESS

The focus on affective illness is, itself, worthy of some note. Only recently have depression and related disorders been grouped together under the category of affective illness (or mood disorder). Previously, each condition was considered separately as either neurosis or psychosis. Since the turn of the century, the dominant principle for classifying nonorganic (or functional) mental illnesses has been the psychotic versus neurotic distinction. This approach had its roots in psychiatry's origin in asylums and other institutions, which were established by society for severely disturbed individuals.

As psychiatrists and other mental health professionals moved from institutional settings to diverse community settings, they treated patients with nonpsychotic features and, increasingly, patients who were never hospitalized—but in the community—who were distressed by symptoms of anxiety and depression, and/or partially or totally disabled by their mental symptoms.

The DSM-III was the first diagnostic system to establish affective disorders as a separate category. This change represented an acknowledgment of important research on the nature of these conditions as well as their treatment. These findings, primarily based on psychopharmacology, had rendered obsolete the psychotic–neurotic distinction. Thus, this volume recognizes and represents an important current trend in mental health professional life and psychopathology; namely, the focus on discrete groups of disorders—eating disorders, sexual dysfunctions, personality disorders—and the increasing differentiation of psychopathology and specificity of hypotheses and theories as to their causation and manifestation.

Grouping these disorders together as affective illness, or mood disorders, does not, however, imply a single causation. Rather, their common feature is the dominant presentation by the patient of symptoms of disturbance in affect or mood—usually depression, but also mania.

As the psychotic–neurotic distinction became less useful, other efforts to understand the nature of affective psychopathology and its treatment emerged. One example is the bipolar–unipolar distinction in depression in the DSM-III.

The affective disorders are among the most prevalent disorders in the community. Recent epidemiologic studies, particularly the Epidemiologic Catchment Area Study (ECA), corroborate that depression and affective disorders are common psychiatric disorders and that the majority of patients with depression are not in treatment. The patients in treatment, particularly in hospitals, represent only a small fraction of the population with these disorders, usually those who are most distressed and disabled.

THE MATURATION OF FAMILY THERAPY

Historically, psychiatry has been concerned, as has most of medicine, with the individual patient and his or her illness, diagnosis, and treatment. After World War II, as the influence of the social and behavioral sciences increased, attention was given to the social context of the patient's illness. Particular concern was with the family, but interest also focused on the neighborhood, society, and culture.

A family orientation represents a direct extension of the concepts of interpersonal psychiatry. The interpersonal school, a distinctively American contribution to mental health, arose in the Washington–Baltimore area, primarily with the writings of Harry Stack Sullivan and clinical applications by gifted therapists such as Freida Fromm-Reichmann and others. Family orientation was rapidly combined with attempts at various forms of family treatment. Through the 1950s and 1960s, new forms of family intervention were proposed and were quickly diffused into clinical practice through writings, workshops, and seminars.

The initial focus was on the families of severely disturbed schizophrenics. The work of Lidz and Fleck, Wynne, Bateson and Jackson, and Bowen drew attention to problems in the interactions and communication of families with a schizophrenic member. Theories of family origin of schizophrenia emerged and became the center of intense discussion, but, unfortunately, of only limited empirical investigation.

It is, perhaps, inevitable that in the early stages of any new field, optimism and exaggerated claims are made. Currently, however, the field of family studies is considerably more modest in its claims and increasingly more systematic and rigorous in its empirical investigations. The claims for etiology are modest, and multiple factors (i.e., biological, cultural, and sociological) are acknowledged. This trend is evident in the area of family studies in "depression affective disorder," as represented in this volume.

THE "NEW WAVE" OF PSYCHOTHERAPY RESEARCH

In the late 1970s, there emerged a "new wave" of research on psychotherapy. Among its characteristics are: (1) increasing emphasis on studies of outcome and an awareness of the importance of public policy in establishing efficacy; (2) use of systematic designs, including comparative and random assignment studies, approximating the methodology in clinical trials originally developed in pharmacology and now increasingly being extended in all of medicine to include nonpharmacologic treatment (such as surgery) and individual and family psychotherapy; (3) increasing specification of the psychotherapy through the development of manuals, which specify and operationalize the therapist's activities; and (4) use of multiple outcome measures to assess various domains of change, including psychopathology, social functioning, interpersonal relations, personality, and intrafamilial patterns of behavior.

These three trends converge in this volume. Not only are there reports of new innovative forms of therapy focused on the family problems of depressed and affectively ill patients; but the approach of the volume is broad, rather than narrow—chapters on combined pharmacologic and family therapy are included, as well as discussions of genetic issues and cognitive and behavioral strategies. Taken together, these chapters reflect the increasing maturation and sophistication of the field and auger well for its combined future growth and development.

Gerald L. Klerman, MD
Cornell University Medical Center

Preface

There is tremendous enthusiasm today among both mental health researchers and practitioners for the development of a more sophisticated differential therapeutics. Due to some of the technological advances of the '70s and '80s, the field is fast approaching this level of sophistication. Developmental milestones include: (1) construction of a more reliable diagnostic system; (2) operationalized definitions of treatment; (3) systematic comparison studies of specific treatments for specific disorders; and (4) progress toward the goal of developing refined algorithms for assigning patients to the most appropriate treatments. This volume represents the integration of knowledge about affective disorders, family interventions, and the most optimal matching of treatment to disorder currently in practice. By way of introduction, we will begin by presenting a few ideas about each of these variables.

DIAGNOSTIC SPECIFICITY

The Diagnostic and Statistical Manual of Mental Disorders (DSM-III) (American Psychiatric Association, 1980) and now DSM-III-R (APA, 1987) is an imperfect but useful instrument which represents a major advance over its predecessors in terms of multiaxial description of the patient with behavioral terms that can be reliably used by clinicians in diverse settings. With its development, clinicians and researchers alike can communicate more effectively via DSM-III-R terminology. This "universal" terminology alone has improved reliability and inter-rater agreement regarding carefully defined patient groups. The multiaxial approach draws the clinician's attention not only to the symptom picture, but also to possible concurrent personality disorders, stressors in the social, family, and work environments, and to the individual's range of psychosocial functioning in the past. Family therapists have had a mixed reaction to the DSM-III-R, having traditionally eschewed a diagnostic focus on a single individual with preference given to viewing a problem from the perspective of the larger family unit. We share their opinion of the value in viewing a disorder within the family or community context. However, we are also impressed with the value of searching for the commonalities of psychiatric disorders—across individuals and family contexts. Efforts to improve accuracy in defining and identifying patient problems can assist in the differential selection of specific family and individual interventions.

PSYCHOTHERAPY RESEARCH

Advances in the field of psychotherapy research have included the development of well-operationalized and descriptive psychotherapy manuals which more clearly define and delimit the therapy under investigation. State-of-the-art psychotherapy research calls for the use of these treatment manuals in the teaching and implementation of an experimental treatment. Many individual therapies have been manualized (e.g., Luborsky, 1984), including several for the individual treatment of affective disorders (Beck, Rush, Shaw, & Emery, 1979; Klerman, Weissman, Rounsaville, & Chevron, 1984). It is hoped that the major family interventions will eventually be manualized and investigated, and that these efforts will assist in training new family therapists and in clarifying approaches for the experienced clinician. In this volume we have included family interventions for affective disorders that are manualized (e.g., Chapters 3 and 6) or which have reached the stage of manual description (Chapters 4 and 5).

DIFFERENTIAL THERAPEUTICS

Finally, differential therapeutics (Frances, Clarkin, & Perry, 1984), that is, the clinical art of appropriately and efficiently matching the treatment to the individual needs and problems of the patient, will profit from both the development of a diagnostic typology and the use of manualized treatments. The work presented in this volume has been selected with the aim of assisting the clinician in choosing the most optimal treatment format (family, marital, group, or individual) and strategies (e.g., cognitive, behavioral, psychoeducational, strategic, etc.) for the individual with affective disorder and his or her family.

As the field progresses toward more precise and reliable diagnostic description of the patient, more detailed description of the treatments, and more optimal matching of patient and treatment, we can identify a "central theme" in this process: the search for specificity. Global notions regarding pathology, family interaction and family dynamics, and family interventions are no longer sufficient. The art of therapeutic intervention with psychiatric difficulties will advance to the science of assessment and intervention by increasing the specificity of both our diagnostic descriptions and the definition of the goals, strategies, and techniques of treatment. This volume represents an effort to advance the field of family treatments for affective disorders.

Chapter 1 surveys the salient dimensions of our theoretical models of affective disorders, many of which are relevant for family interventions. Chapter 2 recommends individual–family assessment procedures which can inform the clinician and researcher's understanding of the affective disorder. Chapters 3 and 4 describe current cognitive–behavioral and strategic marital interventions when one individual in a marital dyad is depressed. Chapters 5, 6, 7, and 8 describe family interventions when the patient is suffering from a major affective disorder, either major depression or bipolar disorder. Chapter 9 provides the clinician with current thoughts on genetic counseling when affective disorder is involved. In Chapter 10, an experienced clinician describes common clinical predicaments that face the family therapist who works with affectively ill families. And finally, in Chapter 11 the status of research evidence in this area is reviewed and comments about the future of research are made.

John F. Clarkin, Gretchen L. Haas, and Ira D. Glick

REFERENCES

American Psychiatric Association. (1980). *Diagnostic and statistical manual of mental disorders* (3rd ed.). Washington, DC: Author.

American Psychiatric Association. (1987). *Diagnostic and statistical manual of mental disorders* (3rd ed., rev.). Washington, DC: Author.

Beck, A. T., Rush, A. J., Shaw, B. F., & Emery, G. (1979). *Cognitive therapy of depression*. New York: Guilford Press.

Frances, A., Clarkin, J. F., & Perry, S. (1984). *Differential therapeutics in psychiatry: The art and science of treatment selection*. New York: Brunner/Mazel.

Klerman, G. L., Weissman, M. M., Rounsaville, B. J., & Chevron, E. S. (1984). *Interpersonal psychotherapy of depression*. New York: Basic Books.

Luborsky, L. (1984). *Principles of psychoanalytic psychotherapy: A manual for supportive-expressive treatment*. New York: Basic Books.

Contents

PART ONE. THE PSYCHOSOCIAL CONTEXT   1

Chapter 1. Affective Disorders and the Family Context   3
Gretchen L. Haas and John F. Clarkin
Introduction, 3
The Family Therapy Field and the Treatment of Schizophrenia, 5
Current Developments in Research on Affective Disorders, 7
Personal Resources, 10
Stressful Life Circumstances, 13
Environmental Resources, 16
Type of Affective Illness and Interpersonal Context, 20
Relationship of Depression to Interpersonal Context, 21
Affective Illness and Indications for Family Intervention, 22
References, 24

Chapter 2. Assessment of Affective Disorders and
Their Interpersonal Contexts   29
John F. Clarkin and Gretchen L. Haas
Introduction, 29
Classification of Affective Disorders, 31
Goals and Targets of Assessment, 32
Interviewing Affectively Disordered Patients and Their Families, 34
Assessment of Affective Disorders, 35
Assessment of the Interpersonal Context, 41
Assessment as Therapeutic Role Induction, 46
References, 47

PART TWO. THERAPEUTIC STRATEGIES WITH COUPLES   51

Chapter 3. Integration of Cognitive Therapy and
Behavioral Marital Therapy   53
Keith S. Dobson, Neil S. Jacobson, and Joyce Victor
The Nature of Depression, 53
Cognitive and Marital Interventions in Depression, 65

Cognitive–Behavioral Marital Therapy and Depression, 72
Summary, 82
Acknowledgment, 83
References, 83

Chapter 4. Strategic Therapy   89
James C. Coyne
Biology, Classification of Depressive Disorders,
     and Marital Therapy, 90
Conceptualizing Depression in a Marital Context, 93
The Rationale for Working with Each Partner Separately, 95
Initial Interviewing, 97
Initial Interventions, 99
Specific Agenda and Focused Interventions, 100
Postscript: Paradox, Dependence on Marriage,
     and Divorce As a Solution, 110
References, 111

PART THREE. THERAPEUTIC STRATEGIES WITH FAMILIES   115

Chapter 5. Behavioral Family Therapy   117
Ian R. H. Falloon, Victor Hole, Lesley Mulroy,
Lynne J. Norris, and Terence Pembleton
Stress, Vulnerability, and Family Coping Behavior, 118
Behavioral Family Intervention Strategies: An Overview, 120
Behavioral Analysis of Affective Disturbance in the Family, 121
Functional Analysis: A Behavioral System, 123
Behavioral Family Intervention during Acute Affective
     Episodes, 125
Prevention of Episodes of Major Affective Disorders, 129
Conclusion, 132
References, 132

Chapter 6. Inpatient Family Intervention   134
John F. Clarkin, Gretchen L. Haas, and Ira D. Glick
Specific Hypotheses of Our Study, 135
Patients and Their Families, 136
Treatment Assignment, 137
Description of IFI, 137
Working Model of Affective Disorders, 138
Treatment Goals and Therapeutic Strategies of IFI, 138

Assessment Procedures, 139
Results, 140
Illustrative Cases, 142
Discussion of Results, 148
Guidelines for Future Research, 150
References, 152

Chapter 7. Combined Use of Pharmacological and
Family Therapy 153
Nathan B. Epstein, Gabor I. Keitner, Duane S. Bishop, and
Ivan W. Miller
Literature Review, 154
Empirical Findings, 154
Rationale of Treatment Approach, 157
Heterogeneity of Clinical Problems, 163
Clinical Experiences, 163
Conclusion, 171
References, 171

Chapter 8. Management of Manic Episodes 173
Yolande B. Davenport and Marvin L. Adland
Introduction, 173
Bipolar Illness and Its Symptomatology, 175
Review of the Literature, 180
Family Issues in the Treatment of Bipolar Patients, 182
The Bipolar Family as Patient, 183
Case Presentations, 187
Treatment Issues: Denial and Dependency, 192
Conclusion, 193
References, 194

Chapter 9. Genetic Issues in Treatment 196
Steven D. Targum
The Components of Psychiatric Genetic Counseling, 197
The Genetics of Depressive Disorders, 200
Clinical Issues in Psychiatric Genetics, 203
Future Prospects for Clinical Psychiatric Genetics, 209
References, 210

Chapter 10. Common Clinical Predicaments 213
Melvin R. Lansky
Mania, 216
Recurrent Unipolar Depression, 220

Borderline Personality Disorders, 224
The Problem of Suicide, 230
Conclusion, 235
References, 237

PART FOUR. ISSUES IN RESEARCH   239

Chapter 11. Family Intervention in Affective Illness:
A Review of Research   241
Gretchen L. Haas and John Docherty
Current Status of Research in the Field, 241
Conclusion, 248
References, 248

Index, 251

AFFECTIVE DISORDERS AND THE FAMILY

PART ONE

THE PSYCHOSOCIAL CONTEXT

The person is a living organism embedded in a complex, dynamic social network. When an affective disorder arises in an individual, it occurs within an interpersonal (marital, family, community) context and has repercussions for the family, friends, neighbors, and community. The practicing clinician must be alert to the psychosocial context of the affective disorder—the interpersonal environment within which the affective symptoms emerge, the dysfunctional patterns of interpersonal interaction associated with affective psychopathology, and the social network that can serve as a transitional supportive structure to facilitate recovery and change processes.

To achieve an integrated clinical approach to diagnosis and treatment, the clinician aims to identify the multiple causes of the condition and to consider various avenues of intervention—including those that involve important others in the individual's interpersonal network. This is nothing new to family therapists, for whom the interpersonal context is a *sine qua non*. What *is* new is the growing technical sophistication and expertise in the interpersonal approach to assessment and intervention with affective disorders. This section begins with a summary of recent advances in the theoretical and empirical literature on the interpersonal context of affective disorders (Chapter 1). The summary is followed by a discussion of tools and strategies for the assessment of the individual, the family, and the affective disorder (Chapter 2).

1

Affective Disorders and the Family Context

GRETCHEN L. HAAS
JOHN F. CLARKIN

INTRODUCTION

Approximately 20% of the people in the United States will experience clinical depression in their lifetime (President's Commission on Mental Health, 1978). Bipolar disorders will affect from 0.4% to 1.2% of the adult population. Many individuals with affective episodes are married, experience marital problems and conflicts, and have difficulty raising children. Yet, there is to our knowledge no volume, prior to this one, exclusively devoted to the topic of affective disorders and the family. Although the family therapy field has seen tremendous advances in the past 30 years, little direct attention, either clinical or empirical, has been paid to affective disorder within a family context—its diagnosis, interaction with family environmental factors, and treatment via family intervention. Why has there been such a lack of interest in affective disorder from the perspective of the patient and his or her family?

Historically, the family theoreticians have been—on both conceptual and procedural grounds—adverse to the practitioner's prominent focus on the individual patient. Individual diagnosis has been seen as the first step down the "royal road" to blaming the individual for what is viewed by family clinicians as essentially a "systems" problem, and to ignoring the contribution of interpersonal factors to the behavior of any one individual. Among family therapists, symptoms are viewed as having communication value and as serving a function in the dynamic balance of the family structure. This functionalist view of individual symptomatology has contributed an important perspective to our understanding of the interface of individual and family pathology. However, family theorists, too, are at risk of having a too narrow and highly particularistic view of symptoms. Most notable are cases in the family literature in which the identified patient rather clearly met diagnostic criteria for major affective disorder, although this was not documented or given prominence in the writing (or thinking?)

3

of the family therapist. Ironically, such insular thinking among family theorists and therapists only reinforces the schism between individual and family perspectives of psychopathology.

A second reason for the apparent neglect of family treatment for affective disorders is that family therapists have traditonally focused on treatment of the child, adolescent, or young adult patient who suffers from behavioral symptoms. Consequently, those patients that have received attention from family therapists have largely included anorectic, delinquent, or drug-abusing adolescents, young adults, and young schizophrenics living at home with family. In contrast to these disorders, which have a relatively early age of onset, affective disorders generally first occur during adulthood—in the early 40s for unipolar depression and in the late 20s for bipolar disorder. It has been only recently that researchers have felt relatively confident in diagnosing depression in children and adolescents, inasmuch as the symptoms are usually not clearly identifiable or exclusive in these age groups. In fact, it has been largely through the treatment of depression in married patients that the family therapist has made an entree into the field of treatment for the affective disorders (Chapters 3 and 4, this volume). Since depression in its clearest form occurs in adults, and since many adults with depression are married and have marital conflicts, it is not surprising that marital treatments are becoming a more frequently used mode of treatment for the depressive disorders.

Why did the early marital therapists not target the treatment of depressed adults and their spouses? The reasons for this developmental delay may be traced back to the specific origins of marital therapy and the environmental "niche" occupied by marital therapists within the larger field of mental health services. Early marital therapists were most frequently located in marriage and family clinics. Their treatments were almost exclusively reserved for problems characterized predominantly by marital conflict, with little emphasis on the singular symptomatology of an individual family member. The phenomenology of depression is such that the disorder appears to be located within the individual. Moreover, depressive symptoms tend to have an isolating effect on the individual. Depressed individuals often turn inward, blame themselves for their condition, and withdraw from interpersonal relations.

Given this general gestalt, depression—either symptom or syndrome— was one of the last problems that family therapists thought to explore from a family systems perspective. Coyne, Kahn, and Gotlib (1986) have noted that traditionally the mental health field as a whole has viewed depression and the other affective disorders as highly individual phenomena. Beck and colleagues (Beck, Rush, Shaw, & Emery, 1979) have conceptualized depression as the product of the individual's faulty perceptions and cognitions. Even behaviorists such as Lewinsohn (Lewinsohn, Hoberman, Teri, & Hautzinger, 1985) have tended to underestimate the interpersonal dimensions of affective disorder by discussing the social skill deficits of the individual, irrespective of the specific nature of environmental contingencies. Both viewpoints ignore the interrelatedness of individual cognitions, social skills, and the interpersonal context in which these skills are actualized.

THE FAMILY THERAPY FIELD AND THE TREATMENT OF SCHIZOPHRENIA

Unlike the affective disorders, schizophrenia was of early interest to major figures in the family movement, such as Bateson and his students, including Jackson, Weakland, Haley, Bowen, and Wynne. One has only to look at an early classic article by Gregory Bateson, D. D. Jackson, Jay Haley, and John Weakland, entitled "Toward a Theory of Schizophrenia" (1956), to see the then revolutionary view of symptoms of a major psychiatric disorder. In this article, the authors gave the outlines of a communication theory of the origin and nature of schizophrenia: Schizophrenia was viewed as the individual outcome of a characteristic pattern of repetitive family interaction. The schizophrenic was seen as an individual who had adapted to an environment where the most familiar sequences of interpersonal interaction were ambiguous and contradictory. The "double-bind" communication was exemplary of this pattern of interpersonal communication. The communication of the schizophrenic was considered by the larger society "unconventional" in nature, but, according to the communication theorists, it was, nonetheless, well adapted to the family context. Psychosis was viewed as the schizophrenic individual's way of coping with the perpetual double-binding communication of an overtly loving, yet subtly negating, mother. It was hypothesized that psychotic communications were sharp, pithy remarks that permitted the patient to transcend the confines of the double-bind situation and assume a position of relative control of the interpersonal situation.

The communication theory of schizophrenia represented a milestone in the history of psychopathology. It translated our understanding of major psychiatric disorders from the perspective of linear causality and disease models to "systems" models, which focused on the interpersonal, ecological, and transactional functions of a disorder. Nonetheless, these systems models also proved overly simplistic, in that they failed to take into account important biological factors that are primary in the etiology of the illness and that influence the behavior of the schizophrenic and his or her family. The thinking of one of the most outspoken students of the communication school of theory, Jay Haley, epitomizes the ecological perspective; he defined schizophrenia as a means of mediating between warring family triangles.

This family systems perspective offered a boon to the interpersonal and psychosocial models of schizophrenia and its treatment. However, the family systems theories failed in several important respects. They failed to explain differences in the patterns of interpersonal interaction associated with various disorders. What we are finally beginning to recognize is that many problem behaviors are not controlled by the family interaction, such that when these behaviors change (as in the case of agoraphobia), the family system does not recoil with a form of family symptoms substitution but instead integrates the new behavior in a positive way (Clarkin & Haas, 1986). To the extent that the communication theory attempts to explain schizophrenia as the outcome of environmental factors and to understand the schizophrenic experience in terms of basic principles of interpersonal behavioral processes common to all individuals, it is reductionistic and limited in perspective.

Despite these shortcomings, the "systems" theories of schizophrenia forced the field to consider ecological factors influencing the nature and course of major psychiatric disorders.

It is interesting to contrast the view of schizophrenia by family systems theorists that was chronicled by Hoffman (1981) (from Bateson and Bowen, to Haley, Weakland, and Wynne, to Dell and Palazzoli) with the current research efforts to specify crucial family interaction variables related to the onset and course of schizophrenia. This latter orientation began with the work of British investigators who in 1962 reported that patients who returned to live with their families following psychiatric hospitalization were more prone to rehospitalization than those patients who went elsewhere, such as to boarding homes and hostels (Brown, Monck, Carstairs & Wing, 1962). To pursue these interesting findings, this group developed the Camberwell Family Interview to quantify aspects of the family environment that impinge on the patient. This interview yields a measure of what the researchers called "expressed emotion" (EE), which is primarily an index of the family's criticism of and overinvolvement with the family member with schizophrenia. In subsequent years, it has been found with British, Indian, and American samples that the percentage of patients in families with high EE who relapse or are rehospitalized is significantly higher than that in low EE families. Though bypassing the issue of the etiology of schizophrenia, this work is elegant in its simplicity and directness in showing that EE has an impact on the course of the schizophrenic condition.

Heavily influenced by the ability of Brown and colleagues to specify variables in the family environment that influence the course of the illness, research groups have been successful not only in replicating the findings on EE but also in launching intervention programs to ameliorate family environmental conditions and thus affect the course of the illness. Investigations of treatment packages would do best to provide not only data on particular intervention strategies but also experimental evidence that EE has some causal relationship to the course of the illness. In the last few years, this work has been carried out in the United States (Anderson, Reiss, & Hogarty, 1986; Falloon *et al.*, 1982) and in England (Leff, Kuipers, Berkowitz, Eberlein-Vries, & Sturgeon, 1982). The major goals of these intervention packages are to decrease the patient's vulnerability to environmental stimuli through maintenance medication, to reduce family guilt about having caused the disorder, to reduce inappropriate family pressure on the patient, and to improve the skills of the family members in coping with the symptoms of the disorder. Strategies utilized to achieve these goals incude psychoeducation for patient and family about the disorder (its symptoms and early signs), and the learning and practice of skills to reduce stress and better cope with the symptoms of the disorder.

In summary, the historical involvement of the family therapy field in the treatment of schizophrenia suggests a number of themes—either prophetic or instructive—in dealing with affective disorders. Early effort was made to understand the symptoms of schizophrenia as a manifestation of the communication patterns in the family environment. Circular rather than linear notions of causality suggested that schizophrenia was not an illness condition but rather, that the behaviors labeled "schizophrenic" were part and parcel of the pattern of family relationships in which the behaviors were embedded, with no one individual the locus of the disorder (Dell, 1980). A second group, usually found in medical school and hospital settings, is now involved in research into the family environmental variables that impinge on the patient (e.g., Goldstein, Rodnick, Evans, May, & Steinberg, 1978) and in intervention with the family and patient using chemotherapy, psychoeducation, and enhancement of family coping skills to assist in ameliorating the course of the condition.

Some would say that the difference between these branches of family therapy today and the roots described by Hoffman is that the latter integrate biological causality into models of the illness. A review of the history of family therapy indicates that this simple dichotomy does not accurately reflect the important differences between old and new family therapy traditions. Rather, the differences may be a growing specificity in the definition of causal relationships, an increased attention to the environmental moderator variables that influence the course of illness, a greater respect for the value of process and outcome data, and an increased therapeutic pragmatism to help families cope with conditions in the most direct and obvious ways.

CURRENT DEVELOPMENTS IN RESEARCH
ON AFFECTIVE DISORDERS

One cannot ignore the symptomatology and/or diagnoses of the individual patient in planning research and in clinical practice. This is not to say that one can ignore the central hypothesis that the family forms a system that has profound influence on the individual. It is precisely because of this untrue assumption that we espouse the use of family and marital intervention in certain situations when an affective disorder is present. In addition, we are not saying that the diagnosis of the individual patient is the only way to organize our thinking for purposes of research on families. It has, however, been the predominant and actually the only fruitful means of describing, selecting, and classifying families in the investigation of family interaction and intervention to date (Gurman, Kniskern, & Pinsof, 1986).

There are a number of practical research reasons why the most productive investigations of family and marital intervention have focused on relatively homogeneous populations formed around the diagnosis of the identified patient:

1. There is no existing family classification scheme that is reliable and valid (Frances, Clarkin, & Perry, 1984a).
2. The individual diagnostic system is the most reliable and useful system currently available.
3. It is the system most widely used by psychotherapy researchers.
4. The use of standard methods of classifying individual patients has served to select relatively homogeneous samples of patients. Thus the generalization of results can be better established, and comparison more readily made across studies.
5. By careful attention to subgroups of affective disorders and their related variants of family interaction patterns, we will acquire necessary detailed information about how to intervene more effectively and efficiently.
6. Finally, investigations of family interaction and family intervention are not ultimately limited to the study of models that assume linear causality. Interactional patterns that reveal multidirectional patterns (e.g., feedback loops) can be investigated. A good example of this kind of work is the model building of Patterson describing the antisocial behaviors of adolescents (Patterson, 1986).

In addition, there are two clinical reasons for the use of the individual diagnostic classification system:

1. Patients come to clinicians requesting treatment for affective symptoms.
2. Certain affective symptoms (depression and mania)—if properly diagnosed—can be most effectively treated with medication (or electroconvulsive therapy [ECT]), so the individual must be assessed for such treatment.

We will summarize here the developments over the past 20 years in the field of affective disorder research as they affect phenomenology, typologies, and treatment, including chemotherapy and psychotherapy. Particularly important to the family and marital clinician is a detailed assessment of the kind of interpersonal relationships experienced by the person who has affective episodes: A functional analysis of the interpersonal network and temporal sequence of interpersonal events prior to, during, and following the episodes is in order. Such assessment focuses especially on the kind and quality of relationships the person establishes with intimate others, such as parents, spouse, and his or her own children.

Research on the Intersection of Family Interaction and Depression

The field of family therapy has contributed little to our theoretical understanding and assessment of the relationship of affective disorders to family dynamics and treatment. On the other hand, there has been an expansion of research in sociology, psychology, and psychiatry that is relevant to the social context of the individual with depression, most of which has direct relevance to assessment and treatment planning. In this chapter, we will review the research along dimensions that may have clinical relevance— dimensions that appear in most models of affective disorders. As others have done for group therapy (Grunebaum, 1975), we will provide a "soft-headed" review of the "hard-headed" research, a review intended to yield concrete, practical information for the clinician who is faced with an individual *or* a family having a member with an affective disorder.

The theoretical models that implicate psychosocial variables in the etiology and course of the affective disorders tend to focus more on depression than on bipolar disorder. Although it is not clear why this is so, it may be due in part to an underlying assumption that bipolar disorder is characterized by a more pronounced and powerful biological component in its etiology and course.

Most models (e.g., Billings & Moos, 1985; Brown & Harris, 1978a; Klerman & Weissman, 1986) emphasize certain primary or secondary variables that are associated with the occurrence of depression: (1) extraordinary life events and stressors; (2) less dramatic, but still stressful, occurrences of everyday life, that is, daily hassles; (3) environmental support, usually seen as interpersonal support emanating from family, friends, the community, and so forth; (4) personal attributes of the individual, such as personality, social skills, and coping style; and (5) biological and genetic predispositions to affective illness.

We will review the salient dimensions of these models here. However, we will not attempt an exhaustive review, since that has been done elsewhere. Furthermore, our focus will not be on the purity of the research designs but on the clinical relevance and applicability of the studies. We do believe that much of the research that has been done on the interpersonal context and course of affective disorders offers important and useful information for the family clinician.

PERSONAL RESOURCES

We will first consider those variables that are attributed largely to, or are characteristic of, the individual, whether they are sex, age, socioeconomic status, personality strengths, personality disorders, coping styles, and so forth. It is well to keep in mind, however, that such variables as personality and coping styles, which in one sense are more characteristic of the individual, may, on the other hand, be strongly influenced by the social setting and context in which such personality and coping styles are played out.

Demographic Characteristics

At some time in the course of their lives, 18% to 23% of females and 8% to 11% of males will experience a major depressive episode (American Psychiatric Association, 1980, 1987). Age of onset can be at any point in the life cycle. Depression can have serious consequences: Six percent of females and 3% of males will be hospitalized with it, and 15% of depressives will commit suicide (Robins & Guze, 1972).

The first manic episode of a bipolar disorder usually occurs before the age of 30 (American Psychiatric Association, 1980, 1987; Smith & Winokur, 1984). From 0.4% to 1.2% of the adult population will experience a bipolar disorder, equally common in women and men. It is a condition with recurring episodes, with the median number of episodes ranging from seven to nine (Angst *et al.*, 1973).

Across many studies, the most robust finding is that affective disorders are more common in women than in men. Many studies have found that young married women who are attending to young children are most at risk (Wing & Bebbington, 1985).

Personality Disorders and Affective Disorders

"Primary affective disorder" refers to an affective syndrome or symptom constellation (on Axis 1) that can come and go; "depressive personality patterns" refer to a "trait" condition, that is, behaviors that are relatively stable and characteristic of the individual over time. Especially important for the family therapist are the trait characteristics enduring over time that describe how the individual relates to others, especially his or her spouse and children. Therefore the relationship between Axis I affective disorder symptoms and episodes and more characteristic personality traits—especially those that describe characteristic interpersonal behaviors—is of both theoretical and clinical significance. Indeed, beginning at least with Kraepelin (1921), the issue of the relationship between affective disorders and related personality issues was raised. Kraepelin conceived of an underlying personality structure that predisposed individuals to affective episodes.

Docherty, Fiester, and Shea (1986) have articulated the possible linkages between syndromal conditions and personality traits. The two can be causally related: That is, the personality configuration can predispose the individual to particular syndromes such as affective illness. The personality disorder can be a *forme fruste* of the syndrome, that is, an expression of the same process that gives rise to the syndromal picture. The personality disorder can be a complication of the syndromal picture: For example, the depression lifts but gives rise to dependent character traits. It may be that the personality disorder and depressive syndrome have a coeffect or correlation with each other but are caused by some independent third variable. And, finally, the two may have an interactional (or synergistic) relationship such that both are independently caused but that when coexistent, they interact in such a manner as to accentuate both the syndrome and the personality traits.

The existing data on the relationship between depressive personality traits and depressive syndromes are limited and do not enable us at present to draw firm conclusions regarding the relationship between syndromal affective disorders and personality disorders. However, there are some data on the simple covariation of specific personality disorders with affective illness that constitute a beginning.

Two clinical studies investigated the prevalence of personality disorders in affectively disordered patients (Charney, Nelson, & Quinlan, 1981; Pfohl, Stangl, & Zimmerman, 1984). Bipolar patients had a 23% prevalence of personality disorders, and depressed patients had a prevalence of 37% to 53%. The prevalence of personality disorders was much higher among nonmelancholic (61%) than among melancholic (14%) depressives. Among the depressives, the most prominent personality disorders were histrionic, dependent, and avoidant (Pfohl *et al.*, 1984). Pfohl also found that 28% of the patients with affective disorders had two or more nonborderline personality disorders.

There is a somewhat more extensive literature on the prevalence of borderline personality disorders in patients with affective disorders. Rates in eight studies (Docherty *et al.*, 1986) vary from 23% to 67%. Again, it was found that the rate of personality disorders was higher in nonmelancholic patients (26%) than in melancholic patients (2%) (Charney *et al.*, 1981).

In addition to the simple prevalence of personality disorders among patients with affective disorders, there is some evidence that the concurrence of the two is correlated with certain treatment and life course factors. Patients with "depressive spectrum disease" as compared to "pure depressives" (Van Valkenburg, Akiskal, & Puzantian, 1983) have been found to have more hospitalizations, more alcohol abuse, and a more extensive history of antisocial symptoms, and they are more likely to have a history of social withdrawal and introversion. Yerevanian and Akiskal (1979) divided 65 "characterological depressives" into two groups: those who responded to tricyclic medication and those who did not. The nonresponders (whose disorder was labeled "character spectrum disorder" by this research group)—as compared to the responders—had been depressed all their lives; were more unstable characterologically, with passive–dependent, immature, impulsive, and manipulative behaviors; and had a greater history of early object loss, more alcohol abuse, and poorer social outcome. Major depressives with personality disorders had an earlier age of onset, poorer social supports, more life stressors, more frequent separation and divorce, and more frequent nonserious suicide attempts than did depressives without concomitant personality disorders (Pfohl *et al.*, 1984). In a treatment study of 100 outpatient female depressives (Weissman, Prusoff, & Klerman, 1978), the most important predictor of treatment outcome was characterological neuroticism as measured on the Maudsley Personality Inventory (and it, in fact, showed a *negative* association with treatment outcome). Certain chronic forms of personality disorder and social maladjustment appear to develop over the course of repeated depressive episodes (Akiskal, Bitar, Puzantian, Rosenthal, & Walker, 1978; Cassano, Maggini, & Akiskal, 1983; Klein, 1974).

General Social Skills in the Interpersonal Sphere of the Affectively Ill

A number of studies have pointed out the social skill deficits of individuals with depression. We are not focusing here on those social skill deficits that appear in marital and family interaction (although they probably appear there also) but on those that have been observed in studies involving patient interactions with strangers or other nonfamily members.

An extensive body of research indicates that depressives have inadequate social problem-solving skills (Dobson & Dobson, 1981; Fisher-Beckfield & McFall, 1982). Specific deficits such as social passivity, dysfunctional interpersonal cognitions, and inadequate verbal and nonverbal communication skills have been noted (e.g., Hammen, Jacobs, Mayol, & Cochran, 1980; Sanchez & Lewinsohn, 1980).

Sense of Environmental Mastery and Coping

In addition to specific interpersonal skill deficits, there may be trait-like characteristics—for example, more broad-spectrum attitudes and coping styles—that are specific to individuals prone to depressive disorders. For example, there may be characteristic ways individuals appraise and cope with life stresses. One of the more general constructs—locus of control—is highly relevant to understanding the phenomenology of depression. An external locus of control, that is, a generalized sense that one cannot master the environment by controlling or coping with events, has been related to serious depression and dysphoria (Costello, 1982; Warren & McEachren, 1983). In contrast, an internal locus of control, or the generalized sense that one can effect change in one's situation, may not only be related to a sense of well-being but also lead to the persistence of active and effective coping behaviors when stress does occur.

Several recent and more prominent models of depression place emphasis upon the effects of relatively stable cognitive styles of the individual that influence the way the individual perceives stressful situations. The learned helplessness model of depression (Seligman, 1975) hypothesizes that a perceived lack of contingency between an individual's coping responses and subsequent environmental outcomes generates a cognitive set that the environment cannot be controlled. Seligman suggests that such perceived noncontingency may be associated with the onset of dysphoria and depression. Abramson, Seligman, & Teasdale (1978) have elaborated further on this model, noting that key attributions—attribution of control to self versus other and the global/focal nature of such attribution—also influence the sense of mastery and coping behavior of the individual.

Beck's (1967) cognitive theory of depression has been ground breaking in the development of effective psychotherapeutic interventions for depression. It emphasizes that depressed individuals have a generally pessimistic view of the future and self-critical, self-blaming attitudes; are more sensitive to negative than positive events; and assume personal responsibility for negative outcomes.

STRESSFUL LIFE CIRCUMSTANCES

Since the pioneering work of Cannon (1939) and Selye (1976), the mental health field has been alert to the impact of life stressors and the disequilibrium they can create in terms of the individual's mental and bodily functioning. At present, there is more empirical data relating stress to depressive symptoms than to bipolar disorder and symptomatology. In this section, the major focus will be on stressors related to the family system—either major life events involving the family (e.g., divorce, death of a family member) or less traumatic, but more chronic, stressors such as marital discord.

If one sets aside the issue of causality for a moment, it is clear that we often find a temporal association between the onset of depression and stressful life events, including marital and family conflict. In a study of

psychosocial stress and depression, depressed patients reported feeling particularly vulnerable to marital and family stressors (Schless, Schwartz,
Goetz, & Mendels, 1974). If we consider the temporal sequence of events, we
find that stressful marital and/or family events often preceded or were
concomitant with the *onset* of depression (Ilfeld, 1977; Paykel *et al.*, 1969;
Paykel & Weissman, 1973; Pearlin & Johnson, 1977; Weissman & Paykel,
1974). In fact, in one study, marital friction was the most common event
reported during the 6 months prior to the onset of depressive symptoms
(Paykel *et al.*, 1969).

Of course, an insidious depressive illness process may lead to the
marital conflict. Alternately, a more complex interaction between the onset
of prodromal symptoms and marital distress may be occurring. For example, marital conflict and disruption could be one manifestation in the
constellation of symptoms and problems characteristic of the affective episode. Briscoe and Smith (1973) attempted to specify the sequence of marital
conflict and depression using an intensive, semistructured interview procedure to investigate an affective episode that occurred before, during, and
following a divorce. In 38% of the sample, the symptoms of depression were
judged to have preceded and contributed to the marital disruption. Those
individuals who had experienced a previous depression were more likely to
suffer a recurrence of depression during the marital disruption. Interesting
also was the observation that women tended to exhibit more depression
during the marriage and that men tended to become depressed during the
separation.

Research on life events suggests that an important factor influencing the
impact of stressful life events is the extent to which the event is contingent
upon, or independent of, the individual's own actions. Similarly, life stressors
can be quite independent of the actions and responsibility of the family unit
(e.g., job loss related to a decline in the economy, or the death of an individual). Alternately, stress can be the *result* of actions on the part of members of
the family unit. For example, one study has yielded evidence that many of the
stressors acting on the depressed spouse may arise out of the actions and/or
verbalizations of the nondepressed spouse (Leff, Roatch, & Bunney, 1970). Of
course, one cannot infer that the spouse actually causes the depression.
However, it appears that there may be some kind of feedback loop between
depression in the patient, the reactions of the spouse and family, and the
emergence of more severe depression in the patient. Given that symptoms of
depression—social withdrawal, decreased motivation, inability to follow
through on tasks, decreased self-esteem, and a sense of despair—are often
experienced as unpleasant or alienating, it is not surprising that spouses of
depressed persons often become frustrated, confused, overly solicitous, or
angry and emotionally withdrawn (Rush, Shaw, & Khatami, 1980). Depressives are likely to elicit critical or rejecting responses from others (Coyne,
1976), and it has been noted that spouses often respond to depressed mates

with what they call "constructive criticism" but what more "objective" observers term "hostility" (McLean, Ogston, & Grauer, 1973).

Although these findings suggest quite clearly that psychological stress is associated with the onset or occurrence of depression, there are still many research design problems that prevent us from drawing clear-cut conclusions regarding the causal linkage between depression and stressful interpersonal interactions (Kessler, Price, & Wortman, 1985). There are problems, too, in the development of assessment instruments designed to differentiate between life event stressors that are independent of the illness process itself and those events that are simply a part of the illness. Furthermore, although there is clear evidence of an association between stressful events and depression, the power of this relationship seems relatively small.

Stressors and Social Support

In their discussion of the interpersonal context of depression, Coyne *et al.* (1986) indicate that on rational grounds, the interaction between two factors—stress and social support—should predict depressions. However, the empirical findings suggest that there is only meager evidence for such interaction. They note that the most robust finding in community surveys is an association between depression and lack of social support (e.g., Andrews, Tennant, Hewson & Vaillant, 1978; Aneshensel & Stone, 1982; Costello, 1982). While depressed individuals residing in the community report that they seek social support more than do nondepressed people, at the same time they perceive themselves as receiving less support (Coyne, Aldwin, & Lazarus, 1981; Schaefer, Coyne, & Lazarus, 1981). Moreover, friends and relatives of depressed individuals report that their ("supportive") conversations tend to be focused on the depressed person's problems, which in turn makes these supportive others feel depressed (Arkowitz, Holliday, & Hutter, 1982).

In a much quoted study, Brown and Harris (1978b) found that in a sample of urban women, involvement in an intimate relationship was relevant to vulnerability to depression. Those women stressed by life events who had an intimate and confiding relationship with a male (either boyfriend or mate) seemed to be buffered from depression. While only 4% of those with an intimate relationship became depressed, almost 40% of the women with life stress but without such a buffer became depressed. This finding has been replicated in other population studies, including community surveys, studies of recent onset psychiatric cases, and surveys of normal population comparison groups (e.g., Slater & Depue, 1981).

In summary, it would appear that certain types of support, especially emotional support from an intimate partner, and the perception that one has access to a range of support if needed act to insulate against the impact of life stress and thereby decrease the risk for depression.

Stress and Coping

There are too few, although a growing number of studies that more carefully assess how the individual actually copes with life's stressors, whether they be unusual and extraordinary ones or common and mundane ones. Coyne *et al.* (1981) found that depressed subjects coped by appraising situations as requiring more information in order to act: They were more likely to seek emotional or informational support and more likely to engage in wishful thinking. It has been suggested (e.g., Kessler *et al.*, 1985) that the coping strategies of depressed individuals are characterized by negative self-preoc-cupations that hamper their ability to cope with confidence, efficiency, and decisiveness. Although it is not clear whether such a coping style leads to the development of the affective disorder or is a result of the disorder, it does suggest that intervention with the coping style may be one aspect in the rehabilitation and prophylactic treatment of individuals who are prone to the affective disorder.

Folkman and Lazarus (1986) have investigated the way depressed individuals appraise the threat or harm of a stressful event and subsequently cope with the stressor. Subjects were married women between the ages of 35 and 45 with at least one child at home. Monthly interviews were conducted to reconstruct the most stressful event during the previous week. As op-posed to subjects low in depressive symptoms, those with a high level of depression (3 males and 15 females) assessed stressful encounters as having a high degree of risk. The depressives used more confrontation, self-control, and escape avoidance in their effects to cope with the situation. They also accepted more responsibility and sought more social support. With regard to their emotional response, the depressive subjects were angrier; more disgusted, worried, and fearful; and less confident and secure. In summary, when confronted with stress, the depressed subjects seemed to perceive a higher degree of vulnerability, and their coping had a hostile but passive character.

ENVIRONMENTAL RESOURCES

Assortative Mating and Influence of Marital Partner Support

Affectively disordered patients tend to select similarly disposed individuals as mates (Merikangas, Bromet, & Spiker, 1983). The social maladjustment of the endogenous depressed patient predisposes such patients to maladap-tive selection of a marital partner and subsequent marital maladjustment (Merikangas *et al.*, 1983). Conversely, the apparent protective functions of an intimate relationship with a normal partner, as described by Brown and

Harris (1978b), are manifest among those endogenous depressed patients who marry a psychiatrically well partner and experience subsequent remission or reduction of their depressive symptoms (Merikangas *et al.*, 1983).

Family Support

Several studies have investigated the dimensions of support that operate within the family environment. Billings and Moos (1982) found that adults residing in families low in cohesion and expressiveness and high in interpersonal conflict reported more depressive symptoms. Compared with matched nondepressed controls, unipolar depressed patients have less supportive marital relationships, and their family environments are characterized by less cohesion and interpersonal expressiveness and more conflict (Billings, Cronkite, & Moos, 1983). In fact, the level of family support has effectively discriminated between depressed and nondepressed women (Wetzel, 1978; Wetzel & Redmond, 1980).

In a community survey (Pearlin & Johnson, 1977), married individuals reported less depression than did unmarried individuals, even after controlling for such variables as gender, age, and ethnicity. Married individuals were less exposed to various life strains than the unmarried. When, however, samples were equated for levels of life strain, married individuals were still less depressed than the unmarried.

Marital and Family Functioning

There is evidence that social dysfunction occurs during the acute phase of the depressive disorder. Using structured interviews, Weissman and Paykel (1974) found that depressed women were most impaired in their roles as wives and mothers. Marriages were characterized by interpersonal friction, poor communication, dependency, and diminished sexual satisfaction. Hostility was frequently overt, and there was a lack of affection toward their mates. Clinically recovered depressed women continued to experience problems functioning in their parental and spousal roles several months after recovery from the depressive symptoms. Interpersonal friction, inhibited communication, and the expression of hostility endured in interpersonal relations over the course of 8 months despite symptom improvement (Paykel & Weissman, 1973). A characteristic lack of autonomy and a tendency to cling to partners have been noted among endogenous depressives (Akiskal *et al.*, 1978). Others have noted a characteristic wish for the partner to be strong and to control or set limits for the depressed spouse. Unipolar endogenous depressed patients tend to have episodes *during* a relationship rather than after separation and breakup, which is more characteristic of nonendogenous depressives (Akiskal, Hirschfeld, & Yerevanian, 1983).

Rounsaville, Weissman, Prusoff, and Herceg-Baron (1979) found that over half of their sample of depressed women reported marital difficulties. In addition, if the marital difficulties persisted as treatment progressed, they were associated with poorer improvement and a greater likelihood of relapse.

Depressives show lower levels of social and marital-role functioning as compared with normal individuals (Birtchnell & Kennard, 1983). In fact, differential levels of depression are associated with good versus poor marital adjustment (Birtchnell & Kennard, 1983). Depression is also associated with disruption of the marital relationship (Bloom, Asher, & White, 1978).

Briscoe and Smith (1973) found that depressed divorced persons were more likely than nondepressed divorced persons to have discovered adultery by their ex-spouses. Coyne *et al.* (1987) found that among the spouses of depressed individuals, 40% were so distressed that they met a criterion for referral for psychotherapy.

Depressed individuals also have difficulties in interactions with their children (Coyne *et al*, 1986). Weissman and Paykel (1974) found that relationships between depressed women and their children were characterized by a lack of involvement and affection, impaired communication, friction, guilt, and resentment. Children of a depressed parent have been found to be at risk for psychological symptoms and behavioral problems. As many as 40% to 50% of children with a depressed parent have diagnosable psychiatric disorders (Cytryn, McKnew, Bartko, Lamour, & Hamvitt, 1982; Decina *et al.*, 1983).

Observational Studies of Interpersonal Interaction

In many ways, investigations that involve the observation and recording of behavioral interaction between affectively disordered individuals and intimate others (e.g., spouses, parents, and/or children) are the most relevant studies for the family theoretician and therapist. From a theoretical point of view, a behavioral record of interaction sequences provides information regarding the functional link or interface between the symptomatology of the patient and the interpersonal context, giving clues as to the sequences that lead to or help maintain the affective disorder. An examination of interpersonal interaction sequences transcends linear models of causality and provides an opportunity to observe how the behavior of each partner correlates with depressive symptoms and behavior patterns. Clinically, such observation can guide intervention schemes to eliminate maladaptive interactional sequences and introduce more helpful ones.

In general, the interaction between a depressed individual and a spouse seems to be characterized by a lack of task orientation, an excessive level of hostility, critical behavior, and a lack of self-disclosure. Depressed psychiatric inpatients verbalize personal subjective experiences more frequently than do control (medical) patients, who tend to be more task oriented in their verbalizations. Depressed couples experience more negative tension than do control couples (Hinchcliffe, Hooper, Roberts, & Vaughan, 1975; Hooper, Roberts, Hinchcliffe, & Vaughan, 1977). Depressed married women display less problem-solving behavior than do their spouses; spouses manifest less self-disclosure; such couples express less facilitative behavior than do control couples, and depression tends to reduce aversive behavior in the spouse (Biglan *et al.*, 1985).

Hautzinger, Linden, and Hoffman (1982) have studied couples seeking marital treatment, including a subset in which one spouse presented with unipolar depression. Conversations between patient and spouse were recorded and scored using an interaction coding system. Couples with a depressed partner exhibited negative and asymmetrical communication, with expression of dysphoric and uncomfortable feelings. Depressed spouses spoke negatively about themselves and positively in regard to their spouses. In contrast, the nondepressed spouses rarely spoke of themselves but evaluated their depressed partners negatively. Since all of the patients in this study had marital conflict, there was no representation of those without marital difficulty. However, Kowalik and Gotlib (1985) compared the interactions of depressed and nondepressed outpatients and of nondepressed nonpsychiatric controls and their spouses in an interactional task. Depressed psychiatric outpatients showed negativity, which was not evident in the nondepressed patient and control couples.

Kahn, Coyne, and Margolin (1985) found that couples with a depressed spouse experienced each other as more negative, hostile, mistrusting, and detached, and as less agreeable, nurturant, and affiliative, than did nondepressed couples. Hooley (1986) has investigated the interaction between depressed individuals and their spouses. Spouses were classified as having high or low EE on the basis of the Camberwell Family Interview. In a 10-minute face-to-face interaction between the patients and their spouses, high EE spouses were more negative and less positive toward their depressed partners, in terms of both verbal and nonverbal behaviors. They made more critical remarks, disagreed with their partners more frequently, and were less likely to accept what their mate said to them. The depressed mates of high EE spouses exhibited low frequencies of self-disclosure and high levels of neutral nonverbal behavior. Thus a high level of negative affectivity and a relative lack of positive, supportive communications seem characteristic of depressed couples.

Control and power issues also surface in the interactions: These may be related to, and/or causitive of, the hostility mentioned previously. Contrary to the theoretical assumptions regarding passivity and dependency of the depressed spouse, Hooper *et al.* (1977) reported that depressed patients in their sample produced substantial control-oriented communication with their spouses during the acute depressive episode—more than during the posttreatment follow-up period. Merikangas, Ranelli, and Kupfer (1979) recorded and rated therapeutic interaction between depressed female inpatients and their spouses. During early sessions, the patient was strongly influenced by the behavior of his or her spouse, but by the last session, there was a more equal balance of power.

Depression in a parent can have a maladaptive influence on interactions between married couples and their children. Biglan *et al.*, (1985) studied the interactions of family members in the presence of a depressed mother. Children of mothers who were depressed displayed significantly more irritability than did controls. The fathers and children reduced their irritated and sarcastic behavior immediately following the mother's displays of dysphoric affect.

In summary, interactional studies promise important clinical information but need to be made more specific and powerful in design. First, many studies fail to take into account the heterogeneity of depressive disorders; investigators simply indicate that the subject was "depressed" according to a cutoff score on some clinical rating scale. We need more specification of the nature of the affective condition and study designs that attempt to control for this heterogeneity. It may well be that endogenous depressives interact differently than nonendogenous depressives. Second, many of the studies do not clearly indicate the stage of the affective illness/episode during which the interaction samples are recorded. It is likely that the patient interacts in different ways depending upon the phase of the affective episode: whether during the prodromal phase, during an illness episode, or during the recovery period. There is also a need for the systematic assessment and study of concurrent personality disorders and of how such chronic behavior patterns influence interaction patterns of patient and spouse. Interpersonal behavior is influenced by *both* the affective symptomatology and the personality styles of the participants.

TYPE OF AFFECTIVE ILLNESS AND INTERPERSONAL CONTEXT

Though depressed patients may appear relatively homogeneous on a symptom-phenomenological level, they show substantial heterogeneity in terms of etiology, current psychosocial context, and so forth. Reliable classification and identification of meaningful subtypes would provide us with a fuller understanding of the affective disorders and enable us to devise well-differentiated treatment planning.

As we have seen in the research literature reviewed earlier in this chapter, the constellation of psychosocial problems manifest in nonendogenous depression contrasts with those of the endogenous depressive disorders. Episodes of neurotic depression are frequently precipitated by the breakup of a conjugal relationship. This is less frequent among cases of endogenous depression, which tend to occur within the context of an intact relationship (Matussek & Feil, 1983). Furthermore, the character of psychosocial deficits differs for the two groups. Among the nonendogenous depressives, mistrust and pseudoindependence or pseudoautonomy occur as a protection against potential frustration or disappointment in interpersonal relations. In contrast, the interpersonal relations of the endogenous unipolar depressive are characterized by overaccommodation, submissiveness, and a lack of self-assertiveness associated with feelings of neediness and dependency. Because of passivity and the fear of abandonment, these patients are likely to be ineffective in coping with interpersonal conflict, to avoid overt expressions of anger, and to lack the capacity to engage in active approaches to interpersonal problem solving. The psychological stress of interpersonal intimacy for these patients may explain the tendency for depressive episodes to occur within the context of a conjugal relationship.

RELATIONSHIP OF DEPRESSION TO INTERPERSONAL CONTEXT

There are a number of possible linkages between affective symptoms in the individual and the psychosocial environment: acute life stresses, chronic stressors in the work or family environment, individual strengths or weaknesses in the patient that influence the pattern of interpersonal relationships and social supports, and characteristics of the family environment (Haas, Clarkin, & Glick, 1985). These can be summarized in terms of four primary "linkage" models:

1. Marital/family stressors may elicit or precipitate the onset of depressive symptoms in a biologically predisposed individual.
2. Marital/family stress or the lack of an intimate relationship may potentiate the effects of other environmental stressors, leading to a depressive episode in a biologically vulnerable individual.
3. Depressive symptoms in one family member may trigger negative responses from other family members, thus acting to elicit marital/family conflict.
4. Subclinical depressive or characterological traits, behavior patterns, and so forth, in one or more family members may potentiate marital/family discord, which, in turn, triggers the onset of a depressive episode.

Linkages 1-4, though different, could all lead to the conclusion that one should introduce family or marital treatment as a major or minor element in a treatment regimen, the timing of which would depend upon the mediating goals of treatment. Linkage 1 would call for chemical treatment concomitant with or followed by marital treatment. Linkage 3 would call for chemical treatment, followed by brief family intervention leading to equilibrium.

AFFECTIVE ILLNESS AND INDICATIONS FOR FAMILY INTERVENTION

The survey of the various linkages of affective disorders to the marital/ family environment persuades us of the need for systematic assessment of affective symptoms/behaviors within the family context, specification of indications for family intervention, and formulation of mediating goals of family/marital therapy. Chapter 2 of this volume presents an approach to assessment when a family member has an affective disorder and suggests the use of particular assessment instruments and procedures that best serve this purpose.

Indications for family/marital intervention with affective disorders follow the guidelines for family intervention in general (Clarkin, Frances, & Moodie, 1979; Frances, Clarkin, & Perry, 1984b). However, when symptoms of an affective disorder are present in one or more family members, the assessment process needs to be more specific. In general, when a family member (be it child, adolescent, or adult) shows affective symptoms, a family evaluation should be done. The focus of the interpersonal evaluation (see Chapter 2) should be on assessment of the linkages (as described previously) between the affective symptoms/behaviors and the interpersonal context.

Type of Family Intervention

At least theoretically, the orientation and focus of the family/marital intervention (when one individual has an affective disorder) will depend upon the specifics of the patient and the family environment. Our review of the literature suggests that there are several key areas for potential intervention with the marital/family system when an affective disorder is involved:

1. *Severity of the affective episodes*. The severity of the affective disorder (indicated by the number and length of episodes, the psychotic versus nonpsychotic nature of symptoms, associated character pathology, and level of functioning between episodes) will be an important factor in determining the need for pharmacotherapy (Chapter 7) and the setting and timing of the

treatment (see Chapter 6 for a discussion of inpatient treatment, and Chapters 3 and 4 for outpatient treatment). When affective symptoms appear as part of a well-circumscribed episode that begins and ends with dramatic changes in functioning (e.g., a clear bipolar manic episode), one would be likely to use psychoeducational approaches (e.g., Chapter 5).

2. *Cognitive factors.* The specific cognitions and cognitive style of the depressed individual may be key in determining the specific focus of intervention. Assessment of the cognitive/attributional styles of the spouse and intimate others can also yield important information regarding the interpersonal context of the affective disorder and functional characteristics of the patient's interpersonal world that need to be utilized or addressed in treatment.

3. *Lack of marital intimacy.* Empirical research indicates that an intimate relationship is a strong buffer against depression. However, the marriages of depressed individuals may be lacking in support, comfort, and other aspects of intimacy. Therapeutic techniques that assist in the development of such intimacy are highly relevant to the treatment of depression and to the prevention of future episodes.

4. *Hostile interaction.* The interactions of depressed individuals with their spouses are characterized by hostility and perceived criticism. Therapeutic strategies and techniques that focus on reducing such behavior and on increasing more supportive interchange have been recommended (e.g., Chapters 3 and 7).

5. *Poor social skills.* The inability to engage effectively in supportive social interaction and the failure to secure positive social reinforcements may be central targets of intervention and skill building (e.g., behavioral marital therapy, Chapter 3).

6. *The coping process.* The problem-solving skills and coping behavior of the depressive-prone individual might be an appropriate and necessary focus of intervention. In addition, the way in which the well spouse perceives and copes with the disorder must be assessed and addressed in treatment. More specifically, some attention must be given to how the individuals in the family cope with the depressive and manic behaviors of the patient. Inpatient family intervention (IFI) for affective disorders (Chapter 6) focuses directly on educating and training the family and patient in coping with the symptoms.

7. *Parenting skills.* Depression and bipolar disorder typically interfere with parenting functions. This can contribute to increased risk for psychiatric illness among the children of parents with affective disorders.

In the chapters that follow, a number of treatment models for affective disorders and the family are described. These models are used in inpatient and outpatient settings. The treatments are alike in that they utilize the family or marital format for intervention. However, the strategies and techniques of intervention vary according to the specific characteristics of the disorder (depression versus bipolar disorder), the severity of the condition, the stage of the illness process, and the theoretical orientation of the authors.

REFERENCES

Abramson, L. Y., Seligman, M.E.P., & Teasdale, J. (1978). Learned helplessness in humans: Critique and reformulation. *Journal of Abnormal Psychology, 87,* 49–74.

Akiskal, H. S., Bitar, A. H., Puzantian, V. R., Rosenthal, T. L. & Walker, P. W. (1978). The nosological status of neurotic depressions: A prospective three- to four-year follow-up examination in the light of the primary–secondary and the unipolar–bipolar dichotomies. *Archives of General Psychiatry, 35,* 756–766.

Akiskal, H. S., Hirschfeld, M. A., & Yerevanian, B, I. (1983). The relationship of personality to affective disorders: A critical review. *Archives of General Psychiatry, 40,* 801–810.

American Psychiatric Association. (1980). *Diagnostic and statistical manual of mental disorders* (3rd ed.). Washington, DC: APA.

American Psychiatric Association. (1987). *Diagnostic and statistical manual of mental disorders* (rev. 3rd ed.). Washington, DC: APA

Anderson, C. M., Reiss, D. J., & Hogarty, G. E. (1986). *Schizophrenia and the family.* New York: Guilford Press.

Andrews, G., Tennant, C., Hewson, D., & Vaillant, G. (1978). Life stress, social support, coping style, and risk of psychological impairment. *Journal of Nervous and Mental Disease, 166,* 307–316.

Aneshensel, C. S., & Stone, J. D. (1982). Stress and depression: A test of buffering model of social support. *Archives of General Psychiatry, 39,* 1392–1396.

Angst, J., Baastrup, P., Grof, P., Hippius, H., Poldinger, W., & Weis, P. (1973). The course of monopolar depression and bipolar psychoses. *Psychiatria Neurologica et Neurochirurgia, 76,* 489–500.

Arkowitz, H., Holliday, S., & Hutter, M. (1982). *Depressed women and their husbands: A study of marital interaction and adjustment.* Paper presented at the meeting of the Association for the Advancement of Behavior Therapy, Los Angeles.

Bateson, G., Jackson, D. D., Haley, J., & Weakland, J. (1956). Toward a theory of schizophrenia. *Behavioral Science, 1,* 251–264.

Beck, A. T. (1967). *Depression: Clinical, experimental and theoretical aspects.* New York: Harper & Row.

Beck, A. T., Rush, A. J., Shaw, B. F., & Emery, G. (1979). *Cognitive therapy of depression.* New York: Guilford Press.

Biglan, A., Hops, H., Sherman, L., Friedman, L. S., Arthur, J., & Osteen, V. (1985). Problem-solving interactions of depressed women and their spouses. *Behavior Therapy, 16,* 431–451.

Billings, A. G., Cronkite, R. C., & Moos, R. H. (1983). Social–environmental factors in unipolar depression: Comparisons of depressed patients and nondepressed controls. *Journal of Abnormal Psychology, 92,* 119–133.

Billings, A. G., & Moos, R. H. (1982). Social support and functioning among community and clinical groups: A panel model. *Journal of Behavioral Medicine, 5,* 295–311.

Billings, A. G., & Moos, R. H. (1985). Psychosocial stressors, coping, and depression. In E. E. Beckham & W. R. Leber (Eds.), *Handbook of depression: Treament, assessment and research* (pp. 940–974). Homewood, IL: Dorsey Press.

Birtchnell, J., & Kennard, J. (1983). Does marital maladjustment lead to mental illness? *Social Psychiatry, 18,* 79–88.

Bloom, B., Asher, S., & White, S. (1978). Marital disruption as a stressor: A review and analysis. *Psychological Bulletin, 85,* 867–894.

Briscoe, C. W., & Smith, J. B. (1973). Depression and marital turmoil. *Archives of General Psychiatry, 29,* 811–817.

Brown, G. W., & Harris, T. O. (1978a). Social origins of depression: A reply. *Psychological Medicine, 8,* 577–588.

Brown, G. W., & Harris, T. O. (1978b). *Social origins of depression: A study of psychiatric disorder in women.* New York: Free Press.

Brown, G. W., Monck, E. M., Carstairs, G. M., & Wing, J. K. (1962). Influence of family life on the course of schizophrenic illness. *British Journal of Preventive & Social Medicine, 16,* 55–68.

Cannon, W. B. (1939). *The wisdom of the body.* New York: W. W. Norton.

Cassano, G. B., Maggini, C., & Akiskal, H. S. (1983). Short-term subchronic and chronic sequelae of affective disorders. *Psychiatric Clinics of North America, 6,* 55–67.

Charney, D. S., Nelson, C. J., & Quinlan, D. M. (1981). Personality traits and disorder in depression. *American Journal of Psychiatry, 138,* 1601–1604.

Clarkin, J. F., Frances, A., & Moodie, L. (1979). Selection criteria for family therapy. *Family Process, 18,* 391–403.

Clarkin, J. F., & Haas, G. L. (1986). Alternative treatment formats: Current research evidence. In S. Sugarman (Ed.), *The interface of individual and family therapy* (pp. 73–83). Rockville, MD: Aspen.

Costello, C. G. (1982). Social factors associated with depression: A retrospective community study. *Psychological Medicine, 12,* 329–339.

Coyne, J. C. (1976). Depression and the response of others. *Journal of Abnormal Psychology, 85,* 186–193.

Coyne, J. C., Aldwin, C., & Lazarus, R. S. (1981). Depression and coping in stressful episodes. *Journal of Abnormal Psychology, 90,* 439–447.

Coyne, J. C., Kahn, J., & Gotlib, I. H. (1986). Depression. In T. Jacob (Ed.), *Family interaction and psychotherapy* (pp. 509–533). New York: Plenum.

Coyne, J. C., Kessler, R. C., Tal, M., Turnbull, J., Wortman, C. B., & Greden, J. F. (1987). Living with a depressed person. *Journal of Consulting and Clinical Psychology, 55,* 347–352.

Cytryn, L., McKnew, D. H., Bartko, J. J., Lamour, M., & Hamovitt, J. (1982). Offspring of patients with affective disorders: II. *Journal of the American Academy of Child Psychiatry, 21,* 389–391.

Decina, P., Kestenbaum, C. J., Farber, S., Kron, L., Gargan, M., Sackeim, H. A., & Fieve, R. R. (1983). Clinical and psychological assessment of children of bipolar probands. *American Journal of Psychiatry, 140,* 548–553.

Dell, P. (1980). Researching the family theories of schizophrenia. *Family Process, 19,* 321–335.

Dobson, D., & Dobson, K. (1981). Problem-solving strategies in depressed and nondepressed college students. *Cognitive therapy and research, 5,* 697–705.

Docherty, J. P., Fiester, S. J., & Shea, T. (1986). Syndrome diagnosis and personality disorder. In A. Frances & R. E. Hales (Eds.), *American Psychiatric Association Annual Review, Volume 5* (pp. 315–354). Washington, DC: American Psychiatric Press.

Falloon, I. R. H., Boyd, J. L., McGill, C., Razani, J., Moss, H., & Gilderman, A. (1982). Family management in the prevention of exacerbations of schizophrenia: A controlled study. *New England Journal of Medicine, 306,* 1437–1440.

Fisher-Beckfield, D., & McFall, R. M. (1982). Development of a competence inventory for college men and evaluation of relationships between competence and depression. *Journal of Consulting and Clinical Psychology, 50,* 697–705.

Folkman, S. & Lazarus, R. S. (1986). Stress processes and depressive symptomatology. *Journal of Abnormal Psychology, 95,* 107–113.

Frances, A., Clarkin, J. F., & Perry, S. (1984a). DSM-III and family therapy. *American Journal of Psychiatry, 141*, 406–409.

Frances, A., Clarkin, J. F., & Perry, S. (1984b). *Differential therapeutics: A guide to the art and science of treatment planning in psychiatry*. New York: Brunner/Mazel.

Goldstein, M. J., Rodnick, E. H., Evans, J. R., May, P. R. A., & Steinberg, M. R. (1978). Drug and family therapy in the aftercare treatment of acute schizophrenics. *Archives of General Psychiatry, 35*, 1169–1177.

Grunebaum, H. (1975). Soft-headed review of hard-nosed research on groups. *International Journal of Group Psychotherapy, 25*, 185–195.

Gurman, A. S., Kniskern, D. P., & Pinsof, W. M. (1986). Research on marital and family therapies. In S. L. Garfield & A. E. Bergin (Eds.), *Handbook of psychotherapy and behavior change* (pp. 565–624). New York: Wiley.

Haas, G. L., Clarkin, J. F., & Glick, I. D. (1985). Marital and family treatment of depression. In E. E. Beckham & W. R. Leber (Eds.), *Handbook of depression: Treatment, assessment and research* (pp. 151–183). Homewood, IL: Dorsey Press.

Hammen, C. L., Jacobs, M., Mayol, A., & Cochran, S. D. (1980). Dysfunctional cognitions and the effectiveness of skills and cognitive–behavioral training. *Journal of Consulting and Clinical Psychology, 48*, 685–695.

Hautzinger, M., Linden, M., & Hoffman, N. (1982). Distressed couples with and without a depressed partner: An analysis of their verbal interaction. *Journal of Behavior Therapy and Experimental Psychiatry, 13*, 307–314.

Hinchcliffe, M., Hooper, D., Roberts, F. J., & Vaughan, P. W. (1975). A study of the interaction between depressed patients and their spouses. *British Journal of Psychiatry, 126*, 164–172.

Hoffman, L. (1981). *Foundations of family therapy: A conceptual framework for systems change*. New York: Basic Books.

Hooley, J. M. (1986). Expressed emotion and depression: Interactions between patients and high versus low EE spouses. *Journal of Abnormal Psychology, 95*, 237–246.

Hooper, D., Roberts, F. J., Hinchcliffe, M. K., & Vaughan, P. W. (1977). The melancholy marriage: An inquiry into the interaction of depression. I. Introduction. *British Journal of Medical Psychology, 50*, 113–124.

Ilfeld, F. W. (1977). Current social stressors and symptoms of depression. *American Journal of Psychiatry, 134*, 161–166.

Kahn, J., Coyne, J. C., & Margolin, G. (1985). Depression and marital conflict: The social construction of despair. *Journal of Social and Personal Relationships, 2*, 447–462.

Kessler, R. C., Price, R. H., & Wortman, C. B. (1985). Social factors in psychopathology: Stress, social support and coping processes. In M. R. Rosenzweig & L. W. Porter (Eds.), *Annual review of psychology* (Vol. 36, pp. 531–572). Palo Alto, CA: Annual Reviews.

Klein, D. (1974). Endogenomorphic depressions: Toward a terminologic revision. *Archives of General Psychiatry, 31*, 447–454.

Klerman, G. L., & Weissman, M. M. (1986). The interpersonal approach to understanding depression. In T. Millon & G. L. Klerman (Eds.), *Contemporary directions in psychopathology: Towards the DSM-IV* (pp. 429–456). New York: Guilford Press.

Kowalik, D., & Gotlib, I. H. (1985). *Depression and marital interaction: Concordance between intent and perception of communications*. Unpublished manuscript, University of Western Ontario.

Kraepelin, E. (1921). *Manic–depressive illness and paranoia*. Edinburgh: E & S Livingstone, Ltd.

Leff, J. P., Kuipers, L., Berkowitz, R., Eberlein-Vries, R., & Sturgeon, D. (1982). A controlled trial of social intervention in the families of schizophrenic patients. *British Journal of Psychiatry, 141*, 121–134.

Leff, M., Roatch, J., & Bunney, L. E. (1970). Environmental factors preceding the onset of severe depression. *Psychiatry, 33*, 298–311.

Lewinsohn, P. M., Hoberman, H. M., Teri, L., & Hautzinger, M. (1985). An integrative theory of depression. In S. Reiss & R. Bootzin (Eds.), *Theoretical issues in behavior therapy*. New York: Academic Press.

Matussek, P., & Feil, W. B. (1983). Personality attributes of depressive patients: Results of group comparisons. *Archives of General Psychiatry, 40*, 783–790.

McLean, P. D., Ogston, K., & Grauer, L. (1973). A behavioral approach to the treatment of depression. *Journal of Behavior Research and Experimental Psychiatry, 4*, 323–330.

Merikangas, K. R., Bromet, E. J., & Spiker, D. G. (1983). Assortative mating, social adjustment, and course of illness in primary affective disorder. *Archives of General Psychiatry, 40*, 795–800.

Merikangas, K. R., Ranelli, C. J., & Kupfer, D. J. (1979). Marital interaction in hospitalized depressed patients. *Journal of Nervous and Mental Disease, 167*, 689–695.

Patterson, G. R. (1986). Performance models for antisocial boys. *American Psychologists, 41*, 432–444.

Paykel, E. S., Myers, J. K., Dienelt, M. N., Klerman, G. L., Lindenthal, J. J., & Pepper, M. P. (1969). Life events and depression: A controlled study. *Archives of General Psychiatry, 21*, 753–760.

Paykel, E. S., & Weissman, M. M. (1973). Social adjustment and depression. *Archives of General Psychiatry, 28*, 659–663.

Pearlin, L. I., & Johnson, J. (1977). Marital status, life strains, and depression. *American Sociological Review, 42*, 704–715.

Pfohl, B., Stangl, D., & Zimmerman, M. (1984). The implications of DSM-III personality disorders for patients with major depression. *Journal of Affective Disorders, 7*, 309–318.

President's Commission on Mental Health. (1978). *Task panel's reports submitted to the President's Commission on Mental Health* (Vol. 4, Appendix). Washington, DC: U.S. Government Printing Office.

Robins, E., & Guze, S. B. (1972). Classification of affective disorders: The primary–secondary, the endogenous–reactive, and the neurotic–psychotic concepts. In T. A. Williams, M. M. Kazt, & J. A. Shield (Eds.), *Recent advances in the psychobiology of the depressive illnesses*. (DHEW Publication No. HSM 70-9053). Washington, DC: U.S. Government Printing Office.

Rounsaville, B. J., Weissman, M. W., Prusoff, B. A., & Herceg-Baron, R. L. (1979). Marital disputes and treatment outcome in depressed women. *Comprehensive Psychiatry, 20*, 483–490.

Rush, A. J., Shaw, B., & Khatami, M. (1980). Cognitive therapy of depression: Utilizing the couples system. *Cognitive Therapy and Research, 4*, 103–113.

Sanchez, V., & Lewinsohn, P. M. (1980). Assertive behavior and depression. *Journal of Consulting and Clinical Psychology, 48*, 119–120.

Schaefer, C., Coyne, J. C., & Lazarus, R. S. (1981). The health-related functions of social support. *Journal of Behavioral Medicine, 4*, 381–406.

Schless, A. P., Schwartz, L., Goetz, C., & Mendels, J. (1974). How depressives view the significance of life events. *British Journal of Psychiatry, 125*, 406–410.

Seligman, M. E. P. (1975). *Helplessness: On depression, development and death*. San Francisco: W. H. Freeman.

Selye, H. (1976). *The stress of life* (rev. ed.). New York: McGraw-Hill.

Slater, J., & Depue, R. A. (1981). The contribution of environmental events and social support to serious suicide attempts in primary depressive disorder. *Journal of Abnormal Psychology, 90*, 275–285.

Smith, R. E., & Winokur, G. (1984). Affective disorders—bipolar. In S. M. Turner & H. Hersen (Eds.), *Adult psychopathology and diagnosis* (pp. 245-262). New York: Wiley.

Van Valkenburg, C., Akiskal, H. S., & Puzantian, V. (1983). Depression spectrum disease or character spectrum disorder? A clinical study of major depressives with familial alcoholism or sociopathy. *Comprehensive Psychiatry, 24*, 589-595.

Warren, L. W., & McEachren, L. (1983). Psychosocial correlates of depressive symptomatology in adult women. *Journal of Abnormal Psychology, 92*, 151-160.

Weissman, M. M., & Paykel, E. S. (1974). *The depressed woman: A study of social relationships*. Chicago: University of Chicago Press.

Weissman, M. M., Prusoff, B. A., & Klerman, G. L. (1978). Personality and the prediction of long-term outcome of depression. *American Journal of Psychiatry, 135*, 797-800.

Wetzel, J. W. (1978). The work environment and depression: Implications for intervention. In J. W. Hawks (Ed.), *Toward human dignity: Social work in practice*. New York. NASW Professional Symposium Service.

Wetzel, J. W., & Redmond, F. C. (1980). A person-environment study of depression. *Social Service Review, 54*, 363-375.

Wing, J. K., & Bebbington, P. (1985). Epidemiology of depression. In E. E. Beckham & W. R. Leber (Eds.), *Handbook of depression: Treatment, assessment, and research* (pp. 765-794). Homewood, IL: Dorsey Press.

Yerevanian, B. I., & Akiskal, H. S. (1979). Neurotic, characterological, and dysthymic depressions. *Psychiatric Clinics of North America, 2*, 595-617.

2

Assessment of Affective Disorders and Their Interpersonal Contexts

JOHN F. CLARKIN
GRETCHEN L. HAAS

INTRODUCTION

In this chapter, we will describe the symptoms of depression and mania, and the characterological traits associated with individuals who suffer affective episodes. We will survey and evaluate the utility of the various instruments utilized to assess affective symptoms, associated personality traits, and the interpersonal context of the patient with an affective disorder. Finally, we will make recommendations for instruments and procedures, reviewing (1) assessment procedures used by practicing family therapists, (2) assessment instruments specifically useful for diagnosis and treatment of affective symptomatology, and (3) a selected battery of instruments that will assist the clinician in identifying and modifying problems related to the interpersonal behavior and context of the affectively disordered patient.

Since the age of onset for affective disorders is in the early to middle adult years, and since most descriptive and intervention research with affective disorders is done with adults, this chapter (and the remainder of this volume) will focus primarily on the adult patient and his or her family. However, since childhood and adolescent depression is of significant occurrence and of special interest to family therapists, we will also include some discussion of assessment issues specific to these age groups.

This chapter is intended to serve a number of purposes. First, it describes the symptomatology of affective disorders—what to look for and how to describe and evaluate possible symptoms. Second, it provides a critical review of methods for the assessment and diagnosis of affective disorders. Third, it discusses research applications in the assessment of the family context of an affective disorder. Fourth, and perhaps most important, this chapter is oriented toward the practicing clinician who is faced with the clinical tasks of assessing and intervening with the affectively disordered patient and his or her family.

Family clinicians do not typically use assessment instruments in their treatments. This is understandable, given clinicians' busy schedules, their lack of clerical backup, and the general orientation of instrument development, which is geared to the individual patient and pays little attention to the family or marital context. However, the assessment scene is changing in some important ways: (1) There are more assessment instruments that include the family or marital dyad as the primary unit of observation and assessment; (2) there are more family-oriented clinicians and clinical researchers who are developing self-report instruments with the family context as the major focus; and (3) with the development of computerized methods of assessment, the clinician is more likely to include assessment procedures in the initial phase of evaluation.

The question of time and cost in the use of assessment instruments bears some examination. The use of self-report instruments that the marital couple and family can complete at home involves little time on the part of the clinician. Many such instruments can be scored quickly and easily by hand or by computer. Computerization is quickly changing the assessment field, and in the very near future, most clinicians' offices may have personal computers at which patients will sit and respond to various standard assessment questionnaires. The computer will score the response record and print out a report within a matter of minutes.

The authors of this chapter are clinicians and clinical researchers. In our family/marital therapy training, little, if any, attention was given to the use of formal assessment instruments. It was out of the demands of clinical research that we began systematically using assessment instruments with patients and their families. In that context, we have come to appreciate the value of assessment instruments in our work with families.

Structured assessment tools with well-operationalized procedures and assessment criteria offer a means of evaluating clinical outcome on a case-by-case or group-comparison basis. The clinician is offered some yardstick by which to compare specific outcomes (on one or more dimensions) of any given case with outcomes (expected or previously observed) from work with the same or other cases. Thus the family clinician can use structured assessment procedures to evaluate progress or treatment outcome in the identified patient and in other members of the family. Clinical outcomes can be evaluated for a single family, comparing pretreatment and posttreatment measures on the dimensions targeted for treatment. A second general use is to compare pretreatment and posttreatment scores with the values one would expect for similar patients and families given the same treatment. This application affords the clinician the opportunity to systematically assess and compare family treatment outcomes using a standard metric, so as to begin to accrue cumulative data on treatment response across a group of cases.

We have also learned that individuals are usually willing to fill out assessment instruments if they do not take an inordinate amount of time. In fact, many family members enjoy completing the forms, want to discuss their responses, and become quite curious about how others in the family have responded. The response to the task of completing assessment questionnaires at the beginning of treatment is usually predictive (diagnostic) of other behavior patterns: For example, families and couples who fail to complete the instruments are often resistive to therapy homework tasks; couples who use the instruments to focus on areas of agreement as well as disagreement are able, later in therapy, to use their strengths to overcome difficulties. In sum, it is our impression that formal assessment procedures offer an effective and efficient means of gathering information. Family clinicians should make more frequent use of assessment devices in their clinical work, especially low-cost ones such as self-report instruments.

CLASSIFICATION OF AFFECTIVE DISORDERS

Issues in the classification of affective disorders have not been resolved empirically, but the specific behavioral symptoms of mania and depression given in DSM-III-R (American Psychiatric Association, 1987) are a step in the right direction, enabling researchers to define (with, at times, very arbitrary terms) relatively homogeneous groups, and clinicians to communicate reliably. Certain distinctions that clinically relevant to the assessment of affective disorders include neurotic–psychotic, reactive–endogenous, primary–secondary, and unipolar–bipolar distinctions. These distinctions and their current research standing are reviewed elsewhere (Leber, Beckham, & Danker-Brown, 1985).

Under the major heading of mood disorders, DSM-III-R distinguishes bipolar disorders (including bipolar disorder and cyclothymia) and depressive disorders (including major depression and dysthymia):

Bipolar disorders
Bipolar disorder
  Manic
  Depressed
  Mixed
Cyclothymia
Bipolar disorder not otherwise specified
Depressive disorders
Major depression
  Single episode
  Recurrent

Dysthymia
Depressive disorder not otherwise specified
Psychotic disorders not elsewhere classified
Schizoaffective disorder
Adjustment disorders
With depressed mood

Symptoms of a major depressive episode, as defined in DSM-III-R, include depressed mood, markedly diminished interest or pleasure in most activities, significant weight loss or weight gain, insomnia or hypersomnia, psychomotor agitation or retardation, loss of energy, feelings of worthlessness or excessive guilt, lack of concentration and/or indecisiveness, and recurrent thoughts of death or suicidal ideation. Distinctions are made between major depression with melancholia and that without melancholia, and for cases having a seasonal pattern.

For a patient with a history of one or more manic episodes with or without depression, the diagnosis of bipolar disorder is made. The symptoms of a manic episode include elevated, expansive, or irritable mood; grandiosity; decreased need for sleep; pressured speech; flight of ideas; distractibility; increased goal-directed activity or psychomotor agitation; excessive involvement in pleasurable activities with painful consequences (e.g., buying sprees); and marked impairment in occupational and social functioning. With a five-digit number, the clinician indicates the severity of the manic episode, ranging from a mild one to one with psychotic features.

GOALS AND TARGETS OF ASSESSMENT

Since affective disorders are heterogeneous with regard to etiology and treatment response, it is essential that the clinician utilize careful assessment procedures in order to tailor an optimal treatment package for the individual patient. The assessment process is instrumental in both describing the nature of the problems and designing a treatment plan. As described in Chapter 1, the environmental factors that contribute to, interact with, or are influenced by the disorder must be specifically identified; a functional assessment of their relationship to the patient's symptomatology can be helpful in designing an intervention strategy.

Hence the goals of assessment are to (1) detail the symptom picture, (2) describe the personality and interpersonal behavior of the patient, (3) assess the family environment and interaction patterns, (4) plan an intervention program tailored to the specific case, (5) pinpoint the areas that treatment should focus on, (6) obtain baseline measures so that progress in treatment can be ascertained, and (7) use the assessment to design an intervention strategy and negotiate a treatment contract with the patient and his or her family.

The domain target for assessment must include more than simply the depressive symptoms in the individual and the general patterns of family functioning. As will become clear in the treatment chapters in the remainder of this volume, the theoretical model of intervention (based on behavioral, systems, and interpersonal models) gives rise to a correlated set of mediating goals in the treatment. Those specific mediating goals are targets of assessment. Thus, depending on the model of intervention, the targets for assessment in affective disorders include the cognitive distortions, dysfunctional attitudes, irrational beliefs, and distorted attributions of the depressed individual, and/or the positive and negative reinforcers in the social environment, the social skills of the patient, the patient's typical coping styles, marital conflict, the degree of interpersonal intimacy, stressors, and poor parenting skills (see Table 2.1).

Table 2.1. Assessment Instruments for Affective Disorders and the Social Content

Instrument	General classification	Description
Diagnostic assessment		
SADS	Semistructured interview	7-point rating scales of symptoms
SCID	Semistructured interview	3-point rating scales of symptoms
Symptoms		
HRSD	Clinical interview	17 items, 3- or 5-point severity scales
CRS	Self-report	52 self-descriptive statements
BDI	Self-report	21 items, 4-point intensity scales
Manic-State Rating Scale	Observer-rated scale	26 items, 5-point scales
Cognitions		
DAS	Self-report	40 items, 7-point scales
Social skills		
SAS-SR	Self-report	42 items, 5-point scales of severity
Suicide potential		
SIS	Self-report	15 items, 3-point categorical scales
Interpersonal context		
Dyadic Adjustment Scale	Self-report	31 items, 4 dimensions
Marital Satisfaction Inventory	Self-report	280 items
FACES	Self-report	6 items on each of 16 subscales
FAS	Self-report	53 items, 5 factors
Family Assessment Device	Self-report	7 dimensions of family functioning

INTERVIEWING AFFECTIVELY DISORDERED PATIENTS AND THEIR FAMILIES

The initial interview process with family and patient must be orchestrated to provide the family therapist with information bearing on three key questions:

1. Does one assess affective symptoms via an individual or a family interview?
2. Does one assign, in the interview process, the "sick role" to the patient?
3. Is there a need for pharmacological treatment of the symptoms, and, if so, how is this treatment to be initiated without identifying the patient as the sole focus of treatment and reinforcing the family's tendency to externalize or scapegoat?

These three questions are closely interrelated. There are many marital and family therapists who would fear that assessing the depressive or manic symptoms of an individual in the presence of the family would be to put the psychiatric stamp of approval on the scapegoating of one family member, thereby reinforcing the pathological system rather than modifying it. There is no empirical data on this issue, and it is our clinical impression that assessing and discussing affective symptoms with the whole family (especially when they are moderate to severe in degree) is both clinically necessary and therapeutically useful. Family members are often helpful in identifying and describing symptoms that the patient has ignored, denied, or—because of serious pathology—been unable to report. This is useful both in terms of obtaining an accurate clinical picture and in helping the patient get a realistic picture of the severity of his or her condition, especially in the cases of hypomania and mania.

If a clinician does not acknowledge affective symptoms in a family member, the patient and his or her family may lose confidence in the clinician, fearing that the symptoms, which probably brought the family in for help, will not be adequately addressed. Based on our clinical experience, we believe that affective symptoms should be assessed *both* in an individual interview with the patient and in an interview with the family, thus enabling a more thorough clinical assessment and promoting an alliance with the family. This is not to suggest that the patient is necessarily assigned the "sick role." It does mean, however, that with patients who have moderate to severe symptomatology—especially those in an inpatient setting—the clinician should begin by acknowledging the condition of the patient and, as the affective episode lifts, gradually shift the focus to the interactional patterns in the family.

ASSESSMENT OF AFFECTIVE DISORDERS

Diagnostic Assessment of DSM-III-R Axis I Disorders

In this era of semistructured interviews for assessment of DSM-III-R Axis I disorders, one can now reliably assess the affective symptoms of the patient and assign a DSM-III-R Axis I diagnosis or categorical statement about the patient's condition. Questions of practical treatment planning involve differential diagnosis (endogenous versus nonendogenous depression, psychotic versus nonpsychotic depression, and chronic versus acute and intermittent pattern). The instruments most frequently used for this purpose are described below.

The Schedule for Affective Disorders and Schizophrenia (SADS; Endicott & Spitzer, 1978) is a semistructured interview guide that enables the clinician to identify and quantitatively assess symptoms during the preceding week, during the worst period of the most recent illness episode, and over the course of the patient's life. The SADS provides a reliable method for the systematic assessment of symptoms related to depression, mania, and schizophrenia. Administration time for the interview ranges between 1 and 2 hours, depending on the patient's age and the severity of his or her disturbance. The interview data enable the clinician to make a reliable assessment of symptomatology and to arrive at a diagnosis based on Research Diagnostic Criteria (RDC; Spitzer, Endicott, & Robins, 1978). The SADS has gained prominence in the research field because of its reliability and usefulness in identifying homogeneous patient groups. Its utility is enhanced by its overlap with the criteria for DSM-III-R diagnosis. It is probably too lengthy for use in routine clinical work, but selective use of various sections may be quite helpful. In addition to yielding a categorization for diagnosis, the SADS provides summary scaled scores for severity of depressive mood and ideation, endogenous features, depressive-associative features, and suicidal ideation and behavior. Such scaled scores may be as useful in treatment planning and assessment of treatment response as is the diagnosis itself.

More recently, Spitzer, Williams, and Gibbon (1987) constructed the Structured Clinical Interview for DSM-III-R (SCID). This is also a semistructured interview format useful for clinicians in determining both Axis I and Axis II diagnoses.

Assessment of Axis II Disorders

As noted in Chapter 1, there is a growing literature on the prevalence of personality disorders in patients with major affective disorder. The most common personality disorders noted in these studies include histrionic, dependent, avoidant, and borderline. Patients with depressive spectrum disorders are more likely to have alcohol abuse, antisocial symptoms, shyness, and introversion.

For research purposes, a semistructured interview such as the SCID can be used to obtain a reliable DSM-III-R Axis II diagnosis on the family member with an affective disorder and/or on other significant family members. Probably more useful clinically because it takes less of the clinician's time is the Millon Clinical Multiaxial Inventory (MCMI; Millon, 1983), which gives scores on both Axis I disorders (including affective disorders) and Axis II disorders. In marital therapy, this instrument can be given to both spouses.

A broader approach to a taxonomy of interpersonal behaviors has been presented by Benjamin and colleagues. They have constructed the Structural Analysis of Social Behavior (SASB; Benjamin, in press), a self-report instrument that classifies interpersonal behaviors and intrapsychic events. A descriptive, taxonomic instrument such as this can be used by the family clinician to guide the focus of family therapy intervention (Benjamin, 1977; 1982).

There are many problems with the DSM-III-R Axis II construction and organization. There is inadequate coverage of typical interpersonal problems and behaviors. The way the criteria are currently grouped into 11 different diagnoses is quite arbitrary, with little empirical support. In fact, careful inspection of the criteria across the 11 diagnoses reveals extensive item overlap.

In Table 2.2, following the helpful lead of Marshall and Barbaree (1984), we have grouped the Axis II criteria into meaningful content areas of interpersonal behavior. Clinically, these areas—inappropriate assertive behavior, interpersonal aversiveness, dominance and submission, social anxiety, dysfunctional affiliation or bonding, and inappropriate affect—are most relevant to the interpersonal context of affective disorders and could be major foci for therapeutic intervention.

Dimensional Assessment of Symptomatology and Functioning

In contrast to the diagnostic or categorical approach to assessment, which emphasizes typology, the multidimensional approach permits a systematic assessment of the severity of various aspects of depression on scalar measures. This approach affords the advantages of quantitative assessment and assessment of change over time, and presumes that variation or change on one dimension can occur independent of change on another (a concept that is *not* shared by a typological or categorical approach to assessment). In this section, we will describe a selected set of instruments useful for dimensional assessment of symptomatology, cognition, social skills, suicide potential,

Table 2.2. Areas of Interpersonal Behavior in DSM-III-R Axis II Criteria

Interpersonal behavior	DSM-III-R Axis II criteria	Relevant Axis II diagnoses
Inappropriate assertive behavior	Excessive emotionality and attention seeking	Histrionic
	Self-centered; acts toward obtaining immediate satisfaction	
	Constantly seeks reassurance, approval, praise	
	Inappropriately sexually seductive	
	Procrastination	Passive–aggressive
	Argumentative when asked to do something	
	Works deliberately slowly or does poorly on tasks	
	Resents useful suggestions from others	
	"Forgetfulness"	
	Unreasonably criticizes those in authority	
Interpersonal aversiveness	Excessively impressionistic style of speech	Histrionic
	Uncomfortable if not the center of attention	
	Constantly seeking reassurance	
	Interpersonal exploitativeness	Narcissistic
	Lack of empathy	
	Reacts to criticism with rage or humiliation	
	Pattern of unstable and intense interpersonal relationships	Borderline
Dominance and submission	Insistence that others submit to his or her way of doing things	Obssessive-compulsive
	Allows others to make his or her important decisions	Dependent
	Agrees with others even when he or she believes they are wrong for fear of being rejected	
Social anxiety	Easily hurt by criticism or disapproval	Avoidant
	Unwillingness to enter into relationships unless certain of being liked	
	Reacts to criticism with rage, shame, or humiliation	Narcissistic
Dysfunctional affiliation	Interpersonally exploitative	Narcissistic
	Frantic efforts to avoid real or imagined abandonment	Borderline
	Social withdrawal	Avoidant
Inappropriate, unstable, or restricted affect	Inappropriate, intense anger or lack of control of anger	Borderline
	Affective instability	
	Restricted expression of affection	Obsessive-compulsive

and interpersonal contextual characteristics of the affectively disordered patient and his or her family.

Symptoms

We will cover here the most useful instruments for the dimensional assessment of affective disorder symptoms.

The Hamilton Rating Scale for Depression (HRSD; Hamilton, 1960) is a frequently used instrument that provides a method for rating the severity of depression in a patient already known to be depressed. Although the HRSD yields reliable ratings by trained clinicians, it is not a semistructured interview and does not provide a standardized method for obtaining the information that is rated. The original HRSD involved 21 items, 17 of which were rated on either a 3-point or a 5-point scale. The 17 items place heavy emphasis on the behavioral and somatic symptoms of depression. Because of its emphasis on somatic symptoms and its relative neglect of the cognitive/affective modes, it may be more useful for the assessment of *severely ill* patients, where indications for somatic treatment must be assessed.

The Carroll Rating Scale for Depression (CRS; Carroll, Feinberg, Smouse, Rawson, & Greden, 1981) is a self-report instrument that in content is closely related to the HRSD. The CRS contains 52 statements to which the patient responds with a forced choice (yes or no), based upon subjective experience of the past few days. Correlations between the CRS and the HRSD range from .71 to .80 (Carroll *et al.*, 1981).

The Beck Depression Inventory (BDI; Beck, Ward, & Mendelson, 1961) appears to be one of the most useful self-report instruments for the measurement of depression it is; helpful in guiding treatment intervention and in gauging therapeutic progress (Fuchs, 1975; Rush, Khatami, & Beck, 1975). The original scale was administered in an interview-assisted manner, but a completely self-administered version has been developed (Beck & Beamesderfer, 1974). The 21 items on the inventory cover the following categories: mood, pessimism, crying spells, guilt, self-hate and accusations, irritability, social withdrawal, work inhibition, sleep and appetite disturbance, and loss of libido. Schwab, Bialow, Clemmons, and Holzer (1966) point out that the content of the BDI emphasizes pessimism, sense of failure, punishment, and self-punitive wishes, consistent with Beck's cognitive view of depression and its causes.

The Minnesota Multiphasic Personality Inventory (MMPI; Hathaway & McKinley, 1951) is probably the most widely used self-report psychodiagnostic instrument and one of the best researched instruments available. The MMPI Depression Scale is one of nine clinical scales contained in this instrument. Of the 60 true–false items constituting the Depression Scale, 11 items were chosen on the basis of their power to discriminate between depressed patients and other psychiatric patients, and the remaining 49 items, on the basis of their power to discriminate among manic depressives, depressives, and normal individuals. The content of the items covers low self-esteem, psychomotor retardation, withdrawal, lack of interest, and physical complaints. The scale has adequate internal consistency, short-term test–retest reliability, and acceptable construct validity, since it correlates with other self-report measures of depression. The MMPI Depression Scale is a useful device for defining depressed populations and for measuring therapeutic outcome.

The Manic-State Rating Scale (Beigel & Murphy, 1971; Beigel, Murphy, & Bunney, 1971) is an observer-rated scale with 26 items covering depression, irritability, impulse control, sexual preoccupation, and so forth. This scale has demonstrated adequate reliability and concurrent validity, and has been used as an outcome measure to evaluate change (Beigel & Murphy, 1971; Janowsky *et al.*, 1978).

Cognitions

Apart from dimensional and categorical assessment of the general phenomenology of depression, there are various aspects of depressive cognition and perception that are seen as critical by cognitive therapists and theoreticians dealing with depression. Beck's intervention, with its focus on changing the cognitive style of the depressed individual, is a prime example. Cognitive distortions and biases in the depressed individual can be measured by such self-report instruments as the Cognitive Bias Questionnaire (Hammen & Krantz, 1976), the Automatic Thoughts Questionnaire (Hollon & Kendall, 1980), the Dysfunctional Attitude Scale (DAS; Weissman & Beck, 1978), the Irrational Beliefs Test (Jones, 1969), the Attributional Style Questionnaire (Peterson *et al.*, 1982), and the Self-Control Questionnaire (Rehm *et al.*, 1981).

As an example of this type of instrument, we will describe the DAS, in that it is relevant to one of the major therapeutic orientations to outpatient depressives (cognitive therapy as defined by Beck and colleagues) and has some good psychometric properties. The DAS is a 40-item self-report instrument that asks the individual to indicate on a 7-point scale the degree to which he or she experiences certain attitudes that are theoretically related to the occurrence of depression. These attitudes relate to such areas as self-esteem, making mistakes and taking risks, and judgments of others. The instrument has adequate internal consistency and stability over time (Hamilton & Abramsom, 1983; Weissman, 1979). Scores correlate with those for the BDI (Weissman & Beck, 1978) and are elevated in depressed inpatient samples in contrast to nondepressed samples (Hamilton & Abramson,

1983). More relevant to treatment planning, the DAS has been shown to predict the outcome of cognitive therapy (Keller, 1983) and to reflect changes from a coping skills treatment for depression (Fleming & Thornton, 1980).

General Social Skills

It has been the behaviorally oriented therapists who have posited and investigated the general social skill deficits in many individuals who complain of depression (e.g., Lewinsohn & Arconad, 1981). These social skill deficits may extend beyond the immediate family environment and arise in social situations in general and in job or school situations. Depressive individuals complain of discomfort and infrequent engagement in social activities (Youngren & Lewinsohn, 1980), discomfort in being assertive, and negative cognitions concerning interpersonal situations. Lewinsohn and Lee (1981) recommend a number of instruments for the assessment of general social skills.

The Social Adjustment Scale—Self-Report (SAS-SR; Weissman & Bothwell, 1976) is a self-report rating of performance and work, social and leisure activities, relationships with extended family, marital and parental activity, and economic independence. Relevant here, too, are a number of social assertiveness inventories, including the Assertion Inventory (Gambrill & Richey, 1975) and the Assertiveness Behavioral Survey Schedule (Cautela & Upper, 1976). A useful, more extensive self-report measure of interpersonal adjustment is the Interpersonal Events Schedule (Youngren, Zeiss, & Lewinsohn, 1975). This is a 160-item inventory tapping interpersonal activities; subjects are asked to rate the frequency and impact of each event. Scaled scores are derived from questions relating to each of the following dimensions: social activity, assertion, cognition, conflict, give positive, receive positive, give negative, and receive negative. In addition, there are a number of role-playing tests of social skills, such as the Interpersonal Behavior Role-Playing Test (Goldsmith & McFall, 1975).

Assessment of Suicide Potential

Clearly, the most important method of assessing suicide potential is conducting a thorough clinical interview with the patient, obtaining complete knowledge of the personality characteristics and social support systems of the patient (Linehan, 1981). As a supplement to the clinical interview, a number of self-report instruments might provide helpful ancillary data. Not only the content and scores that these instruments yield but also a discussion with the patient of the specific responses may be clinically useful.

The Suicide Intent Scale (SIS; Beck, Schuyler, & Herman, 1974) elicits information concerning prior suicide attempts, including information regarding preparation for the attempt, method, and expectation for rescue. The Beck Hopelessness Scale (Beck, Weissman, Lester, & Trexler, 1974) has been found to be a better predictor of future suicide attempts than of depressive episodes. A third scale developed by Beck and colleagues (Beck, Kovacs, & Weissman, 1979) is the Scale for Suicidal Ideation, which is designed to measure the intensity of current self-destructive thoughs and/or wishes.

In a clinically important examination of positive attitudes (the other side of the coin), Linehan, Goldstein, Nielsen, and Chiles (1983) devised the Reasons for Living Inventory. This self-report instrument measures primary reasons for living, including survival and coping beliefs, responsibility to family, child-related concerns, fear of suicide, fear of social disapproval, and moral objections. In general samples of people surveyed at shopping centers and in a sample of psychiatric patients, individuals who scored high on the inventory in the areas of survival and coping, responsibility to family, and child-related concerns were less likely to attempt suicide.

ASSESSMENT OF THE INTERPERSONAL CONTEXT

As we have pointed out elsewhere (Haas, Clarkin, & Glick, 1985) the family context in relationship to an affective disorder can be conceived of as presenting three different possibilities: (1) a history of relatively good family functioning, with current good coping with the ill member; (2) a history of good family functioning but poor coping with the ill member while in affective episodes; and (3) chronic poor family functioning, with moderate to poor handling of the affective episodes. When the family context is seen in relationship to the type of depression, one has an overall perspective on the important areas for assessment and treatment planning (Table 2.3.).

Stuart (1980) has outlined five criteria for adequate and appropriate marital (and family) assessment. First, the assessment should be parsimonious, so as not to slow down the treatment process. There is little need to gather information in the assessment process that will not be used in the treatment.

Second, the assessment should be multidimensional; that is, several instruments involving different methods of gathering information (patient self-report, observer ratings, etc.) should be utilized in order to achieve some convergent validity in the assessment process. An overlap of content areas by two instruments, each of which has a different method of obtaining data, gives one a firmer clinical footing.

Third, the assessment should be linked to a theory of intervention. It seems only obvious and logical that the assessment process should be directly related to the mediating and final goals of the treatment. Or, from the other point of view, the results of the assessment of relevant patient and

Table 2.3. Differential Treatment Planning for Depression

| Family context | Types of depression | | |
	Endogenous	Nonendogenous	Nonendogenous with life stress
Cooperative family environment; adequate coping with present episode	Combined pharmacotherapy and brief family psychoeducation	Individual therapy; consider pharmacotherapy	Individual or family therapy depending on nature of stresses; consider pharmacotherapy
Inadequate or poor reaction to current depressive episode	Combined pharmacotherapy and brief family therapy, including psychoeducation	Brief family therapy and psychoeducation; consider pharmacotherapy	Brief family therapy; consider pharmacotherapy
Chronically hostile and intrusive interactions	Combined pharmacotherapy and family intervention; attention to children at risk	Family intervention; consider pharmacotherapy	Family intervention; consider pharmacotherapy

family variables should lead to the differential assignment of the patient and family to a treatment that will address the specific areas of pathology (Frances, Clarkin, & Perry, 1984). For the clinician interested in the family and marital aspects of an affective disorder, this usually means that the assessment must cover the patient's social skills and family interactional behaviors around affective symptoms.

Fourth, the assessment must be situation specific. The assessor cannot assume that the behavior of an individual in one context is the same as that in another context. Systems theorists emphasize this point in arguing that what might be perceived as "personality traits" may actually be specific behaviors of an individual in a particular family system.

And, finally, Stuart (1980) notes that participation in the assessment process must be of value to the couple as an end in itself. Many couples are doing an assessment themselves of whether or not to continue to work with the assessor and to continue therapy for their problem. If they come away from the assessment process with some beginning alliance with the assessor and increased self-knowledge, they are more likely to pursue intervention. The assessment process should help develop a therapeutic alliance and involve an active negotiation with the family around the appropriate mediating and final goals of intervention.

There are, as far as we know, no existing instruments that measure interactional attributes, styles, or dimensions that are exclusive to affective disorders and to families coping with them. Indeed, there may be no dysfunctional family interactions that are specific to affective disorders, that is, no specific interactions that are likely to trigger an affective disorder or give specific stress to an affectively vulnerable individual. Coping with a depressed or manic individual, as opposed to coping with an individual with schizophrenia, or with diabetes, may, however, call for specific coping strategies.

Marital Satisfaction and Commitment

There are a number of brief and useful self-report measures of overall marital adjustment and satisfaction. The Dyadic Adjustment Scale (Spanier, 1976) is a 31-item self-report measure intended to assess the quality of marital or dyadic relations. It measures the specific dimensions of satisfaction, cohesion, consensus, and affectional expression. A more extensive, albeit lengthy (280 items), self-report instrument, the Marital Satisfaction Inventory, was developed by Snyder, Willis, and Keiser (1979). There are two forms of inventory, one for couples with children and one for childless couples. This scale is notable for its inclusion of a measure of social desirability, a virtue that the frequently used Locke-Wallace Marital Adjustment Test does not have. Finally, the Marital Status Inventory (Weiss & Cerreto, 1980) is a self-report instrument consisting of 14 items that ask about specific behaviors leading to divorce.

Marital Interaction

In the clinical assessment of marital interaction, Jacobson, Elwood, and Dallas (1981) suggest giving the couple a problem-solving task, with the therapist as observer, and rating the couple on a variety of dimensions relevant to communication effectiveness as codified in, for example, the Marital Interaction Coding System (MICS; Weiss, Hops, & Paterson, 1973). Simply reviewing the dimensions of the MICS can help the clinician pinpoint the specific couple's difficulties.

As another alternative (Jacobson *et al.*, 1981), it has been recommended that the practicing clinician utilize the Verbal Problem Checklist (Thomas, 1977). With this instrument, the clinician, as the observer of marital interaction, can rate 49 categories of verbal behavior (e.g., fast talk, slow talk, obtrusions, excessive question asking).

Although Lewinsohn does not do marital intervention, he does assess the interpersonal skills and the interpersonal reinforcers that operate with the depressed individual. Two self-report scales, the Pleasant Events Schedule and the Unpleasant Events Schedule, are used to assess reinforcers. An Interpersonal Events Schedule (Youngren & Lewinsohn, 1980) is used to assess engagement in, and the impact of, interpersonal events.

The clinician can also utilize the observations of each spouse in order to complete the assessment of marital interaction. Though it can be argued that spouses' observations might be inaccurate, it is eminently useful for the clinician to know in what areas a spouse's observations seem biased and distorted. Thus, comparing the observations of one spouse with those of the other and with those of the clinician is quite helpful in planning for treatment focus.

Developed by the Oregon Research Institute (Patterson, 1976), the Spouse Observation Checklist covers 12 categories of behavior, including companionship, affection, consideration, sex, communication, coupling activities, child care and parenting, household responsibilities, financial decision making, employment–education, personal habits and appearance, and self and spouse independence. Each spouse is told to check all behaviors engaged in by the spouse during the previous 24 hours and to indicate only those behaviors that were experienced as either pleasing or displeasing. The data can be used to pinpoint displeasing behaviors, to provide a baseline for pretherapeutic efforts, and to focus interventions on increasing positive behavior.

The Areas-of-Change Questionnaire, developed by Weiss and associates (Patterson, 1976; Weiss *et al.*, 1973), asks each spouse to list behaviors of the mate in which change would be desirable. It asks for an indication of major areas for change, including a prediction of what change the partner will desire. The questionnaire score is highly correlated with the score on the Locke-Wallace Marital Adjustment Test and provides information on target areas of treatment.

The Marital Precounseling Inventory (Stuart & Stuart, 1972) was developed to elicit material from both spouses on an extensive range of marital issues: identification of target problems, common interests, satisfaction with communication, rules for decision making, reinforcement power, general satisfaction, and optimism regarding the future. This self-assessment packet is quite extensive and is seen as one of the most comprehensive and thorough self-report packages for behavioral marital intervention (Jacobson *et al.*, 1981).

The Sexual Interaction Inventory (LoPiccolo & Steger, 1974) is a self-report measure that yields specific behavioral information regarding the quality of the couple's sex life and preference for various sexual activities.

Marital Assessment Packages

Several authors recommend a particular combination of instruments for assessing the marital relationship. For example, for pretreatment assessment, the University of Washington Psychology Clinic utilizes the Areas-of-Change Questionnaire, portions of the Marital Precounseling Inventory, the

Marital Status Inventory, the Marital Activities Inventory, the Dyadic Adjustment Scale, and the Sexual Interaction Inventory (Jacobson *et al.*, 1981).

Weiss and Margolin (1977) describe the assessment package utilized by the Oregon group: self-report instruments (the Locke-Wallace test, the Areas-of-Change Questionnaire, the Marital Activities Inventory, the Marital Status Inventory, a 28-item problem checklist, and the Pleasing and Displeasing Spouse Observation Checklists) and two 10-minute samples of problem-solving behavior rated by the MICS.

Family Interaction

The Family Assessment Device (Epstein, Baldwin, & Bishop, 1983) is a self-report measure that assesses seven dimensions of family functioning seen as central in one model of family functioning. This measure has been used in studies of intervention with families having a member suffering from major depression and reflects dysfunction of the families as well as change following family intervention (see Chapter 6, this volume). It appears to be a promising instrument in guiding the focus of intervention.

The Family Adaptability and Cohesion Evaluation Scales (FACES; Olson, Portner, & Bell, 1982) provides and index of family structure and adaptability.

Moos and Moos (1976) have developed a self-report measure tapping the quality of the patient's family environment, a measure that can be used to assess inferentially the possible contribution of family environmental variables to the affective disorder.

A self-report version of the SAS-SR (Weissman & Bothwell, 1976) provides a measure of interpersonal functioning, including family and marital relations, and parental role functioning.

Family Attitude toward the Affective Disorder

One of the assumptions we make is that the affective disorder is not under the total control of the family system. This assumption is not always shared by family therapists either overtly or covertly. However, there is a growing movement to consider major psychiatric disorders, such as schizophrenia and affective disorders, as having many causes and contributing factors, including biological and psychosocial variables. Given this assumption, it follows that a family clinician would want to assess the family's attitude toward the individual with the affective disorder and toward the disorder itself.

The spouse's observation and *evaluation* of the affectively ill patient probably constitute a crucial area for prognosis and intervention, as suggested by the work with expressed emotion Camberwell Family Interview (CFI; Brown & Rutter, 1966) has been used to evaluate family attitudes toward the patient (including criticism, hostility, and overinvolvement). Empirical study of CFI-generated responses shows that patients with spouses who express hostile attitudes toward them are more likely to have future depressive episodes. The CFI is a 1-hour semistructured interview of a significant family member. An audiotaped recording of the interview is rated for overinvolvement, criticality, and hostility. Because the CFI rating requires relatively extensive training, the CFI cannot be easily adopted for typical clinical practice. However, the CFI research literature has yielded information regarding a clinically relevant construct in the treatment of affective disorders—critical attitudes—and assessment of such family attitudes should be considered when interviewing the spouse alone or with the affectively ill spouse present. On a more positive note, utilization of the spouse's observation of the affective symptoms of the mate could be crucial not only to diagnosis but also to catching early signs of relapse in the future.

The Family Attitude Scale (FAS; Haas *et al.*, 1986) is a 53-item, self-report scale assessing family members' attitudes toward the patient and toward psychiatric care. Items for the FAS were either generated by our research group or culled from existing scales, such as the Patient Rejection Scale by Kreisman, Simmens, and Joy (1979), which measures family expressed emotion, and the Family Evaluation Form (Spitzer, Gibbon & Endicott, 1971), developed to measure the impact of the patient on the family. A principal components analysis of responses from a sample of family members of 134 inpatients gathered both at the time of hospital admission and at discharge yielded five factors that possessed moderate to high internal reliability (Crombach's alpha ranging from .63 to .91) and substantial internal stability over time as assessed by independent principal components analysis for data at three times of assessment. The five factors are as follows: (1) family attitude toward the patient, (2) willingness to accept professional help, (3) emotional involvement with the patient, (4) perceived family disruption/burden, and (5) family reliance upon social support. The FAS scales have successfully detected the effects of an inpatient family intervention on the attitudes of family members of chronic schizophrenics, patients with major affective disorders, and patients falling under mixed diagnostic categories.

ASSESSMENT AS THERAPEUTIC ROLE INDUCTION

Much of family intervention is predicted on the assumption that it is the entire system, not the individual patient, that is dysfunctional. Furthermore, an essential part of the induction of the family into family therapy is to communicate, either overtly or covertly, that the patient with affective symptoms is not the sole source of the family's problems but that there are larger family issues that are a necessary part of the intervention focus. The assessment procedure, including the initial assessment interviews and any testing, can serve as an important tool in the role induction process in family treatment. For example, when the husband of a depressed wife is asked to fill out a questionnaire regarding his perception of the marital interaction, the focus on his perceptions and feelings can help remove an exclusive focus on the wife and her symptoms. It can also contribute significantly to the development of a strong working alliance between both members of the dyad.

In summary, we consider systematic assessment of three major domains as an integral part of family/marital treatments for affective disorders:

1. *Evaluation of individual symptomatology, cognition, and role functioning* is essential during the early phase of work with the affectively disordered patient and his or her family. This clinical assessment of the affective syndrome and related personality traits and behavior is important in helping to identify the specific type of affective disorder and in determining any need for adjunct pharmacotherapy.

2. *Assessment of the illness-related perceptions, cognitions, and behaviors of the spouse and other family members* can provide fundamental information regarding the family's response to the patient's symptoms. It can assist in identifying maladaptive family attitudes and behaviors that serve to reinforce or maintain the affective disorder. In addition, it can help pinpoint specific targets for intervention and means of enlisting family involvement in the family/marital therapy process.

3. *Identification of maladaptive interpersonal communication patterns and problem-solving behaviors* is important because they may contribute to or maintain the affective disorder within the context of family and/or spousal relations. Observational assessment procedures can be especially useful in detecting the specific patterns of interpersonal interaction that limit more adaptive functioning and/or contribute to the negative and self-defeating cognitions and behaviors of the patient with affective symptoms.

In our view, systematic, targeted assessment of these three domains is not only informative but also therapeutic and facilitative in the induction and alliance-building phase of treatment.

REFERENCES

American Psychiatric Association. (1987). *Diagnostic and statistical manual of mental disorders* (rev. 3rd ed.). Washington, DC: APA.

Beck, A. T., & Beamesderfer, A. (1974). Assessment of Depression: The Depression Inventory. In P. Pichot (Ed.), *Psychological measurement in psychopharmacology. Modern problems in pharmacopsychiatry* (Vol. 7). Basel, Switzerland: Karger.

Beck, A. T., Kovacs, M., & Weissman, A. (1979). Assessment of suicidal intention: The Scale for Suicidal Ideation. *Journal of Consulting and Clinical Psychology, 47*, 343–352.

Beck, A. T., Schuyler, D., & Herman I. (1974). Development of suicidal intent scales. In A. T. Beck, H. L. P. Resnick, & D. J. Lettieri (Eds.), *The prediction of suicide.* Bowie, MD: Charles Press.

Beck, A. T., Ward, C. H., & Mendelson, M. (1961). An inventory for measuring depression. *Archives of General Psychiatry 4*, 561–571.

Beck, A. T., Weissman, A., Lester, D., & Trexler, L. (1974). Measurement of pessimism: The hopelessness scale. *Journal of Consulting and Clinical Psychology, 42*, 861–865.

Beigel, A., & Murphy, D. (1971). Assessing clinical characteristics of the manic state. *American Journal of Psychiatry, 128*, 44–50.

Beigel, A., Murphy, D., & Bunney, W. (1971). The Manic-State Rating Scale: Scale construct, reliability, and validity. *Archives of General Psychiatry, 25*, 256–262.

Benjamin, L. S. (1977). Structural analysis of a family in therapy. *Journal of Consulting and Clinical Psychology, 45*, 391–406.

Benjamin, L. S. (1982). Use of Structural Analysis of Social Behavior (SASB) to guide interventions in psychotherapy. In D. Kiesler & J. Anchin (Eds.), *Handbook of interpersonal psychotherapy.* New York: Pergamon Press.

Benjamin, L. S. (in press). Construct and content validity of SASB. In L. S. Benjamin (Ed.), *Interpersonal diagnosis and treatment: The SASB approach.* New York: Guilford Press.

Brown, G. W., & Rutter, M. L. (1966). The measurement of family activities and relationships. *Human Relations, 19*, 241.

Carroll, B. J., Feinberg, M., Smouse, P. E., Rawson, S. G., & Greden, J. F. (1981). The Carroll Rating Scale for Depression I. Development, reliability, and validation. *British Journal of Psychiatry, 138*, 194–200.

Cautela, J. R., & Upper, D. (1976). The Behavioral Inventory Battery: The use of self-report measures in behavioral analysis and therapy. In M. Hersen & A. S. Bellack (Eds.), *Behavioral assessment: A practical handbook* (pp. 77–110). Elmsford, NY: Pergamon Press.

Endicott, J., & Spitzer, R. (1978). A diagnostic interview: The Schedule for Affective Disorders and Schizophrenia. *Archives of General Psychiatry, 35*, 837–844.

Epstein, N., Baldwin, L., & Bishop, D. S. (1983). The McMaster Family Assessment Device. *Journal of Marriage and Family Therapy, 9*, 171–180.

Fleming, D. M., & Thornton, D. W. (1980). Coping skills training as a component in the short-term treatment of depression. *Journal of Consulting and Clinical Psychology, 48*, 652–654.

Frances, A., Clarkin, J. F., & Perry, S. (1984). *Differential therapeutics: A guide to the art and science of treatment planning in psychiatry.* New York: Brunner/Mazel.

Fuchs, C. Z. (1975). *The reduction of depression through the modification of self-control behaviors. An instigation group therapy.* Unpublished doctoral dissertation, University of Pittsburgh.

Gambrill, E., & Richey, C. (1975). An assertion inventory for use in assessment and research. *Behavior Therapy, 6*, 550–561.

Goldsmith, J. B., & McFall, R. M. (1975). Development and evaluation of an interpersonal skill-training program for psychiatric inpatients. *Journal of Abnormal Psychology, 84*, 51–58.

Haas, G., Clarkin, J. F., & Glick, I. D. (1985). Marital and family treatment of depression. In E. Beckham & W. Leber (Eds.), *Handbook of depression: Treatment, assessment, and research.* Homewood, IL: Dorsey Press.

Haas, G. L., DiVittis, A. T., Levitt, M., Spencer, J. H., Clarkin, J. F., & Glick, I. D. (1986, May). *Preliminary validation of a family attitude scale.* Paper presented at the meeting of the American Psychiatric Association, Washington, DC.

Hamilton, M. (1960). A rating scale for depression. *Journal of Neurology, Neurosurgery and Psychiatry, 23*, 56–61.

Hamilton, E. W., & Abramson, L. Y. (1983). Cognitive patterns and major depressive disorders: A longitudinal study in a hospital setting. *Journal of Abnormal Psychology, 92*, 173–184.

Hammen, C. L., & Krantz, S. E. (1976). Effects of success and failure on depressive cognitions. *Journal of Abnormal Psychology, 85*, 577–586.

Hathaway, S. R., & McKinley, J. C. (1951). *MMPI manual* (rev.). New York: The Psychological Corporation.

Herz, M. I., Endicott, J., & Gibbon, M. (1979). Brief hospitalization: Two year follow-up. *Archives of General Psychiatry, 36*, 701–705.

Hollon, S., & Kendall, P. (1980). Cognitive self-statements in depression: Development of an automatic thoughts questionnaire. *Cognitive Therapy and Research, 4*, 383–396.

Jacobson, N., Elwood, R., & Dallas, M. (1981). Assessment of marital dysfunction. In D. Barlow (Ed.), *Behavioral assessment of adult disorders* (pp. 439–479). New York: Guilford Press.

Janowsky, D., Judd, L., Huey, L., Rochman, N., Parker, D., & Segal, D. (1978). Naloxone effects on manic symptoms and growth-hormone levels. *The Lancet, 2*, 320.

Jones, R. G. (1969). A factored measure of Ellis' irrational belief system, with personality and maladjustment correlates. *Dissertation Abstracts International, 29*, 11–13.

Keller, K. E. (1983). Dysfunctional attitudes and cognitive therapy for depression. *Cognitive Therapy and Research, 7*, 437–444.

Kreisman, D. E., Simmens, S. J., & Joy, V. D. (1979). Rejecting the patient: Preliminary validation of a self-report scale. *Schizophrenia Bulletin, 5*, 220–222.

Leber, W. R., Beckham, E. E., & Danker-Brown, P. (1985). Diagnostic criteria for depression. In E. E. Beckham & W. R. Leber (Eds.), *Handbook of depression: Treatment, assessment, and research*, (pp. 343–371). Homewood, IL: Dorsey Press.

Lewinsohn, P., & Arconad, M. (1981). Behavioral treatment of depression: A social learning approach. In J. F. Clarkin & H. I. Glazer (Eds.), *Depression: Behavioral and directive intervention strategies*, (pp. 33–67). New York: Garland STPM Press.

Lewinsohn, P., & Lee, W. (1981). Assessment of affective disorders. In D. Barlow (Ed.), *Behavioral assessment of adult disorders*, (pp. 129–179). New York: Guilford Press.

Linehan, M. M. (1981). A social–behavioral analysis of suicide and parasuicide: Implications for clinical assessment and treatment. In J. F. Clarkin & H. I. Glazer (Eds.), *Depression: Behavioral and directive intervention strategies*, (pp. 229–294). New York: Garland STPM Press.

Linehan, M. M. Goldstein, J. L., Neilson, S. L., & Chiles, J. A. (1983). Reasons for staying alive when you are thinking of killing yourself: The Reasons for Living Inventory. *Journal of Consulting and Clinical Psychology, 51*, 276–286.

LoPiccolo, J., & Steger, J. C. (1974). The Sexual Interaction Inventory: A new instrument of assessment of sexual dysfunction. *Archives of Sexual Behavior, 3*, 585–595.

Marshall, W. L., & Barbaree, H. E. (1984). Disorders of personality, impulse, and adjustment. In S. M. Turner & M. Hersen (Eds.), *Adult psychopathology and diagnosis*, (pp. 406–449). New York: Wiley.

Millon, T. (1983). *Millon clinical Multiaxial Inventory* (3rd ed.). Minneapolis: Interpretive Scoring Systems.

Moos, R. H., & Moos, B. S. (1976). A typology of family social environments. *Family Process, 15*, 357–371.

Olson, D. H., Portner, J., & Bell, R. (1982). *FACES II. Family Adaptability and Cohesion Evaluation Scales.* Family Social Science, University of Minnesota, St. Paul, MN.

Patterson, G. R. (1976). Some procedures for assessing changes in marital interaction patterns. *Oregon Research Institute Bulletin, 16*(7).

Peterson, C., Semmel, A., Von Baeyer, C., Abramson, L. Y., Metalsky, G. I., & Seligman, M. E. P. (1982). The Attributional Style Questionnaire. *Cognitive Therapy and Research*, *6*, 287–300.

Rehm, L. P., Kornblith, S. J., O'Hara, M. W., Lamparski, D. M., Romano, J. M., & Volkin, J. I. (1981). An evaluation of major components in a self-control therapy program for depression. *Behavior Modification*, *5*, 459–489.

Rush, A. J., Khatami, M., & Beck, A. T. (1975). Cognitive and behavior therapy in chronic depression. *Behavior Therapy*, *6*, 398–404.

Schwab, J. J., Bialow, M. R., Clemmons, R. S., & Holzer, C. E. (1966). The affective symptomatology of depression in medical inpatients. *Psychomatics*, *7*, 214–217.

Snyder, D. K., Willis, R. M., & Keiser, T. W. (1979). Empirical validation of the Marital Satisfaction Inventory: An actuarial approach. *Journal of Consulting and Clinical Psychology*, *49*, 262–268.

Spanier, G. B. (1976). Measuring dyadic adjustment: New scales for assessing the quality of marriage and similar dyads. *Journal of Marriage and the Family*, *38*, 15–28.

Spitzer, R., Endicott, J., & Robins, E. (1978). Research Diagnostic Criteria: Rationale and reliability. *Archives of General Psychiatry*, *35*, 773–782.

Spitzer, R., Gibbon, M., & Endicott, J. (1971). *Family Evaluation Form*. New York: Biometrics Research Department, New York State Department of Mental Hygiene.

Spitzer, R., Williams, J., & Gibbon, M. (1987). *Instruction manual for the Structured Clinical Interview for DSM-III-R* (SCID, 4/1/87 rev.). New York: Biometrics Research Department, New York State Psychiatric Institute.

Stuart, R. (1980). *Helping couples change*. New York: Guilford Press.

Stuart, R. B., & Stuart, F. (1972). *Marital Precounseling Inventory*. Champaign, IL: Research Press.

Thomas, E. J. (1977). *Marital communication and decision-making*. New York: Free Press.

Weiss, R. L., & Cerreto, M. C. (1980). The Marital Status Inventory: Development of a measure of dissolution potential. *American Journal of Family Therapy*, *8*, 80–85.

Weiss, R. L., Hops, H., & Patterson, G. R. (1973). A framework for conceptualizing marital conflict, technology for altering it, some data for evaluating it. In L. A. Hamerlynck, L. C. Handy, & E. J. Mash (Eds.), *Behavior change: Methodology, concepts, and practice*. Champaign, IL: Research Press.

Weiss, R. L., & Margolin, G. (1977). Assessment of marital conflict and accord. In A. R. Ciminero, K. D. Calhoun, & H. E. Adams (Eds.), *Handbook of behavior assessment*. New York: Wiley.

Weissman, A. N. (1979). *The Dysfunctional Attitude Scale: A validation study*. Unpublished doctoral dissertation, University of Pennsylvania.

Weissman, A. N., & Beck, A. T. (1978). *Development and validation of the Dysfunctional Attitude Scale: A preliminary investigation*. Paper presented at the meeting of the American Educational Research Association, Toronto.

Weissman, M. M., & Bothwell, S. (1976). Assessment of social adjustment by patient self-report. *Archives of General Psychiatry*, *33*, 111–115.

Youngren, M. A., & Lewinsohn, P. M. (1980). The functional relationship between depression and problematic interpersonal behavior. *Journal of Abnormal Psychology*, *89*, 333–341.

Youngren, M. A., Zeiss, A. M., & Lewinsohn, P. M. (1975). *The Interpersonal Events Schedule*. Unpublished mimeo, University of Oregon.

PART TWO

THERAPEUTIC STRATEGIES WITH COUPLES

Family and marital treatments are often thought of as therapeutic *strategies*, when, in fact, the term "marital therapy" more accurately refers to the *format* of treatment, defined by the constellation of participants in the therapeutic interaction rather than by the therapeutic techniques or theory of action. This section of the book focuses on the application of marital treatments for the couple when one spouse has an affective disorder. The two chapters in this section highlight two very different treatment approaches, including comprehensive strategies and techniques for use within a marital treatment format.

In Chapter 3, Dobson, Jacobson, and Victor review the theoretical foundations of cognitive–behavioral marital treatments for depression. They present innovative strategies for treating depression when it is accompanied by marital distress.

In Chapter 4, Coyne presents a description of strategic marital therapy for couples with a depressed spouse. He elaborates further on the relationship between marital problems and depression; problematic marital interactions are viewed as ineffective efforts to cope with the depressive symptoms. Included in this chapter is a series of illustrative clinical vignettes.

3

Integration of Cognitive Therapy and Behavioral Marital Therapy

KEITH S. DOBSON
NEIL S. JACOBSON
JOYCE VICTOR

Although it has been recognized for some time that depression and marital distress tend to co-occur (Hinchcliffe, Hooper, Roberts, & Vaughan, 1975; Lewinsohn, 1974; Weissman & Paykel, 1974), it is only recently that theorists and therapists have addressed themselves to developing integrated strategies for the treatment of depressed persons in their marital context. This chapter presents one model of treatment for depressed persons that uses the marital system as a vehicle for change but that also makes use of interventions that have been developed for treating individual depressed persons. The treatment is therefore an integrated model, drawing from behavioral marital therapy (Jacobson, 1984a; Jacobson & Margolin, 1979) and cognitive therapy (Beck, 1976; Beck, Rush, Shaw, & Emery, 1979; DeRubeis & Beck, 1988) in the treatment of marriages where one person is depressed.

THE NATURE OF DEPRESSION

Clinical depression has repeatedly been noted to be a multivariate problem (American Psychiatric Association, 1980; Craighead, 1980). The diagnosis of depression rests upon the identification of a number of symptoms that can be roughly divided into cognitive, behavioral, affective, and physiological categories. Available treatment models for depression tend to reflect the major categories of symptomatology in depression, as evidenced by the existence of cognitive (Beck et al., 1979) behavioral (Lewinsohn, Munoz, Youngren, & Zeiss, 1978), and physiological (e.g., Bassuk & Schoonover, 1978) therapies. Within this complex series of problems and treatment approaches, our model focuses upon two aspects of depressive functioning, namely, the cognitive component of depression and behavioral (interpersonal) functioning.

Cognitive Aspects of Depression

There is a large body of literature that addresses cognitive aspects of depression. Although some of the research attempts to document differences between depressed and nondepressed persons on cognitive tasks (see Miller, 1975, for a review), much of it is based upon Beck's model of depression (Beck, 1976; Beck et al., 1979; Kovacs & Beck, 1978). In brief, the cognitive model of depression states that individuals become depressed and maintain their depression as a result of certain negative patterns of thinking that lead to dysphoric mood, inhibited behavior, and the other symptoms of depression. Also, while depressed persons may initially respond to some negative, aversive event in their lives, the cognitive model asserts that these persons are also likely to distort the nature of their experience in a depressive fashion, through one of a series of possible cognitive distortions. Based upon these distorted perceptions of interactions and events, depressed persons may experience events as worse than they are, and through their response to these experiences, they may further exacerbate the depression through inappropriate reactions. For example, a woman who misperceives her husband's lateness from work as a sign that he no longer cares for her (when, in fact, his boss detained him for some extra work) may react with anger and sadness; reactions that are not based on an accurate understanding of the situation.

There have been many research attempts to document the distortion hypothesis in depression. The overwhelming body of evidence suggests that depressed persons, compared to similar but nondepressed persons, do tend to view events as somewhat more stark and negative. This finding has been documented in the areas of life events (Miller, Klee, & Norman, 1982; Paykel et al., 1969), ambiguous feedback after performance (DeMonbreun & Craighead, 1977; Dobson & Shaw, 1981; Nelson & Craighead, 1977), and memory for interpersonal feedback (Gotlib, 1983), as well as in other areas. Thus it is tempting to conclude that depressives do negatively distort events and experience. However, there is also evidence in some situations that nondepressed persons may distort experience in a positive fashion (Lewinsohn, Mischel, Chaplin, & Barton, 1980), perhaps in an effort to maintain self-esteem. In any event, it does appear that depressed people experience events in a more negative fashion than nondepressed persons, and whether this negative experience is due to a negative distortion of the event, or to the failure of depressives to distort events in a positive fashion so as to maintain positive self-esteem, the depressive nature of depressed person's cognitions is not in much doubt (Coyne & Gotlib, 1983; Dobson, 1986).

A second area in which cognitive phenomena in depression have been highlighted is in attributions for events. With the change of the original learned helplessness model of depression (Seligman, 1975) into the attributional reformulation (Abramson, Seligman, & Teasdale, 1978), many studies examined the nature of explanations for outcomes given by depressed persons. In general, these studies have shown that depressed persons tend to explain negative outcomes in terms of internal and stable attributions (i.e., they blame themselves), but provide more external and unstable attributions for success (i.e., they attribute success to luck). These patterns of causal attributions have been examined in terms of this impact on self-esteem and mood, and the therapeutic implications of these patterns have also been explored (Beach, Abramson, & Levine, 1981).

Another area of research on the cognitions of depressives concerns the cross-situational beliefs and assumptions that depressives may hold that might predispose them to negative distortions of specific events. These hypothesized assumptions, or schemas, are thought to be organized systems of cognitions that actively filter and organize the information a person gleans from the environment. For example, Beck *et al.* (1979) present the case of a person who held the assumption that "not being loved leads automatically to unhappiness" (p. 260). Presumably, a person with such an active assumption would strive, in his or her interpersonal interactions, to be loved, or failing this, might become depressed. Thus a number of specific situations might lead to unhappiness through the operation of this one assumption. Research attesting to the depressive nature of assumptions is sparse, but it does appear that depressed persons tend to endorse assumptions that are more depressive (Dobson & Breiter, 1983; Eaves & Rush, 1984; Weissman & Beck, 1978). Also, at least one study has found that negative assumptions may be predictive of relapse of depressive symptoms following treatment (Simons, Lustman, Wetzel, & Murphy, 1985). Thus, though the causal nature of these assumptions is still speculative, the evidence does support negative thinking styles in depression.

Interpersonal Relationships and Depression

In addition to the extensive research that exists on the cognitive component of depression, there is a large body of literature focusing on the behavioral component. This literature can be conceptualized as examining three different areas of interpersonal relationships: the behavior of the depressed persons themselves, the social response that depressed persons engender, and intimate relationships and depression.

The interpersonal behavior of depressed persons has been examined largely in terms of skill deficits that they may have that lead to unsatisfying interpersonal interactions and lower rates of positive reinforcement for their interpersonal behavior, leading, in turn, to withdrawal, social avoidance and isolation, and the other symptoms of depression (Lewinsohn, 1974; Lewinsohn & Arconad, 1981; McLean, 1981). Included among the behavioral skills that have been identified as possible causes of problems for depressed persons are communication skills (McLean, 1981), assertiveness skills (Lewinsohn & Arconad, 1981; Lewinsohn et al., 1978), problem-solving skills (Gotlib & Asarnow, 1979), and other social skills (e.g., time management) (Epstein, 1985). Because of the identification of these potential behavioral skill deficits, a number of therapies for depression have incorporated skill training in their treatment packages (Beck et al., 1979; Klerman, Weissman, Rounsaville, & Chevron, 1984; Lewinsohn et al., 1978).

The social response engendered by depressives was highlighted by Coyne (1976b). He suggested that depressed persons initially receive support and a show of concern when they express depressive behavior, but that if this depression does not soon remit, its negative aspects soon become aversive to those around them, and the social interactions will tend to become more negative and potentially hostile. The depressed person, perceiving this hostility, tends to become more despondent, which, in turn, leads to further rejection and more depression, in what Coyne labeled a "deviation amplifying process" (p. 18). A number of studies have been conducted that support the contention that depressed persons are socially rejected. These findings have been found with telephone contacts (Coyne, 1976a), intercom speakers (Hammen & Peters, 1977), and confederate depressives (Howes & Hokanson, 1979). Gotlib and Robinson (1982), while failing to find social rejection of depressed college students in their study, did find that depressed persons received more negative verbal comments and fewer positive comments in the 15-minute interactions used in their study. Although there have also been failures to find the social rejection phenomenon (King & Heller, 1984), the general consensus appears to be that depressed persons do engender a negative response in those with whom they are interacting, such that they appear to have more unsatisfying interactions (Strack & Coyne, 1983), and that other people are less likely to want to interact with them in the future. Thus, though it is not clear exactly what it is about the behavior of depressed persons that leads to this negative social response, the social rejection of depressed persons does appear to occur, supporting Coyne's original hypothesis (1976b).

The marital consequences of depression have been documented by a number of investigators (Coleman & Miller, 1975; Epstein, 1985; Heins, 1978; Hinchcliffe, Hooper, & Roberts, 1978a, 1978b; Jacobson, 1984b; Weissman & Paykel, 1974). As has been noted elsewhere (e.g., Epstein,

1985), most of the studies that examine depression and marital adjustment have been cross-sectional and correlational. As such, the causal primacy of depression for marital disturbance, or of marital disturbance for depression, has not been adequately demonstrated. For example, in one of the first major investigations of the interpersonal relationships of depressed persons, Weissman and associates studied the social adjustment of 40 depressed women. As Weissman and Paykel (1974) reported, the social adjustment of these women was markedly worse than that of a control group of 40 nondepressed women, and this social maladjustment was most pronounced in the areas of marital relationships and parent and worker roles. In a 4-year follow-up of a subsample of women from the depressed group who were free from depressive symptoms, Bothwell and Weissman (1977) reported much less social maladjustment than previously, although this group was still less well-adjusted than the nondepressed control group in the areas of interpersonal friction and marital role adjustment. These results support the contention that interpersonal maladjustment and depression tend to co-occur and that marital maladjustment may be relatively stable in individuals who have been depressed. Since prospective data were not collected, it is not possible to make an etiological argument for marital dysfunction and depression.

A number of observational studies have also been conducted to examine the marital interaction patterns of couples when one spouse is depressed. The first of these studies was a series conducted by Hinchcliffe, Hooper, and Roberts (1978a, 1978b). Couples with a depressed spouse demonstrated more tension than control couples, who consisted of surgical patients and their spouses. Depressed couples also interrupted their spouses more and exhibited less fragmented speech than their nondepressed counterparts. Other differences included more negative tension releasers, less laughter, and more personal references in depressed couples. In short, the interactions between depressed patients and their spouses were generally negative, highly emotional, formal, uneven, and disruptive.

These and several other, unpublished studies failed to control for marital distress in their comparisons between depressed couples and controls. Since depression and marital distress are highly correlated, it is entirely possible that the differences found in the Hinchcliffe *et al.*, 1978a, 1978b) study were due to marital distress *per se* rather than to depression in particular. The first study to control for marital distress was conducted by Hautzinger, Linden, and Hoffman (1982), who included two maritally distressed groups, one of which also had a depressed spouse. The nondepressed partners of depressed spouses expressed more hopefulness for the future, more statements of positive well-being, and more positive self-evaluations than did their depressed spouses. Nondepressed spouses were also higher on negative partner evaluations, demands for help, self-exclusions, initiations, and disagreements than their depressed partners. When compared to the nondepressed spouses with nondepressed partners, the nondepressed spouses of depressed partners cried more, spoke less positively about their own somatic and psychological well-being, evaluated their partners and their relationships more negatively and themselves more positively, agreed less often with their partners, and offered more help to their partners. Overall, these results indicate that the nondepressed partner is positive when evaluating himself or herself but negative when evaluating his or her depressed spouse.

In another recent study (Biglan *et al.*, 1985), the interactions of normal married couples were compared to those of depressed couples with and without marital distress. Normal couples used more self-disclosure than either of the two clinical groups, while distressed/depressed couples exhibited the least amount of facilitative behavior. The clinical groups also tended to engage in more aggressive behavior than did the normal couples. Finally, husbands in distressed/depressed relationships offered more solutions to their problems than did their wives; this tendency was also found in the depressed-only couples.

Thus far, we have discussed mainly the data on the nondepressed partners of depressed patients. Many of the studies we have cited also report data on the behavior of the depressed spouses themselves. For example, in the Hinchcliffe *et al.* (1978a, 1978b) study, depressed patients were more expressive and showed more tension than did control-group subjects. They also exhibited more negative tension release and used more pauses and interruptions than did control subjects. In the Hautzinger *et al.* (1982) study, depressed people were more negative in their self-evaluations and expressed greater pessimism about the future than did control subjects. Relative to their partners, they were more positive in their evaluations of the relationship but also were more demanding, and, when compared to control couples, they were more likely to agree with their partners' statements. Biglan *et al.* (1985) found that depressed wives exhibited more depressive behavior (e.g., complaining, ignoring, self-derogating, any statement with dysphoric affect).

In one of only two studies using sequential analyses, to examine the behavior of depressives and their spouses, Biglan *et al.* (1985) found that in depressed/distressed relationships, the wives' depressive behavior was functional in reducing the probability of subsequent aggressive behavior on the part of the husbands. Among these couples, the wive's aggressive behavior decreased the probability of the husbands' problem-solving proposals, and the wives' facilitative behavior led to increased facilitative behavior from the husbands. Other findings of note were that in depressed-only couples, wives' facilitative behavior increased hsubands' subsequent dysphoric behavior; aggressive behavior on the part of the husbands was associated with a greater reduction in the wives' subsequent depressive behavior; and facilitative behavior of husbands in the depressed-only group also increased the wives' facilitative behavior to a greater extent than was the case among normal couples.

Finally, Hooley and her associates (Hooley, 1985; Hooley & Hahlweg, 1985, in press) looked at two groups of couples with a hospitalized depressed spouse. In the group where couples scored high on expressed emotion (EE), the nondepressed spouse's, when interviewed alone, made many critical remarks about their partners, whereas nondepressed spouses in the low EE group offered few criticisms of their depressed partners. In a sequential analysis based on the researchers' data, positive escalation patterns were found more often in the low EE couples, whereas in high EE couples, there was a higher probability of negative escalation. In low EE relationships, the patient was responsible for keeping the positive escalation process going, whereas in high EE relationships, the nondepressed spouse controlled both positive and negative escalation sequences.

Within the general observation that depression and marital conflict tend to coexist, a number of more specific related sets of problems can be identified. At both the behavioral and the cognitive levels, research has shown that similar deficits emerge in both depression and marital conflict. At a behavioral level, communication skills have been implicated in depression (Lewinsohn, 1974; Lewinsohn & Arconad, 1981), and several therapy programs for depression incorporate communication and social skill training. Similarly, communication deficits have been widely acknowledged in marital distress, and communication timing is almost universally applied in the treatment of couples (Baucom, 1984; Jacobson & Margolin, 1979; L'Abate, 1981).

More recently, attention has been given to cognitive correlates of depression and marital distress. For example, while it has been acknowledged for some time that depressed persons tend to have attributional patterns that contribute to maintaining their depressed status, recent research has begun to analyze the attributional patterns of distressed couples, and attempts are being made to devise attribution-based therapy interventions. Much of this research has been spurred by an interest in the addition of mediational variables to behavioral models of marital dysfunction and therapy (Doherty, 1982; Eidelson & Epstein, 1982; Jacobson, Follette, & McDonald, 1982; Jacobson, Waldron, & Moore, 1980).

In general, the focus of this research in distressed couples has been on the identification of patterns of attributions that may lead to or maintain disturbed relationships. One of the major predictions in this vein has been that distressed couples will be marked by a tendency to attribute negative or aversive behavior in their partners to internal causes, and positive or caring behavior to external causes. This prediction suggests that distressed couples will, therefore, tend to see their partners in a negative light and to blame them for unpleasant interactions. In an investigation of attributional patterns in distressed couples, Jacobson, McDonald, Follette, & Berley (1985) had 49 nondistressed and 23 distressed couples attempt to solve a hypothetical problem wherein one of the partners had previously been instructed to act in either a positive or a negative fashion. Following the interactions, attributional ratings for the partner's behavior confirmed the experimental prediction: whereas nondistressed couples tended to attribute negative behavior to external causes, a strong group-by-partner-behavior interaction emerged as a result of the distressed couples' attributing negative behavior to internal causes.

Becaue of the existence of studies that have failed to find the internal attribution for negative behavior in distressed couples (cf. Fincham & O'Leary, 1983), Fincham (1985) conducted a study in which 18 distressed and 19 nondistressed couples made a series of attributions for actual marital difficulties. The results of this investigation revealed that distressed couples were more likely to attribute marital difficulties to their partners or to the relationship, although no group differences emerged for self-attributions or "circumstance" attributions for marital difficulties. Fincham suggests that these data contradict the use of unipolar internal versus external ratings of attributions, as were employed in other studies. In addition, Fincham (1985) found evidence for more global attributions in distressed couples, suggesting that such couples tend to view their problems in a nonspecific, vague manner.

Finally, Holtzworth-Munroe and Jacobson (1985) extended this literature by attempting to replicate previous studies and answer two additional questions: First, to what extent are couples likely to engage in attributional activity when such attributions are not directly solicited by psychologists, and second, what kinds of attributions are produced spontaneously when they do occur? Thus, in addition to studying the content of causal attributions in both distressed and nondistressed couples, Holtzworth-Munroe and Jacobson developed an indirect probe in order to look at the volume of spontaneously occurring attributional activity as a function of distress level, valence of behavior (positive and negative), and frequency of behavior in the relationship. One of the most interesting findings was a distress-by-sex interaction, such that husbands in unsatisfying relationships reported a greater tendency to engage in attributional activity than did happily married husbands, whereas wives in the two groups did not differ. Across levels of distress, negative behavior was more likely to produce attributional activity than was positive behavior. Finally, in the indirect as well as in the more traditional direct probes, the content differences found in previous studies were replicated: Distressed couples, compared with their nondistressed counterparts, were particularly likely to report "distress-maintaining" attributions and particularly unlikely to report "relationship-enhancing" attributions. In short, distressed couples tended to attribute their partners' negative behavior to internal, global, stable, and intentional factors, whereas positive behavior was written off as specific, unstable, external, and unintentional.

The preceding research supports the tendency in distressed couples to explain negative behavior or marital problems in terms of their partners—in effect, to blame them for the distress and problems (Baucom, Bell, & Duhe, 1982; Berley & Jacobson, 1984; Revenstorf, 1984). The existence of this attributional tendency has been used to argue for the development of cognitive–behavioral models and interventions in marital therapy for distressed couples (Berley & Jacobson, 1984; Epstein, 1985; Jacobson, 1984a, 1984b). More specifically, it has been argued that some of the reattribution interventions developed in the context of cognitive–behavioral therapy for depression may be useful in dealing with marital attributions. One question, however, that requires exploration before such techniques can be adopted for marital therapy is the extent to which depression in the marriage may interact with the attributional tendencies that occur in the context of depression. As previously noted, the attributional bias that has been most often discussed in depression is the tendency to attribute failure to internal, causal factors, and to attribute success to external, unstable factors. Nondepressed persons, on the other hand, have demonstrated a tendency to attribute failure to more external causes, in what has been termed an "illusory glow." As such, nondepressed persons in distressed marital relationships should theoretically behave in an entirely consistent attributional fashion. For them, a problem in the marriage can be attributed to external factors, such as the partner's behavior or some environmental circumstance, thereby enabling them to maintain their current level of self-esteem, even if disparaging the partner or relationship somewhat. Depressed persons in distressed relationships are more likely to demonstrate a more confused or complex pattern of attributions for events than their partners. For example, if a positive event occurs in the relationship, depressed persons are not likely to attribute it to themselves, since, this action would not be concordant with their depressed self-view. They are not, however, likely to attribute the event to their partners, since this would be inconsistent with attributional biases seen in distressed relationships. As such, depressed persons in distressed relationships are most likely to demonstrate an extreme external, unstable attribution. In the context of therapy, positive partner behavior may be "explained" by depressed persons as being due to the demands of the therapist or the therapy situation.

If a negative event occurs in a relationship, depressed persons in distressed relationships are also likely to exhibit a complex pattern of attributions. On the one hand, their depression would make it more likely for them to attribute negative events to themselves. On the other hand, being in a distressed relationship appears to make it more likely that they would attribute the negative event to their partners. On the basis of these two "attributional pulls," one may expect that depressed persons will demonstrate erratic attributions for the negative events in their relationships, at times blaming themselves and thus exacerbating their depression, and at times blaming their partners and thus contributing to negative feelings about their partners and to marital distress.

In summary, though several interpersonal aspects of depression have been researched, a number of questions remain with respect to the relationships of depressed persons. It appears, for example, that depressed persons tend to receive negative reactions from those with whom they interact (Coyne, 1976a; Gotlib & Robinson, 1982; Hammen & Peters, 1977), although the nature of this negative reaction requires further investigation. Inasmuch as some studies have reported behavioral signs of a negative response but not a self-reported rejection, other studies have reported a self-report rejection of depressed persons, and a few studies have failed to find a social rejection of depressives (Doerfler & Chaplin, 1985). A second general conclusion is that depressed persons appear to exhibit a number of deficiencies in interpersonal performance relative to nondepressed persons, at least while the depressive episode is ongoing (Lewinsohn & Arconad, 1981; McLean, 1981). These deficiencies include problem-solving deficits, social problems, and other, more specific interpersonal difficulties (cf. McLean, 1981; Miller, 1975). It also appears that depressed persons are more likely to have interpersonal friction in their marriages (and presumably in their families), marital problems, problems with child rearing, and problems with the extended family. It is not clear, based upon the literature to date, to what extent these various deficiencies and problems predate the depressive problems, or to what extent the development of a depressive reaction in a person leads to various types of interpersonal deficiencies and problems, including potential marital distress. Since the vast majority of research in the area of depression tends to be correlational and cross-sectional, the temporal sequencing of interpersonal difficulties and severity of depression is an area that requires much further research.

An Interactive Model of Depression

Based upon the studies to date, it appears that both cognitive and interpersonal aspects of functioning are implicated in depression. It is equally clear that marital dysfunction is related to depression inasmuch as: (1) the two phenomena tend to co-occur and (2) some of the same interpersonal and attributional processes can be presumed to be operative for each phenomenon. Thus, though undoubtedly there are distressed relationships in which neither partner is depressed, and nondistressed relationships in which one or both partners are depressed, the clinical experience is that these two difficulties often go hand in hand. Feldman (1976) has noted this linkage between depression and marital interaction. His systems model of depression argues that both depression-eliciting and depression-maintaining feedback loops may operate within a marital relationship, and that both the actual valence of the marital behavior (positive vs. negative) and the cognitive schema and resultant perception of behavior by the depressed person require elucidation to enable us to understand how the depression develops or is maintained. Although he makes no reference to the attributional style literature, Feldman (1976) again argues for a complex attributional pattern in the depressed person when negative events occur: "The depressed spouse vacillates between states of acutely painful, conscious self-depreciation and periods of passive or active other-directed hostility" (p. 392). Again, what Feldman has observed clinically matches what has since been formalized in the depression and marital dysfunction research on attributional processes (Berley & Jacobson, 1984).

Coyne (1976b) has also made observations about what he perceives as the interpersonal process that initiates depression. He suggests that some initial insult or loss is experienced by the person who eventually becomes depressed, followed by a shift of affect in the individual and by his or her expression of this affective shift. The family members or marital partner initially respond to this affective shift with attention and support, but Coyne suggests that rather than having a curative effect, and therefore enabling the depressed person to reduce his or her depressed affect, this initial response of positive attention reinforces the depressive shift. As such, the depressed person continues to exhibit a depressed mood and may even start to hold the perception that he or she is "depressive" in nature. Eventually, the concern that family members have shown becomes less available, in that they continue to verbally express their concern for the individual who is becoming depressed, but nonverbally give signs that they are less interested, or even becoming hostile. For example, a family member may say something like "You know we will be there when you need us," but when telephoned late at night, will give some other response. This type of double message is interpreted by the depressed person, according to Coyne, in line with the nonverbal behavior, and this person perceives the social rejection that he or she is in fact receiving.

In contrast to the positions taken by Feldman and Coyne, Rush, Shaw, and Khatami (1980) hold that a depressed person in a relationship initiates and maintains the depression based on his or her own intrapsychic distortions and beliefs. Thus their model is firmly rooted in Beck's cognitive theory and therapy of depression. As a concrete example, Rush *et al*. (1980) would suggest that if a husband of a depressed woman comes home late from work and his wife reacts in a negative manner, this reaction on the part of the wife is probably based on her belief about the importance of coming home at a predetermined time and on her misinterpretation of her husband's lateness as a sign that he no longer cares for her, that the relationship is in serious difficulty, or even that he may have a secret lover. Not surprisingly, Rush *et al*. have also suggested that such distortions and misperceptions may lead to communication difficulties between the family or marital partners, and that this family disruption can in turn feed back into selective attention and misperception of other interpersonal interactions. Additionally, Rush *et al.* note that in some instances, partners may actually lack the requisite social skills to change this pattern of negative communication and interaction once it occurs, and that in these select instances, some form of social skill training may be required. In general, however, they advocate examining the communication of the interacting members, and further scrutinizing the cognitions of the members for negative thinking and faulty ideation. Rush *et al.* also suggest that once the depressed member of the family has been able to overcome some of his or her depressive symptomatology, it is important to examine the beliefs that may have predisposed the individual to depression.

Each of the preceding three positions argues strongly that depressed individuals who are in marriages need to be seen and treated within the context of the marital relationship. As such, each of the theorists of these positions argues for a marital approach to treating depression and has provided a descriptive account of what form that treatment might take. It is of note, though, that very little, if any, research has been generated in an attempt to document the impact of seeing the couple in the context of depression. Further, what research has been completed has been generated mostly by researchers interested in improving marital relationships *per se* rather than in treating depression by involving the couple.

For example, Beach and O'Leary (in press) reported on eight couples with wives who met criteria for major depressive disorder who were treated with conjoint behavioral marital therapy, individual cognitive therapy, or a waiting-list control condition. Their results suggest that depression and marital discord were effectively treated with the conjoint behavioral marital therapy, that depression was effectively alleviated with cognitive therapy, and that both of these results were significantly better than those for the wait-list control condition. They argue, therefore, that a marital therapy approach for the treatment of individuals who are depressed and in a relationship may be of value. Unfortunately, the small sample size and the limited nature of the therapy make firm conclusions impossible, but there is reason to believe, based upon these results, that some form of combined cognitive–behavioral marital therapy, or some form of cognitive therapy combined with marital therapy, may be of benefit to persons in marital relationships in which one of the spouses is depressed.

It is proposed, therefore, that a combination therapy, or some form of highly developed cognitive–behavioral marital therapy, may be the form of therapy that would best suit couples with depressed partners. The remainder of this chapter will begin to develop the nature of this form of therapy and will present some early anecdotal experience with a combined cognitive–behavioral marital therapy intervention for depressed individuals in a marital relationship. Thus, though what is presented must be considered formative and still in development, we hope that some of our suggestions will prove researchable and that some clinical developments may derive from this work.

COGNITIVE AND MARITAL INTERVENTIONS
IN DEPRESSION

Cognitive Therapies

Although many cognitive–behavioral therapies exist for the treatment of depression, perhaps the most well articulated and researched is that developed by Beck and associates (Beck *et al.*, 1979). Beck's model, which focuses on the psychosocial processes within the depressed individual, has been developed over the last two decades or so and has been empirically examined in a number of research outcome studies. Evidence attesting to the efficacy of this type of therapy has been substantial (Blackburn, Bishop, Glenn, Whalley, & Christie, 1981; Murphy, Simons, Wetzel, & Lustman, 1984; Rush, Beck, Kovacs, & Hollon, 1977), and the general conclusion that appears warranted at this time is that it is a highly effective mode of intervention for a depressed individual.

In general, the therapy focuses on idiosyncratic patterns of distorted thinking that an individual may have that would either enable him or her to become depressed in the first instance or to maintain a depressed response once it had been initiated. Included in this conceptualization of depression are two different types, or levels, of thinking. First, there are the more day-to-day modes of thinking which Beck has labeled "automatic thoughts," These automatic thoughts are the momentary ideas, images, and evaluations that individuals have of the ongoing activities in their environment. The focus of cognitive therapy is on idiosyncratic negative automatic thoughts that may distort an event into a negative, potentially depressing type of situation. In this vein, Beck has identified a number of types of cognitive distortions, such as overgeneralization, magnification, minimization, and arbitrary inference, all of which are examples of distorted thinking that may be depressive. A second, more general and less situation-specific type of thinking that Beck has discussed is the level of assumptive, or schema-based, thinking. Schematic thinking is generally of the same form as automatic thinking, but it has fewer situation-specific referents. For example, a depressive type of assumption may be "Everyone either hates me or loves me." Persons who hold this type of assumption will generally evaluate their interpersonal relationships along this love–hate dimension. Thus, this type of assumption will predispose individuals to categorize along this dimension specific people they meet, and it may predispose them to such automatic thoughts as "They hate me" or "They love me," without allowing for variations between the two extremes. Such preexisting assumptions interact with specific interpersonal relationships to engender automatic thoughts that may be of a depressive nature. It is important to note in this context that it is equally likely for automatic thoughts and assumptions to be nondepressive in nature. For example, it is possible for someone to hold the belief that "everyone either loves me or hates me" but also to have a predispositional bias toward believing that everyone loves him or her. This pattern of nondepressive thinking has been viewed as a self-serving bias (Lewinsohn *et al.*, 1980), and there is some discussion in the social psychological literature about persons who may exhibit a self-enhancing illusory cognitive style.

As previously mentioned, Beck's model of depression has been extended into the area of marital interactions (Rush *et al.*, 1980). Even within the marital context, however, the focus of intervention is still on the individual's appraisals of and cognitions about the interpersonal partner. A key cognitive intervention that becomes possible when the marital partner is present is that of the individual's identifying and testing the validity of his or her misperceptions about the partner. For example, suppose that the depressed husband of a woman who decides to go on a holiday to visit her own family determines that she is going out of a desire to abandon him or to try to ignore him. If the therapist can see this couple together, it may allow him or her to ask the husband to question his wife directly on this point and thereby gather evidence about the truthfulness of his belief. The major difference between this type of intervention and the intervention that would be used if the husband were being seen as an individual client is that in the former instance, the wife is present and can directly answer the husband's questions about her perception of the relationship and her potential desire to leave him. Had the wife not been present, it would have been necessary to ask the depressed husband to question his wife between therapy sessions. This type of "homework," though commonly employed in cognitive therapy, is fraught with potential difficulties, not the least of which include the husband's clear understanding of the homework, his ability to conduct the homework properly, his wife's potential decision not to answer his question if he asks it, his selective attention to and reporting of her response to his question, and his ability to recall the entire question-and-answer sequence when he sees the therapist at the next session. Obviously, the immediate presence of the wife enables the therapist to conduct the cognitive inervention in a much briefer and less ambiguous manner than would be possible if he saw the depressed husband alone.

Beyond the obvious advantage of using the marital partner as a source of information about potential misperceptions and attributional distortions of the depressed person, Rush *et al.* (1980) make relatively few other specific suggestions about how the marital relationship can be used in a cognitively oriented therapy. Thus, although they refer to communication training as a specific form of therapeutic intervention with the couple, they make this reference only in a general form. They do not explicitly state why this type of communication training may be important for the depressed individual or whether this training needs some kind of patterning or organization within an overall therapeutic framework. Further, there has been no specific test of the predictions made by Rush *et al.* about the utility of a cognitive approach with the marital partner present. Thus comparative studies between cognitive therapy for individuals and cognitive therapy for couples have been wanting. Although the promise for a cognitively oriented marital therapy is certainly great, few theorists have attempted to make developments of this type (Epstein & Eidelson, 1981).

Behavioral Marital Therapy

Early formulations of behavioral marital therapy tended to derive their therapeutic principles from direct extensions of the behavioral model. Stuart (1969) recognized the role of social exchange processes and reciprocal reinforcement in relationship creation and maintenance and developed some of the pioneer intervention techniques based upon exchange and reinforcement processes. Behavioral marital therapy (BMT) has since been elaborated by Weiss, Hops, and Patterson (1973), O'Leary and Turkewitz (1978), Jacobson and Margolin (1979), and Stuart (1980), with each author and time period bringing its own advances.

The beneficial effects of BMT on distressed relationships have been repeatedly observed. It has been demonstrated that BMT is significantly superior to a waiting-list (Jacobson, 1977; Jacobson & Follette, 1985; O'Leary & Turkewitz, 1981) or an attention placebo condition (Jacobson, 1978). Further research has attempted to define and test the benefits of the major components of BMT (O'Leary & Turkewitz, 1981), which, generally, include "having spouses clearly and specifically state their desires; teaching them communication skills that are seen as prerequisites for successful negotiation; and using contingency contracting, in which explicit rewards or penalties are associated with particular behaviors designated in written agreements" (p. 159). These treatment components have been referred to as problem solving (which involves problem specification, communication about personal reactions to the problem, brainstorming of solutions, solution implementation, solution revision, and problem resolution) and behavior exchange, which includes contingency contracting but also encompasses any effort to instigate increases in the mutual exchange of positive behaviors at home.

In an early attempt to assess the impact of BMT components, Jacobson (1979) treated six couples in highly distressed relationships with problem-solving training. All six couples improved over the course of therapy, although the specific impact of the training was demonstrable in only three cases. In another attempt to examine component effects, O'Leary and Turkewitz (1981) contrasted BMT as a package (involving primarily contingency contracting, but with some communication training) versus a highly developed communication training intervention. Their results, based upon use of the interventions with moderately distressed couples, revealed no overall advantage to one intervention over the other. They themselves caution, however, that the design of the study was less than ideal, since their BMT condition included a communication training component that tended to make the contrast less than ideal.

Jacobson (1984b; Jacobson & Follette, 1985) has presented an in-depth report of the treatment effectiveness of "behavior exchange" (BE; a contingency contracting approach) and "communication/problem-solving training" (CPT). Sixty distressed couples were randomly assigned to one of four conditions: BE, CPT, complete treatment (CO), or a waiting-list condition. Investigations of average group change as well as measures of clinical significance (Jacobson, Follette, & Revenstorf, 1984; Jacobson, Follette, Revenstorf, Baucom, Hahlweg, & Margolin, 1984) were employed to analyze the dependent measures, which included marital satisfaction (Spanier, 1976) and areas of change (Weiss & Perry, 1979). With respect to the marital satisfaction scores, the pretest-to-posttest comparison indicated that an average of 72.1% of the couples improved across three BMT conditions versus 17.6% of the couples assigned to a waiting list. At a 6-month follow-up, however, the three BMT conditions showed quite variable results. Most dramatic in this regard is that 71% of the BE couples showed deterioration in marital satisfaction versus 14% of the CPT couples and 20% of the CO couples. These dramatic deterioration rates for BE couples make sense when considered in light of the fact that BE is a very present-oriented behavior change technique. Therefore many of the skills that may be predicted to be more important for long-term marital satisfaction (general communication skills and problem-solving techniques) were not given to this treatment group, and its high relapse rate simply reflects this lack of maintenance skills for therapy gains. The results of this study therefore suggest that BE alone is a powerful *short-term* intervention technique.

The scores on the Areas-of-Change Questionnaire suggested a pattern comparable to that for the marital satisfaction scores, although the improvement rates were not as large in the pretest-to-posttest comparison, and the dramatic deterioration seen in the BE group for marital satisfaction did not emerge based on the areas-of-change information. For example, the average rate of improvement across the three BMT conditions from pretest to posttest was only 62.8%, compared to 23.5% for the waiting-list condition. Also, though the deterioration rate for BE was still the highest among the BMT conditions, it was only 28.6%, considerably lower than for the marital satisfaction scores. Discussion of the areas-of-change data, though, raises some cautions about this measure (see also Margolin, Talovic, and Weinstein, 1983), and the authors conclude that "these reports may suggest limitations to the AC [areas of change] as an outcome measure" (Jacobson & Follette, 1985, p. 260).

More recently, 1-year and 2-year follow-up data were collected on the same sample of couples (Jacobson, Follette, Follette, Holtzworth-Munoe, Katt, & Schmaling, 1985; Jacobson, Schmaling, & Holtzworth-Munroe; 1986). Although these data generally showed that the CO couples were doing reasonably well, very high relapse rates predominated in the other two conditions. Moreover, even CO couples had begun to relapse by the 2-year follow-up. At that time, only 50% of the couples in the CO category could have been considered nondistressed based on our clinical significance criteria (Jacobson, Follette, & Revenstorf, 1984).

In summary, the outcome research regarding BMT uniformly suggests a positive change associated with the two components of BE and CPT, although comparisons involving a CO package show an overall BMT approach to have the most dramatic and long-term benefits. Theorists and therapists in BMT have now begun to direct their attention to conceptually more refined issues and to adjunctive aids to maximize treatment efficacy. It has been suggested, for example, that variability in treatment outcome (Jacobson, Follette, & Elwood, 1984; Jacobson & Follette 1985; Jacobson, Follette, & Pagel, in press), and even treatment failure (Jacobson, Follette & Revenstorf, 1984; Jacobson, Berley, Melman, Elwood, & Phelps, 1985), can provide information about what BMT *does not do*—information that might lead to ultimate greater efficacy. A second area of investigation concerns the provision of standardized versus flexible intervention strategies. The predominant research strategy has been to contrast one structured intervention plan (usually formalized in a treatment manual) against another. This degree of therapy precision is necessary for replicability of independent variables (i.e., treatments) across studies but has been criticized because of the more regimented, artificial, and less externally valid nature of these treatments. This issue, though of great theoretical and practical importance, has not been adequately researched to date. A third area requiring further investigative efforts is that of measurement. Although measurement issues are certainly more settled today than they have been in the past (Baucom, 1984; Jacobson, Elwood, & Dallas, 1981), there is a continuing need to evaluate the theoretical and psychometric utility of assessment measures applied to martial dysfunction (Jacobson, Follette, & Revenstorf, 1984).

Cognitive–Behavioral Marital Therapy

One recent development has been the introduction of cognitive components into the practice of BMT (Baucom, 1984; Berley & Jacobson, 1984; Jacobson, 1984b). Cognitive–behavioral marital therapy (CBMT) represents a formal declaration of the importance of cognitive processes for marital satisfaction (Baucom, 1984; Jacobson, 1984b) and allows for the therapeutic development of interventions based upon cognitive formulations of marital distress. A number of CBMT interventions have already been devised, most of which are oriented toward the modification of cognitions in distressed couples. In marital dysfunction, there are at least four general areas in which cognitive distortions or negative thinking can arise:

1. *Problem definition.* Traditional BMT has employed problem-solving strategies as one of its primary treatment components. The format of this intervention generally consists of problem identification, brainstorming of solutions (usually through BE), solution implementation, solution verification, and recycling, if necessary. Less likely is any probing about the cognitions that lie behind the identification of the problem (e.g., "Why is this a problem?"). In fact, a traditional BMT therapist would likely discourage discussion about the problem as identified, since he or she would not want to undermine the "complaining" spouse's authority to identify a problem. Further, it is through problem identification and the brainstorming of compromise solutions that BMT achieves many of its effects. Having the therapist stop the problem identification phase might, therefore, seem a questionable suggestion. Nonetheless, questioning about the ideas behind the problem's identification can be important for at least three reasons that are sound in terms of cognitive intervention: (1) Asking about the nature of the problem may in and of itself lead the "complainant" to recognize that the problem is not as troublesome as he or she had first thought (i.e., the individual had magnified it); (2) asking why a concern is a concern may lead to the identification of less specific beliefs (e.g., a wife who complains about her husband's regular lateness from work may have derived this problem from an underlying fear of his being "somewhere else" or from the idea that one day he will not come home); (3) problems shift and change over the course of therapy, but if the cognitive processes that led to problem development (e.g., magnification) stay constant and are assessed, then these processes themselves may be targeted for change.

2. *Expectancies for self and one's spouse.* Baucom and others (Berley & Jacobson, 1984; Eidelson & Epstein, 1982; Jacobson, 1984b) have recognized the importance of assessing expectations held by spouses for themselves and their partners. Assessment of expectations is relevant both for situation- or problem-specific behaviors and for more general behavior patterns. The therapist may want to intervene when negative and/or distorted expectancies are found. For example, a husband who consistently expects his wife to complain about his cigarette smoking may alter his smoking behavior *in expectation* of his wife's complaints. This behavior change may create inconvenience and resentment on the part of the husband, even though he has reacted only to his expectation. His wife may be quite willing to negotiate, or even to forgive his smoking, if dealt with openly.

3. *Beliefs about change.* A specific type of expectancy that requires general assessment early in therapy and specific assessment throughout

therapy is that of beliefs regarding change. Initially, a couple must be asked about the degree to which they believe each of them can change. In the extreme, this question can be translated into the question "Can this marriage be saved?" The couple's response is necessarily related to how hard they will attempt to make personal changes and to their level of positive expectancy for the therapy. Of particular importance here are the specific expectancies each partner has for himself or herself *and* for his or her spouse, and the identification of potential misperception of the possibility for change. This misperception can occur in two ways. One partner may expect little or no change compared to the other, thereby leading to early resentment and a lack of effort in complying with therapy; or, one partner may expect more change than the other, potentially leading to an overzealous attempt to change too much too soon, and eventually leading to disappointment and despair about the partner. It is critical in this regard that the CBMT therapist clearly assess general expectancies for change at the initiation of therapy. Equally important is the continued assessment of expectancies for specific contracted behavior changes throughout the course of therapy.

4. *Attributions for behavior.* The first three areas in which cognitions must be assessed are areas that are evaluated before behavior change; however, it is critical that therapists pay attention to what spouses make of behavior change after it has occurred (Berley & Jacobson, 1984). Thus, spouses causal explanations, or attributions, for behavior change must be assessed and, if necessary, changed. It has already been stated in this chapter and elsewhere that couples in distress demonstrate a "disturbed" pattern of attributions. More specifically, they tend to attribute their partners' negative behaviors to internal, stable causes, and the positive behaviors to external, unstable causes. These attributional tendencies have previously been recognized (Berley & Jacobson, 1984; Jacobson, 1983; Jacobson & Margolin, 1979), and they necessitate attention by the CBMT therapist if they are inaccurate and potentially injurious to the relationship.

At a broader level, the awareness of a negative attributional pattern in dysfunctinal couples has lead to modifications in BMT. Jacobson (1983) has written about the "decline of contingency contracting." Included in this decline are the less frequent use of explicit reinforcers, the increased use by marital partners of a variety of options that will fulfill behavioral contracts (i.e., negotiated behavior changes are general, allowing greater flexibility in achieving behavioral goals), and the increasing ability of the person whose behavior needs to be changed to give direction to the change rather than reflexively responding to a request for behavior change. This shift in the technique of contingency contracting has been hypothesized to result in a more positive pattern of attributions for behavior change. Whereas traditional *quid pro quo* behavioral exchange allows spouses to explain their partner's positive behavior change in terms of external, unstable factors (i.e., "You only did this because you told Dr. X you would, and we have our next appointment tomorrow"), a less explicit, more general, and partner-directed form of contingency contracting makes such dysfunction-maintaining cognitions less likely. Indeed, using the modified contingency contracting scheme now favored is likely to promote a causal attribution pattern that is inconsistent with marital dysfunction (Berley & Jacobson, 1984).

There are a number of therapy techniques that distinguish CBMT from BMT. Berley and Jacobson (1984) have identified the six main interventions of CBMT as (1) challenging myths, expectations, and beliefs; (2) relabeling; (3) behavioral enactment; (4) mood and affect modification; (5) strategic interventions;* and (6) telling stories that may present therapeutic principles and rules. Although some of these interventions are theoretical and have not yet been empirically validated, the range of techniques suggests the expanded scope of BMT into CBMT.

COGNITIVE–BEHAVIORAL MARITAL THERAPY AND DEPRESSION

One area that continues to require attention is the application of BMT and CBMT to specific populations. It is clear that depression has many interpersonal consequences and that certain modifications must be made in "standard" CBMT issues and techniques when dealing with couples for whom depression is a problem. Unfortunately, there are, to date, no completed studies upon which to rely, and so what we offer here constitutes clinical suggestions based on cognitive–behavioral therapy with depressed individuals (who may be married) and on CBMT with distressed couples (either or both of whom may be depressed). Also, research at the University of Washington is under way to pilot test "combined" individual cognitive therapy *and* CBMT for couples for whom depression is a problem. Because of the formative nature of much of this work, what we present here is more in the way of working ideas than finished therapy prescriptions. For purposes of clarity, the following discussion of areas that may be amenable to CBMT when one of the spouses is depressed will use the same general target areas used in our previous discussion of CBMT.

1. *Problem definition.* When one member of a couple is depressed, it is likely that the depressed spouse's definition of the scope and severity of their problems will be more austere than is warranted (cf. Beck *et al.*, 1979). As

---

*The use of the label "strategic" here is not the same as what appeared elsewhere (Haley, 1976; Minuchin & Fishman, 1981). Berley and Jacobson (1984) define "strategic interventions" as "attempts on the part of the therapist to induce behavior changes that will indirectly promote desirable changes in attributions as well" (p. 46). As such, the CBMT innovations in contingency contracting discussed in the preceding section would qualify as "strategic."

such, the depressed partner is more likely than the nondepressed spouse to see more problems in the relationship and to see these problems as insurmountable. The therapist must ensure that the spouses contract to deal with problem areas that are important to *both* of the spouses but must not overwhelm the depressed partner in the process. As has been suggested in the cognitive therapy of depressed persons, a graduated task approach may be beneficial—an approach in which smaller, but more manageable, areas for change are identified and worked on early in therapy. As change begins to occur, the importance of the problems may be enlarged, with the eventual goal of dealing with the major presenting problems.

We reiterate that while it is important to solve specific problems over the course of therapy, it is in some respects more important to elicit the cognitions surrounding the problems as a way of (1) determining the perceived implications and meanings of the problems and (2) examining the cognitive–behavioral processes that led to the development of the problems. Particularly when perceived implications or meanings or problems appear to be based upon cognitive distortions, the CBMT therapist will need to conduct some cognitive assessment and cognitive restructuring around problems before problem resolution may proceed.

2. *Expectancies.* Much has been written in the literature on depression about the lowered outcome expectancies that depressed people have (Beck, 1976; Dobson, 1986). It also is clear that depressed patients who hold negative expectancies will believe these expectancies without supportive evidence. For example, a young woman who believes she will not have any fun at a party may well avoid that party and therefore create a self-fulfilling prophecy. In the context of marital difficulties, it may sometimes be difficult to determine whether a negative expectancy derives from depressive pessimism or from past negative marital interactions. Practically, though, making this distinction is less important than the therapeutic intervention. Based upon both individual (Beck *et al.*, 1979) and couple (Berley & Jacobson, 1984) therapies, we propose that negative expectancies be dealt with in a three-stage intervention: (1) The client who maintains the expectancy should be ,asked for the evidence that is consistent with his or her prediction. Inconsistent information may be contrasted with that material so as to balance the picture and see if the original negative prediction is still maintained. (2) In some instances, the prediction may appear valid to the client, even though he or she will acknowledge that not all of the important or possible information is known. In this case, homework may be assigned to the individual or couple in order to obtain the critical piece(s) of information. (3) It may be that some negative expectancies are valid or, at least, that the evidence supports the client's negative expectancy. In such an instance, the therapist may have the client label the issue not as an expectancy but as a problem, and then attempt to deal with the problem through a problem-solving approach (e.g., Beck *et al.*, 1979).

3. *Beliefs about change.* Again, it is not so much that depressed persons in distressed marital relationships are likely to have different types of negative beliefs about change compared to nondepressed persons as it is that they are likely to exhibit a stronger degree of negative belief than their nondepressed counterparts. As was stated before, client beliefs about change must be assessed because of the effect that such beliefs may have on efforts to change. It is also important to assess both partners' beliefs about their own and the other partner's ability to change. When dealing with a depressed person, it is particularly important to be sensitive about the person's negatively toned belief about the person's negatively toned belief about his or her own potential for change. Whereas distressed relationships are marked by critical, negative ideas about the partner, depression involves critical ideas about one's self as well, and the therapist must take care not to endorse predictions that change is not possible.

The therapist's stance that change is possible may be particularly difficult to express if the client equates the depression with being hopeless. Especially in cases where one of the spouses has been referred for the treatment of depression, the other marital partner may be quite discouraged about the possibility of change. The therapist must be sensitive to the discouragement felt by that person but at the same time must not join him or her in castigating the depressed spouse. In the extreme, it is possible that the partner of the depressed person in a maritally distressed relationship will be so negative and hostile toward that person that marital therapy will need to be postponed until the depressed individual can be treated alone and can start to make clear, objective gains that can be recognized by his or her partner. These signs of progress can then be employed by the therapist to undermine the partner's belief about the impossibility of therapeutic change (cf. Jacobson & Margolin, 1979).

4. *Attributions for behavior.* Much has been written about attributional processes in depression (Coyne & Gotlib, 1983; Peterson & Seligman, 1984; Peterson, Villanova, & Raps, 1985) and in marital distress (Berley & Jacobson, 1984; Jacobson, 1983; Jacobson & Margolin, 1979). As suggested previously, what is known about attributional processes leads to the conjecture that different attributional processes are likely to occur based on the valence of the behavior (positive or negative) and on which marital partner is making the attribution. Because of these differential predictions regarding attributions, hypothetical patterns for depressed and nondepressed spouses will be discussed separately, as will the respective recommendations for intervention.

The nondepressed spouse in a maritally distressed relationship is most likely to display a clear attributional pattern. Consistent with both the nondepressed status and the problems in the relationship, he or she should tend to attribute negative outcomes in the relationship to external (i.e., to the depressed partner) and stable factors. Thus the nondepressed spouse is most likely to blame the depressed partner for marital problems and to have little appreciation of his or her own role in the interpersonal issues at hand. Consistent with the available research and with his or her nondepressed status, the nondepressed spouse should tend to attribute positive outcomes to self-related factors. Although this attributional pattern may maintain or enhance self-esteem, it also carries the risk of minimizing the depressed partner's role in obtaining the positive outcome. The therapeutic implications of this attributional pattern in the nondepressed spouse are straightforward. The therapist should attempt, first, to have the nondepressed spouse begin to realistically evaluate his or her contribution to the marital distress. This can be done through Socratic questioning of the nondepressed spouse regarding the evidence for his or her attribution or by asking him or her for another, alternative attribution, therefore necessitating a resolution (which is likely to necessitate a less extreme attribution by the nondepressed spouse). Second, the therapist should attempt to train both partners to record positive behaviors of the depressed partner. This focus will potentially lead to a more external attribution for positive aspects of the marriage (i.e., the nondepressed spouse may begin to see his or her partner's role in positive aspects of the marriage).

While the attributional patterns of the nondepressed spouse are relatively predictable, the depressed spouse is likely to vacillate between self-blame (consistent with depression) and blaming the partner (consistent with marital dysfunction), or to adopt both simultaneously. In either instance, the therapist must be cognizant of potential distortions that support these attributions. If such distortions exist, the therapist's task is to work with the couple to obtain a more reasonable interpretation of the event in question, thereby minimizing dysfunction-maintaining cognitions. If the data are insufficient for making a judgment, the presence of the nondepressed spouse in CBMT affords the therapist the opportunity to obtain a contradictory (or corroborative) point of view. It will be most useful to obtain this second viewpoint if the issue is a matter of fact rather than of opinion, since the depressed spouse may feel personally challenged if the therapist invites the nondepressed partner to offer his or her opinions on the validity of the depressed spouse's ideas. In cases where the depressed spouse has ideas about his or her partner's concerns, appraisals, ideas, and so forth, having the partner right there to directly express himself or herself can be an invaluable asset and can bypass the necessity of assigning homework to collect this information, as would be necessary in individual therapy for depression. Again, training in how to divide responsibility reasonably will assist both spouses in making less extreme, less unfounded, and less dysfunctional explanations for interpersonal outcomes.

5. *Special considerations.* When attempting to integrate BMT with cognitive therapy for the depressed spouse alone, the exact nature of the combination will depend upon characteristics of the couple. Thus far, we

have been able to discern four different types of depressed/distressed couples, and each type requires a somewhat different combination of cognitive–behavioral therapy and BMT.

First, there is the *classic* couple. These are couples who present with complaints of both depression and marital distress. They are probably the couples who are best suited for a combination treatment. For many of these couples, the two component treatments will have interactive and synergistic effects on one another, and a treatment plan might involve approximately a 50–50 split between them.

Second, there are *denial* couples. These couples present with complaints of depression on the part of one spouse, and deny the existence of marital distress, but are judged, on the basis of a marital assessment, to be distressed nonetheless. These couples are difficult to treat with a combination format, because at least one of the partners tends to react negatively to the suggestion that the relationship may require some work. Yet a combination treatment can be quite beneficial for these couples, because the likelihood of relapse among recovered depressives within this group is high if no attention is paid to improving the quality of the marital relationship. Therefore the dilemma in treating these couples involves how to engage them in therapy without directly confronting their nondistressed relationship presentation.

The solution to this dilemma, and consequently the key to treating these couples effectively, involves the sequencing of cognitive–behavioral therapy and BMT as well as the rationale presented to these couples for a relationship-focused treatment. The early sessions tend to be cognitive–behavioral therapy for the depressed spouse, augmented by some contact with the nondepressed partner. With this type of sequencing, the nondepressed partner can gradually become accustomed to therapy rather than being suddenly asked to participate as an equal partner. The early focus makes it less likely that the participation of the nondepressed partner will be seen as a sign that the therapist views the relationship as the cause of the depression. Moreover, when the marital distress is, in fact, secondary to the depression and a reaction to the depression, marriages can spontaneously improve, at least to some degree, with an early emphasis on cognitive–behavioral therapy. Finally, quite often the early sessions lead to less self-blame on the part of the depressed spouse and to more anger being directed toward the nondepressed partner. This results in a reduced tendency to deny marital distress and leads to a smooth transition into BMT, if necessary. It seems as if these couples often move into a transition phase, which involves an overt acknowledgment of marital distress, prior to marital therapy having its beneficial effects. If marital therapy sessions were concentrated at the beginning, prior to this transition phase, they would be less powerful and/or produce more resistance.

The rationale is presented in such a way that emphasis stays on the depression; in other words, there is no attempt to redefine the problem as a marital problem. Rather, the nondepressed partner is asked to participate as a resource, and efforts are made to empathize with the frustration he or she must experience in living with a depressed spouse.

Third, there are the *systemic* couples. These couples are relatively rare in a clinic specializing in the treatment of depression but are quite common in clinics specializing in marital and family therapy. They present with complaints of marital distress, but on careful diagnostic assessment, it becomes clear that one or both spouses suffer from major depression. This depressive disorder may have been caused by the marital discord, or it may have triggered the marital discord. In either case, these couples have no problem accepting the rationale for BMT, but they may balk at the need for individual cognitive–behavioral therapy sessions. With some of them, it may indeed be the case that maximal emphasis on BMT will be most useful. In some instances, individual cognitive–behavioral therapy will be important adjunct to the marital therapy.

Finally, there are the *social support* couples. These couples present with complaints of depression on the part of one spouse, deny the existence of marital distress, and indeed look nondistressed on the basis of a marital assessment. Despite the existence of depression, the relationship has remained strong. Certainly, with these couples the emphasis should be on cognitive–behavioral therapy, but at least a few BMT sessions can be useful in enhancing the social support potential of the relationship. For example, even in a nondistressed couple, depression in one spouse almost invariably means that little attention is devoted to relationship quality during the depressive episode. Behavior exchange procedures can be useful in helping the couple cease their preoccupation with the depression and begin concentrating on the relationship. As another example, problem-solving training can often correct the tendency toward slippage in instrumental family-related tasks that occurs during a depressive episode. Parenting, household responsibilities, and financial tasks can be disrupted even in the best of marriages when clinical levels of depression intrude. In short, there is usually plenty of work to do even in nondistressed relationships, although the bulk of the therapeutic effort with "social support" couples may involve cognitive–behavioral therapy.

CASE EXAMPLE

Cognitive–behavioral therapy alone with the depressed spouse does not help couples deal with changes in the relationship that occur as the depressed spouse recovers. As we have already mentioned, not only does the wife often begin to become more assertive with and angry at her husband, but the husband often becomes more assertive and angry. (Although the sexes could be reversed, we are relying on the example of a depressed wife and a nondepressed husband because that is the focus of our current research.)

The husband's anger results in part from his wife's challenging him to a greater degree than she has in the past, but also because he now perceives her as less fragile and therefore not as "safe." In short, as the depression lifts, the marriage often becomes more distressed. On the other hand, the combination of cognitive–behavioral therapy and marital therapy can have a positive synergistic effect. Through cognitive–behavioral work with the depressed wife, she may become more accepting of herself, and this self-acceptance can be enhanced by the increased responsiveness and attentiveness from the husband that results from the marital work. These points are illustrated in the following example:

Sally and Ken were seen for 20 sessions over a 5½-month period. He is a scientist and she is a novelist. They are well educated and in their early 30s. Their marriage of 7 years was the first for both of them. They had met when they were college students, and both felt that the marriage and Sally had been fairly happy until the death of their first child at age 2½. The child died 2½ years prior to the beginning of therapy. Although Sally was very depressed at the time she entered treatment, the spouses presented as a happily married couple.

He was quiet and soft-spoken, often pausing before he responded verbally and then speaking slowly and with a paucity of words. She, on the other hand, was sloppily dressed and extremely overweight, and spoke quickly and effusively on all topics. While she easily identified and expressed her emotions, he had a much milder response to situations and was not used to identifying feelings.

Both of them perceived the cause of her depression to be the unresolved grief for their daughter. However, they both agreed that there were areas that could be improved in their marriage, and the husband expressed a willingness to do his best to help. The areas that they identified as needing work included differing styles of communication, lack of pleasurable activities together, anger and irritability on her part and withdrawal on his, lack of sex and affection between them, and unresolved hurt about their differing ways of dealing with their daughter's death. Privately, Ken expressed fears about Sally's fragility. He was afraid that if he upset her too much, she might become crazy, suicidal, and very angry.

During individual cognitive–behavioral therapy sessions, Sally identified the following problem areas:

1. She felt responsible for the death of her daughter. Even though she knew that this was not rational, she still believed it.
2. During the last months of her daughter's life, when the child had had a colostomy, Sally developed what she called "explosive diarrhea." This progressed into irritable bowel syndrome—a serious enough case that Sally had fecal incontinence about once a month in a public place. She believed that the disease made it permanently

impossible for her to lead a normal life, including holding down a job. She blamed herself for the bowel trouble with thoughts like, "I'm responsible for this disease because I can't handle stress, if I were a stronger person, I could handle stress." She also believed that because of the illness, she could not diet and so could not lose weight. And she felt awkward in public weighing 250 pounds—80 of which she had gained since her daughter's death.

3. She was critical of herself as a mother to their second child and was tormented by fantasies of the son dying and her husband dying or leaving her.

4. At home Sally described herself as angry, hostile, irritable, and easily losing her temper. Prior to the depression, she thought she had been fairly cheerful and pleasant, not involved in finding fault with her husband.

5. Her house was so dirty and messy that she preferred to leave home for many hours with her son rather than trying to live in the litter. She felt unable to clean the house. Because her house was so messy, she believed that she was unable to write, and thus she felt incapable of sustaining a major source of pride and satisfaction.

The first ten sessions of therapy with Sally focused on several goals. One was to work on her exaggerated ideas of responsibility, and another was to help her function more effectively on a daily basis. A plan was developed for organizing and cleaning her house, which included hiring a housecleaning service to get the process started. Sally's automatic thoughts included, "My responsibilities are overwhelming. . . . I'll never have any friends because I am too ashamed to have them over. Ken will leave me because of my housecleaning. . . . People won't think I can accomplish anything else because my house is such a mess." So the therapist reviewed with her what she could get done at home, and eventually alternative responses to her automatic thoughts emerged. One of these was, "Nobody is going to catch anything in my bathroom."

A plan was developed for more child care so that she could start an exercise class and then get back to her writing. And several sessions were spent on her practical problems with fecal incontinence and on her beliefs about the limitations that the irritable bowel syndrome put on her life. Although she made some progress, Sally continued to have thoughts that she was responsible for her own illness and for her daughter's death. Because of this lingering issue, she began to become discouraged by the sixth session. She thought she had made no progress in feeling better and that the most important issues were not being addressed.

During alternating marital sessions, spouses and therapist experimented with ways that Ken could lighten her mood. When Ken paid attention every day to things Sally was doing around the house and praised her, she felt that he noticed and appreciated her. This improved her mood. In many couples with a depressed wife, the increase in positive attention from the husband on a daily basis, combined with an increase in sex and affection, has a powerful positive effect on the wife's mood. This is one way in which behavior exchange has been particularly useful with depressed couples.

In addition to the behavior exchange, with its particular emphasis on which behaviors affected depression, marital sessions focused on communication training. For most couples with a depressed spouse, paraphrasing is very difficult because the depressed wife tends to hear the spouse in a distorted way; she may interpret comments as criticisms or accuse the husband of distorting what she is saying. This phenomenon occurred with Sally: When the therapist challenged her regarding these distortions, she accused the therapist of taking sides against her. Nevertheless, this exercise can provide the therapist with valuable information about cognitive distortions that can be used in future sessions.

Depressed couples also often need help in planning their week together. This focus complements the early emphasis in cognitive–behavioral therapy on the relationship between activities and mood. When couples learn to plan their weeks ahead of time, they schedule in the activities most essential to marital satisfaction and to an improved mood on the part of the depressed spouse. This process also teaches the wife to express her needs directly, in the context of the relationship. When Sally and Ken planned their weeks in advance, she made arrangements for him to take their son so that she could exercise, and he made arrangements with her to have lunch with him once a week.

During the tenth session, the course of therapy shifted dramatically. This type of shift occurs with some predictability, particularly with couples who initially present themselves as happily married. Sally had a very significant session. She was able to challenge her assumption that she was responsible for her daughter's death. First, she remembered hearing from her mother that she should never be a parent, that she could even destroy a child should she become a parent. Sally believed that because she should never have been a parent, she had caused her daughter's death. After she unraveled this connection and saw it to be untrue, there was a dramatic improvement in her mood, and she remained virtually nondepressed for the remainder of therapy. She developed more realistic ideas about parenting her second child; she stopped letting her bowel problems be so limiting and became active in teaching; and she developed some new strategies for interacting with her parents.

But she became extremely angry at Ken between the tenth and eleventh sessions. And he became angry at her. There were no new issues. But she no longer accepted the blame for their problems, nor was she afraid that he would leave her for her inadequacies. She was so angry that within several weeks, she wanted to leave the marriage unless he shaped up right away and met more of her demands for conversation and physical contact.

Most commonly, we respond to this by now predictable phenomenon in two steps. First, we normalize this new development in the couple's relationship. One can say, "It is normal for couples to have more conflict when the wife is feeling better. You can expect that this may go on for a while. If you are both willing to keep working on the relationship, you can get through this into a better relationship with some new patterns." Second, the therapist should supplement continued support of the wife with additional support to the husband, to help him deal with the increased demands from his wife. This may be difficult when the husband blames the therapist for the wife's increase in self-expression. As another husband said to one of us at the point when his wife started to feel better, "Well, you cured her but you ruined the marriage."

With this couple, the marital sessions were quite acrimonious at times. They continued to practice problem solving, communication, and behavior exchange in a more focused way as the significant issues became clearer. So, for example, in the 14th session, they came in describing a particularly severe argument. The therapist helped them develop a set of communication behaviors that they could both practice during the week. Sally agreed to practice (1) not asking Ken why he did things the way he did them, (2) not using their companionship time to discuss problems, (3) not interrupting Ken when he was slow to make his points, and (4) not having to determine who is right in an argument. Ken's list included (1) setting aside time to be together, (2) responding in some way when she asked him a question, (3) letting her know clearly when he was not available for communication, and (4) responding more to her feelings and less to whether she is right or wrong. All these behaviors addressed their fundamental "dance"; she wanted to interact more with him, and he wanted more separate quiet times. She would try to engage him in lengthy conversation, and he would become slow and vague in an attempt to distance himself, which would only irritate her more, so that she tried even harder to involve him in intense interaction, which led to more withdrawal from him. During a corresponding cognitive–behavioral therapy session, she focused both on her impatience with his slower way of talking and on his need for less verbal interactions than she wanted.

By experimenting with him being more physically affectionate with her, another dramatic shift occurred. She began to be much less angry and to require less talking from him, and her depression score on the Beck Depression Inventory (BDI) dropped close to zero. So gradually, this couple learned new ways to work through conflict, and by the end of therapy they seemed to have a new sense of strength in, and commitment to, their marriage.

In the final marital session, their original problem areas were reviewed, as were their primary mechanisms for interrupting their "dance." They also

discussed possible signs that might indicate that she was becoming depressed again and things that they could do about this right away.

In the final cognitive–behavioral therapy session, Sally expressed
amazement that her thinking had changed. She saw herself as a good parent.
She felt more securely married, without fear that Ken might leave her. She
still felt sad about her daughter but no longer took responsibility for her
death. She was working on both her novel and her teaching. She had lost
some weight and was in a regular exercise program. She was making new
friends. She had improved her grooming. She was sleeping well and was less
irritable. Finally, Sally used the notes that she kept of key cognitions to help
her deal with destructive thoughts and composed a final letter to herself for
the last session. This exercise provides a good basis for reviewing the last
session and something tangible for the client to use as a tool in remembering
both helpful ideas and the progress made.

When the therapist asked for feedback, the husband said that he had
not realized prior to therapy that he had such a powerful impact on her
mood. She said that it had been helpful to normalize their differences in
style and to hear that even happily married couples have conflict between
them. Her expectations of their relationship had been unrealistic. As of the
6-month follow-up, her BDI score was still a zero, and they were just as
satisified with the marriage as they had been at the time of termination.

SUMMARY

This chapter has focused on the role of cognitive and interpersonal dynamics in the maintenance of disturbance, both within a depressed individual
and within a disturbed marital relationship. Our discussion has relied on
existing research and clinical experience, but it also extrapolates somewhat
in terms of the specific applicability of CBMT to treating relationships in
which one spouse is depressed. In general, there is much room for optimism
in this area, because of the proven efficacy of using both BMT (from which
CBMT has evolved) and cognitive–behavioral interventions in depression,
and there exist good theoretical reasons to combine these approaches. In
doing so, however, theorists and clinicians need to monitor the progression
of interventions and to continue to be aware of outcomes for interventions
that are developed.

At present, very little is known about the appropriateness of combining
individual and marital therapy sessions in the treatment of depression, but
the inherent logic of helping depressed persons increase their behavioral
rates, alter their negative distortions, and begin to enhance their self-esteem
before attempting to shift interpersonal communication and problem-solving patterns is compelling. Questions that require clinical and research
attention include the following: (1) When is a depressed person's behavior so

disturbed that marital therapy is impossible? (2) When are a partner's negative attitudes and ideas about the hopelessness of the depressed person so overwhelming that the depressed person must be seen alone? (3) If treating the depressed person alone, when and how should the partner be introduced into therapy? (4) If the therapist treats both the depressed individual *and* the couple, who is his or her client? Is there a possibility of a conflict of interest between what is best for the depressed individual and what is best for the couple? (5) What are the relative marital effects of seeing the depressed person alone versus seeing the couple together? (6) What are the relative effects on depression of seeing the depressed person alone versus seeing the couple together? (7) What are the therapeutic goals? Do these goals tend to favor individual or marital therapy? These and numerous other questions require examination and response on the part of clinicians and researchers.

ACKNOWLEDGMENT

We would like to thank Liz McCririck and Brenda Partlo for their assistance in manuscript preparation.

REFERENCES

Abramson, L. Y., Seligman, M. E. P., & Teasdale, J. D. (1978). Learned helplessness in humans: Critique and reformulation. *Journal of Abnormal Psychology*, 49–74.

American Psychiatric Association. (1980). *Diagnostic and statistical manual of mental disorders* (3rd ed.). Washington, DC: APA.

Bassuk, E. L., & Schoonover, S. C. (1978). *The practitioner's guide to psychoactive drugs.* New York: Plenum.

Baucom, D. H. (1984). The active ingredients of behavioral marital therapy: The effectiveness of problem solving/communication training, contingency contracting, and their combination. In K. Hahlweg & N. S. Jacobson (Eds.), *Marital interaction: Analysis and modification* (pp. 73–88). New York: Guilford Press.

Baucom, D. H., Bell, W. G., & Duhe, A. (1982, November). *The measurement of couples' attributions for positive and negative dyadic interactions.* Paper presented at the meeting of the Association for the Advancement of Behavior Therapy, Los Angeles.

Beach, S. R. H., Abramson, L. Y., & Levine, F. M. (1981). Attributional reformulation of learned helplessness and depression: Therapeutic implications. In J. F. Clarkin & H. I. Glazer (Eds.), *Depression: Behavioral and directive intervention strategies* (pp. 131–166). New York: Garland STPM Press.

Beach, S. R. H., & O'Leary, D. K. (in press). The treatment of depression occurring in the context of marital discord. *Behavior Therapy.*

Beck, A. T. (1976). *Cognitive therapy and the emotional disorders.* New York: International Universities Press.

Beck, A. T., Rush, A. J., Shaw, B. F., & Emery, G. (1979). *Cognitive therapy of depression.* New York: Guilford Press.

Berley, R. A., & Jacobson, N. S. (1984). Causal attributions in intimate relationships: Toward a model of cognitive-behavioral marital therapy. In P. Kendall (Ed.), *Advances in cognitive-behavioral research, 3* (pp. 168–209). New York: Academic Press.

Biglan, A., Hops, H., Sherman, L., Friedman, L. S., Arthur, J., & Osteen, V. (1985). Problem solving interactions of depressed women and their spouses. *Behavior Therapy, 16*, 431–451.

Blackburn, I. M., Bishop, S., Glenn, M. I., Whalley, L. J., & Christie, J. E. (1981). The efficacy of cognitive therapy in depression: A treatment trial using cognitive therapy and pharmacotherapy, each alone and in combination. *British Journal of Psychiatry, 139*, 181–189.

Bothwell, S., & Weisman, M. M. (1977). Social impairment four years after an acute depressive episode. *American Journal of Orthopsychiatry, 47*, 231–237.

Coleman, R. E., & Miller, A. G. (1975). The relationship between depression and marital maladjustment in a clinical population: A multitrait-multimethod study. *Journal of Consulting and Clinical Psychology, 43*, 647–651.

Coyne, J. C. (1976a). Depression and the response of others. *Journal of Abnormal Psychology, 85*, 186–193.

Coyne, J. C. (1976b). Toward an interactional description of depression. *Psychiatry, 39*, 28–40.

Coyne, J. C., & Gotlib, I. H. (1983). The role of cognition in depression: A critical appraisal. *Psychological Bulletin, 94*, 472–505.

Craighead, W. E. (1980). Away from a unitary model of depression. *Behavior Therapy, 11*, 122–128.

DeMonbreun, B. G., & Craighead, W. E. (1977). Distortion of perception and recall of positive and neutral feedback in depression. *Cognitive Therapy and Research, 1*, 311–329.

DeRubeis, R., & Beck, A. T. (1988). Cognitive therapy of depression. In K. S. Dobson (Ed.), *Handbook of cognitive-behavioral therapies* (pp. 273–306). New York: Guilford Press.

Dobson, K. S. (1986). The self-schema in depression. In L. M. Hartman & K. R. Blankstein (Eds.), *Perception of self in emotional disorders and psychopathology* (pp. 187–218). New York: Plenum.

Dobson, K. S., & Breiter, H. J. (1983). Cognitive assessment of depression: Reliability and validity of three measures. *Journal of Abnormal Psychology, 92*, 107–109.

Dobson, K. S., & Shaw, B. F. (1981). The effects of self-correction on cognitive distortions in depression. *Cognitive Therapy and Research, 5*, 391–403.

Doerfler, L. A., & Chaplin, W. F. (1985). Type III error in research on interpersonal models of depression. *Journal of Abnormal Psychology, 94*, 227–230.

Doherty, W. J. (1982). Attributional style and negative problem solving in marriage. *Family Relations, 31*, 201–205.

Eaves, G., & Rush, A. J. (1984). Cognitive patterns in symptomatic and remitted unipolar major depression. *Journal of Abnormal Psychology, 93*, 31–40.

Eidelson, R. J., & Epstein, N. (1982). Cognitive and relationship maladjustment: Development of a measure of dysfunctional relationship beliefs. *Journal of Consulting and Clinical Psychology, 50*, 715–720.

Epstein, N. (1985). Depression and marital dysfunction: Cognitive and behavioral linkages. *International Journal of Mental Health, 13* (3–4), 86–104.

Epstein, N., & Eidelson, R. J. (1981). Unrealistic beliefs of clinical couples: Their relationship to expectations, goals and satisfaction. *American Journal of Family Therapy, 9*(4), 13.

Feldman, L. B. (1976). Depression and marital interaction. *Family Process, 15*, 389–395.

Fincham, F. D. (1985). Attribution processes in distressed and nondistressed couples: 2. Responsibility for marital problems. *Journal of Abnormal Psychology, 92*, 183–190.

Fincham, F. D., & O'Leary, K. D. (1983). Causal inferences for spouse behavior in maritally distressed and non-distressed couples. *Journal of Social and Clinical Psychology, 1*, 42–57.

Gotlib, I. H. (1983). Perception and recall of interpersonal feedback: Negative bias in depression. *Cognitive Therapy and Research, 7*, 399–412.

Gotlib, I. H., & Asarnow, R. F. (1979). Interpersonal and impersonal problem-solving skills in mildly and clinically depressed university students. *Journal of Consulting and Clinical Psychology, 47,* 86–95.

Gotlib, I. H., & Robinson, L. A. (1982). Responses to depressed individuals: Discrepancies between self-report and observer-rated behavior. *Journal of Abnormal Psychology, 91,* 231–240.

Haley, J. (1976). *Problem-solving therapy.* San Francisco: Jossey-Bass.

Hammen, C. L., & Peters, S. D. (1977). Differential responses to male and female depressive reactions. *Journal of Consulting and Clinical Psychology, 45,* 994–1001.

Hautzinger, M., Linden, M., & Hoffman, N. (1982). Distressed couples with and without a depressed partner: An analysis of their verbal interaction. *Journal of Behavior Therapy and Experimental Psychiatry, 13,* 307–314.

Heins, T. (1978). Marital interaction in depression. *Australian and New Zealand Journal of Psychiatry, 12,* 269–275.

Hinchcliffe, M. K., Hooper, D., & Roberts, F. J. (1978a). *The melancholy marriage: Depression in marriage and psychosocial approaches to therapy.* New York: Wiley.

Hinchcliffe, M., Hooper, D., & Roberts, F. (1978b). The melancholy marriage: An inquiry into the interaction of depression. III. Responsiveness. *British Journal of Medical Psychology, 51,* 1–13.

Hinchcliffe, M., Hooper, D., Roberts, .F., & Vaughan, P. (1975). A study of the interaction between depressed patients and their spouses. *British Journal of Psychiatry, 126,* 164–172.

Holtzworth-Munroe, A., & Jacobson, N. S. (1985). Causal attributions of married couples: When do they search for causes? What do they conclude when they do? *Journal of Personality and Social Psychology, 48,* 1398–1412.

Hooley, J. M. (1985). *Expressed emotion and depression: Interactions between patients and high versus low EE spouses.* Manuscript submitted for publication.

Hooley, J. M., & Hahlweg, K. (1985). *Expressed emotion and depression: (2) Sequential analysis of the interactions of high and low EE dyads.* Unpublished manuscript.

Hooley, J. M., & Hahlweg, K. (in press). The marriages and interaction patterns of depressed patients and their spouses: Comparing high and low EE dyads. In M. J. Goldstein, K. Hahlweg, & I. Hand (Eds.), *Treatments of schizophrenia family assessment and intervention.*

Howes, M., & Hokanson, J. (1979). Conversational and social responses to depressive interpersonal behavior. *Journal of Abnormal Psychology, 88,* 625–634.

Jacobson, N. S. (1977). Problem solving and contingency contracting in the treatment of marital discord. *Journal of Consulting and Clinical Psychology, 45,* 92–100.

Jacobson, N. S. (1978a). Specific and nonspecific factors in the effectiveness of a behavioral approach to the treatment of marital discord. *Journal of Marriage and Family Counseling, 46,* 442–452.

Jacobson, N. S. (1979). Increasing positive behavior in severely distressed marital relationships: The effects of problem-solving training. *Behavior Therapy, 10,* 311–326.

Jacobson, N. S. (1983). Clinical innovations in behavioral marital therapy. In K. Craig & R. McMahon (Eds.), *Clinical behavior therapy* (pp. 179–191). New York: Brunner/ Mazel.

Jacobson, N. S. (1984a). Marital therapy and the cognitive–behavioral treatment of depression. *The Behavior Therapist, 7,* 143–147.

Jacobson, N. S. (1984b). The modification of cognitive processes in behavioral marital therapy: Integrating cognitive and behavioral intervention strategies. In K. Halweg & N. S. Jacobson (Eds.), *Marital interaction: Analysis and modification* (pp. 285–308). New York: Guilford Press.

Jacobson, N. S., Berley, R. A., Melman, K. N., Elwood, R., & Phelps, C. (1985). Failure in behavioral marital therapy. In S. Coleman (Ed.), *Failures in family therapy* (pp. 91–134). New York: Guilford Press.

Jacobson, N. S., Elwood, R. W., & Dallas, M. (1981). Assessment of marital dysfunction. In D. H. Barlow (Ed.), *Behavioral assessment of adult disorders* (pp. 439–479). New York: Guilford Press.

Jacobson, N. S., & Follette, W. C. (1985). Clinical significance of improvement resulting from two behavioral marital therapy components. *Behavior Therapy, 16,* 249–262.

Jacobson, N. S., Follette, W. C., & Elwood, R. W. (1984). Outcome research on behavioral marital therapy: A methodological and conceptual reappraisal. In K. Hahlweg & N. Jacobson (Eds.), *Marital interaction: Analysis and modification* (pp. 113–132). New York: Guilford Press.

Jacobson, N. S., Follette, V. M., Follette, W. C., Holtzworth-Munroe, A., Katt, J. L., & Schmaling, K. B. (1985). A component analysis of behavior marital therapy: One-year follow-up. *Behavior Research and Therapy, 23,* 549–555.

Jacobson, N. S., Follette, W. C., & McDonald, D. W. (1982). Reactivity to positive and negative behavior in distressed and non-distressed married couples. *Journal of Consulting and Clinical Psychology, 50,* 706–714.

Jacobson, N. S., Follette, W. C., & Pagel, M. (in press). Predicting who will benefit from behavioral marital therapy. *Behavioral Marital Therapy.*

Jacobson, N. S., Follette, W. C., & Revenstorf, D. (1984). Psychotherapy outcome research: Methods for reporting variability and evaluating clinical significance. *Behavior Therapy, 15,* 336–352.

Jacobson, N. S., Follette, W. C., Revenstorf, D., Baucom, D. H., Hahlweg, K., & Margolin, G. (1984). Variability in outcome and clinical significance of behavioral marital therapy: A reanalysis of outcome data. *Journal of Consulting and Clinical Psychology, 52,* 497–504.

Jacobson, N. S., & Margolin, G. (1979). *Marital therapy: Strategies based on social learning and behavior exchange principles.* New York: Brunner/Mazel.

Jacobson, N. S., McDonald, D. W., & Follette, W. C., & Berley, R. A. (1985). Attributional processes in distressed and nondistressed married couples. *Cognitive Therapy and Research, 9,* 35–50.

Jacobson, N. S., Schmaling, K. B., Holtzworth-Munroe, A. (1986). *Component analysis of behavioral marital therapy: Two-year follow-up and prediction of relapse.* Manuscript submitted for publication.

Jacobson, N. S., Waldron, H., & Moore, D. (1980). Toward a behavioral profile of marital distress. *Journal of Consulting and Clinical Psychology, 48,* 696–703.

King, D. A., & Heller, K. (1984). Depression and the response of others: A reappraisal. *Journal of Abnormal Psychology, 93,* 477–480.

Klerman, G. L., Weissman, M. M., Rounsaville, B. J., & Chevron, E. S. (1984). *Interpersonal psychotherapy of depression.* New York: Basic Books.

Kovacs, M., & Beck, A. T. (1978). Maladaptive cognitive structures in depression. *American Journal of Psychiatry, 135,* 525–533.

L'Abate, L. (1981). Skill training programs for couples and families. In A. S. Gurman & D. P. Kniskern (Eds.), *Handbook of family therapy* (pp. 631–661). New York: Brunner/Mazel.

Lewinsohn, P. M. (1974). Clinical and theoretical aspects of depression. In K. S. Calhoun, H. E. Adams, & M. M. Mitchell (Eds.), *Innovative treatment methods in psychopathology* (pp. 67–111). New York: Wiley.

Lewinsohn, P. M., & Arconad, M. (1981). Behavioral treatment of depression: A social learning approach. In J. F. Clarkin & H. I. Glazer (Eds.), *Depression: Behavioral and directive intervention strategies* (pp. 33–67). New York: Garland STPM Press.

Lewinsohn, P. M., Mischel, W., Chaplin, W., & Barton, R. (1980) Social competence and depression: The role of illusory self-perceptions. *Journal of Abnormal Psychology, 89*, 203-212.

Lewinsohn, P. M., Munoz, R., Youngren, M. A., & Zeiss, A. M. (1978). *Control your depression*. Englewood Cliffs, NJ: Prentice-Hall.

Margolin, G., Talovic, S., & Weinstein, C. D. (1983). Areas of change questionnaire: A practical approach to marital assessment. *Journal of Consulting and Clinical Psychology, 51*, 920-931.

McLean, P. (1981). Remediation of skills and performance deficits in depression: Clinical steps and research finding. In J. F. Clarkin & H. I. Glazer (Eds.), *Depression: Behavioral and directive intervention strategies* (pp. 179-204). New York: Garland STPM Press.

Miller, I., Klee, S., & Norman, W. (1982). Depressed and nondepressed inpatients' cognitions of hypothetical events, experimental tasks and stressful life events. *Journal of Abnormal Psychology, 91*, 78-81.

Miller, W. R. (1975). Psychological deficits in depression. *Psychological Bulletin, 82*, 238-260.

Minuchin, S., & Fishman, H. C. (1981). *Family therapy techniques*. Cambridge, MA: Harvard University Press.

Murphy, G. E., Simons, A. D., Wetzel, R. D., & Lustman, P. J. (1984). Cognitive therapy and pharmacotherapy, singly and together, in the treatment of depression. *Archives of General Psychiatry, 41*, 33-41.

Nelson, R. E., & Craighead, W. E. (1977). Selective recall of positive and negative feedback: Self-control behaviors and depression. *Journal of Abnormal Psychology, 86*, 379-388.

O'Leary, K. D., & Turkewitz, H. (1978). The treatment of marital disorders from a behavioral perspective. In T. J. Paolino & B. S. McGrady (Eds.), *Marriage and marriage therapy: Psychoanalytic, behavioral and systems therapy perspectives* (pp. 114-143). New York: Brunner/Mazel.

O'Leary, K., & Turkewitz, H. (1981). A comparative outcome study of behavioral marital therapy and communication therapy. *Journal of Marital and Family Therapy, 7* 159-176.

Paykel, E. S., Myers, J. K., Dienelt, M. N., Klerman, G. L., Lindethal, J. J., & Pepper, M. P. (1969). Life events and depression: A controlled study. *Archives of General Psychiatry, 21*, 753-760.

Peterson, C., & Seligman, M. E. P. (1984). Causal explanations as a risk factor for depression: Theory and evidence. *Psychological Review, 91*, 347-374.

Peterson, C., Villanova, P., & Raps, C. S. (1985). Depression and attributions: Factors responsible for inconsistent results in the published literature. *Journal of Abnormal Psychology, 94*, 165-168.

Revenstorf, D. (1984). The role of attribution in marital distress and therapy. In K. Hahlweg & N. S. Jacobson (Eds.), *Marital interaction: Analysis and modification* (pp. 325-336). New York: Guilford Press.

Rush, A. J., Beck, A. T., Kovacs, M., & Hollon, S. (1977). Comparative efficacy of cognitive therapy and pharmacotherapy in the treatment of depressed outpatients. *Cognitive Therapy and Research, 1*, 17-37.

Rush, A. J., Shaw, B., & Khatami, M. (1980). Cognitive therapy of depression: Utilizing the couples system. *Cognitive Therapy and Research, 4*, 103-113.

Seligman, M. E. P. (1975). *Helplessness: On depression, development and death*. San Francisco: W. H. Freeman.

Simons, A. D., Lustman, P. J., Wetzel, R. D., & Murphy, G. E. (1985). Predicting response to cognitive therapy of depression: The role of learned resourcefulness. *Cognitive Therapy and Research, 9*, 79-89.

Spanier, G. B. (1976). Measuring dyadic adjustment: New scales for assessing the quality of marriage and similar dyads. *Journal of Marriage and the Family, 38*, 15-28.

Strack, S., & Coyne, J. C. (1983). Social confirmation of dysphoria: Shared and private reactions to depression. *Journal of Personality and Social Psychology, 44*, 798-806.

Stuart, R. B. (1969). Operant interpersonal treatment of marital discord. *Journal of Consulting and Clinical Psychology, 33,* 657–682.

Stuart, R. B. (1980). *Helping couples change.* New York: Guilford Press.

Weiss, R. L., Hops, H., & Patterson, G. R. (1973). A framework for conceptualizing marital conflict, a technology for altering it, some data for evaluating it. In L. A. Hamerlynck, L. C. Handy, & E. J. Mash (Eds.), *Behavior change: Methodology, concepts and practice* (pp. 67–79). Champaign, IL: Research Press.

Weiss, R. L., & Perry, B. A. (1979). *Assessment and treatment of marital dysfunction.* Eugene, OR: Oregon Marital Studies Program.

Weissman, A., & Beck, A. T. (1978, May). *Development and validation of the Dysfunctional Attitudes Scale: A preliminary investigation.* Paper presented at the meeting of the American Educational Research Association, Toronto.

Weissman, M. M., & Paykel, E. S. (1974). *The depressed woman: A study of social relationships.* Chicago: The University of Chicago Press.

4

Strategic Therapy

JAMES C. COYNE

Depression is a heterogeneous phenomenon, and depressed persons can be expected to differ widely in their complaints, interpersonal circumstances, and outcomes. Yet depression tends to be a disorder of the married and formerly married. The modal depressed patient is a married woman, and difficulties in her marriage are likely to be among the most frequently discussed issues in therapy and often her presenting problem (McLean, 1976). Furthermore, a large body of literature now documents the importance of marriage and marital problems in the etiology, course, and outcome of depression, as well as the negative impact of depression on the wellbeing of the spouse and the quality of marriage. (For a review, see Coyne, Kahn, & Gotlib, 1987).

It would seem, then, that marital therapy holds considerable promise for the treatment of depression, whether as the primary treatment or as an adjunct to antidepressant medication. Indeed, there has been a growing interest in this approach. However, couples with a depressed spouse typically pose a number of problems for the conducting of conventional couples therapy. The therapist cannot assume that both partners are committed to therapy or the preservation of the marriage. Often, spouses of depressed persons refuse to come to therapy or will come only if their presence is seen as assistance for their ailing partner rather than as marital therapy. There may be little agreement concerning goals, with depressed persons implicating the quality of the marriage in the persistence of their depression and with their partners accusing them of jeopardizing what would otherwise be a good relationship with their distress, complaints and dysfunction. Conjoint interviews or enactment of problematic interactions can prove counterproductive, in that there is a tendency for couples with a depressed spouse to get locked into a destructive pattern of conflict involving hostile attacks, displays of distress, and withdrawal, with little constructive problem solving (Kahn, Coyne, & Margolin, 1985). Consistent with this, some recent outcome data suggest that efforts narrowly focused on increasing the intimacy and sharing of emotion in couples with a depressed spouse may produce negative therapeutic effects (E. Waring, personal communication, 1984).

The brief, strategic therapy approach described in this chapter represents an attempt to come to terms with both the difficulties and the opportunities that marriages of depressed persons pose. It is a pragmatic, goal-oriented, short-term approach that focuses on how the couple's miscarried coping efforts are perpetuating their problems and how these efforts can be redirected. Goals are typically modest, but strategic changes in this behavior are intended to instigate change of a more general nature. Therapeutic sessions are seen mainly as an opportunity to prepare the couple for this change in their everyday life rather than as the primary site of change.

Extensive use is made of extratherapy task assignments, often of a paradoxical nature and often utilizing *reframing* (Coyne, 1985; Watzlawick, Weakland, & Fisch, 1974). In reframing, the therapist works to grasp the language the couples uses to describe a problem, actively acknowledges an acceptance of their perspective, and then extends or turns it in a direction that allows new behavior to be initiated. Another distinctive feature of the strategic approach is its emphasis on splitting sessions and working with the individual spouses. In the typical session, the therapist meets with each spouse separately and follows this with a briefer conjoint meeting in which an extratherapy task assignment is suggested.

Before describing this approach further, it would be useful to address some issues that bear upon the acceptance of marital therapy for depression by mental health professionals. Namely, there is currently widespread confusion about the implications of advances in both the biology and the classification of depressive disorders for psychotherapeutic approaches to depression. As a result, biologically oriented psychiatrists have not recognized the potential contribution of marital therapy. Marital therapists, on the other hand, have done little to challenge these misperceptions and have developed a few of their own.

BIOLOGY, CLASSIFICATION OF DEPRESSIVE DISORDERS, AND MARITAL THERAPY

Discussions of the significance of recent advances in the biology and classification of depression have been dominated by reductionism and dualism (Coyne, 1986a). It has been suggested that because depression is an illness with an established biological basis, it should be treated medically and not with psychotherapy. The alternative argument has also been made that some depressions are biological and should be treated medically and that other depressions are reactive or psychological and should be treated with psychotherapy. Neither extreme position is warranted.

There is evidence that during an episode, at least some, but certainly not all, depressed persons show biological abnormalities such as nonsuppression of cortisol production in response to an oral dose of dexamethasone. Yet, this does not preclude either a role for their interpersonal circumstances in the onset of their episode or the usefulness of marital therapy in its resolution. Dolan, Calloway, Fonagy, DeSouza, and Wakeling (1985) found that antecedent life events were associated with both the onset of a first episode of depression and its severity but not with patient status derived from the dexamethasone suppression test (DST). As part of a larger study of spouses' reactions to their depressed partners (most of whom had been DST nonsuppressors), we found that spouses accepted a strong biological component to the patients' disturbance but that they were nonetheless quite angry at them for being symptomatic (Coyne, Kessler, Tal, Turnbull, Wortman, & Greder, 1987). Whether hostility in the marital relationship preceded or was precipitated by the patients' depression, it could be expected to retard recovery and foster relapse (Hooley, Orley, & Teasdale, 1986).

In recent decades, there have been unambiguous demonstrations of the efficacy of antidepressant medication (Noll, Davis, & DeLeon-Jones, 1985). Yet, rather than obviating the need for marital therapy for depression, the literature concerning antidepressant medication can be interpreted as strengthening the case for developing such a psychotherapeutic approach.

First, although probably at least two thirds of all depressed patients could potentially benefit from antidepressant medication, there continue to be problems with refusal, nonadherence, intolerance of side effects, and relapse. As many as a third of all patients given antidepressants do not adequately adhere to treatment or drop out (McLean & Hakstian, 1979). In one study, 82% of the outpatients who had received antidepressants were depressed at 1-year follow-up as a result of nonimprovement, incomplete recovery, or relapse (Kovacs, Rush, Beck, & Hollon, 1981). Alternative approaches need to be available. Nonadherence to medication is substantially reduced when patients are provided with interpersonally oriented psychotherapy as well (DiMascio *et al.*, 1979). Further, a number of studies have shown that brief, problem-focused psychotherapy can prove more effective than antidepressants with outpatients (McLean & Hakstian, 1979; Rush, Beck, Kovacs, & Hollon, 1977).

Second, the marital problems that many depressed persons present are a negative prognostic indicator in treatment with antidepressant medication (Rousanville, Weisman, Prusoff, & Heraey-Baron, 1979). Those patients whose marriages improve show as good a response to medication as patients with satisfactory marriages, but the evidence is that medication has little direct effect upon the quality of depressed persons' involvement in their marriages (Weissman *et al.*, 1979). The negative influence of marital problems on the outcome of treatment with antidepressants may be the reason for the surprising finding that persons who are in intact marital relationships have a poorer prognosis than depressed persons who are not (Keller *et al.*, 1984).

Undoubtedly, depressed persons vary in their responsiveness to psychotherapy and to marital therapy in particular, but proven selection criteria are generally lacking. The success of lithium and the lack of evidence for the effectiveness of psychotherapy suggest that therapy should best be seen only as adjunctive treatment for manic–depressive or bipolar disorder (Rush, 1982). Yet, even recognizing these limits, marital therapy may prove to be important as part of a larger treatment package for bipolar disorder. Adherence in treatment with lithium remains disappointingly low, so marital treatment that reduces conflict and engenders support may prove beneficial in increasing adherence. Furthermore, even among patients who adhere to treatment and achieve adequate serum lithium levels, there is a treatment failure rate of 20% to 30%, and among patients with adequate lithium levels, positive involvement in social relationships predicts a favorable outcome (O'Connell, Mayo, Eng, Jones, & Gabel, 1985).

In the treatment of unipolar depression, the relevance of particular aspects of being depressed to the marriage and vice versa will vary, as will the appropriateness of marital therapy. Yet here, too, definitive selection criteria are lacking, and existing diagnostic frameworks do not provide much guidance for decisions about treatment. Contrary to clinical folklore, recent stressful life events do not distinguish between endogenous and reactive depressions (Lowry, 1985), and careful interviewing will generally reveal considerable stress in the lives of endogenously depressed patients (Leff, Roach, & Bunney, 1970). Such patients often have maladjusted marriages, and one study found that their marital problems generally preceded the onset of their depression (Birchnell & Kennard, 1983).

The limited data concerning the effectiveness of marital therapy for depression do not address the question of differential effects on endogenous depression. It may be that endogenous or vegetative features of depression are less responsive to therapy than other complaints. If this proves to be the case, marital treatment may still be the most effective way to deal with complaints about marital functioning, even in the presence of endogenous features. This is just one of the many areas in which controlled research is sorely needed.

Future developments in the classification of unipolar depression may have greater implications for decisions about marital therapy, and assessment of the quality of patients' involvement in their marriages may even be usefully incorporated into diagnostic criteria. For instance, among depressed women, stormy close relationships are one important way of identifying depressive spectrum disorder, a diagnostic distinction that has been validated against other criteria (Winokur, 1986). These women may prove to be particularly appropriate for marital therapy.

In sum, advances in our understanding of the biology of depression certainly do not reduce the necessity of considering the interpersonal circumstances of depressed persons, particularly their married lives. There are indications that it would not be appropriate to rely exclusively on psychotherapy for the treatment of bipolar disorder, although marital therapy may have a currently unrealized potential as an adjunctive treatment. Beyond that, "there is currently no evidence to support strict adherence to either a psychotherapeutic or pharmacological model of treating outpatient depression" (Beckman & Leber, 1985, p. 328). Given this state of affairs, pharmacotherapists would do well to consider the influence of marital factors on treatment outcome and the apparent inefficacy of antidepressants for marital problems. Marital therapists, for their part, should be prepared to seek consultation from pharmacotherapists when vegetative symptoms predominate or when marital therapy is failing to have a positive effect. Given our current state of knowledge about the treatment of depression, humility, a sensitivity to the limitations of any one approach, and a willingness to collaborate are in order.

CONCEPTUALIZING DEPRESSION IN A MARITAL CONTEXT

We can anticipate that couples with a depressed spouse will vary in their problems, goals, and attempted solutions, but some common themes recur. Depression and marital disturbance often occur in the same couples, although their temporal patterning varies. Marital difficulties may precipitate a depressive episode, yet depression may also trigger or potentiate marital problems (Briscoe & Smith, 1973). Strategic marital therapy does not assume any invariant relationship between marital problems and the onset of depression. Rather, the working hypotheses are that marital interactions are relevant to both the persistence and resolution of a depressive episode, and that the behavior of depressed persons and the responses of their spouses are likely to become interwoven and concatenated over time. Tracking the precise nature of this patterning in a given case is one of the fundamental tasks of the strategic therapist. There is less interest in the reasons why someone is depressed than in how depression may be perpetuated by the miscarried coping or attempted solutions of the depressed person and his or her spouse. Therapy is focused on interdicting or modifying these efforts and thereby remedying the circumstances maintaining the patient's distress.

Depression or depressive interactions frequently arise in the mismanagement of life transitions or in the accumulated mishandling of daily stress or hassles (DeLongis, Coyne, Dakof, Folkman, & Lazarus, 1982). One or both partners have been unable or unwilling to make an adaptation to these challenges that is mutually satisfying. It may be that distressing circumstances have required that one or both of them rely more heavily upon the marriage, and they may become disillusioned or less willing to accept what has previously been a bearable, but basically unfulfilling or unsatisfying, marriage. Alternatively, one partner's becoming depressed for any reason impinges on the marital relationship in important ways. Depressed persons may make demands or depend on their marriages and spouses differently than in the past, and spouses may feel that their needs are not met, resist the coping efforts of the depressed persons, or otherwise react negatively.

Depressed persons' distress, dependency, inhibition, and difficulties in dealing with hostility do not occur in a vacuum. These problems may very likely reflect their involvement in a marital situation that is distressing and insecure and that is not conducive to renegotiating expectations, to overt disagreement, or to the direct expression of negative affect. On the other hand, the behavior of depressed persons is aversive, powerful in its ability to induce negative moods in others, and also guilt inducing and inhibiting (Coyne, 1976). Spouses, for their part, may reduce the aversiveness of depressed persons by seemingly providing what is being asked for, even while communicating impatience, hostility, and rejection. The subtle and overt hostility and rejection that depressed persons receive elicits further expression of distress, strengthening the pattern. Troublesome in itself, such a pattern can be expected to interfere with a couple's ability to have positive interactions, maintain a household, solve problems, or renegotiate their relationship.

Even when depressed persons are not experiencing marital problems, the recovery process generally necessitates a renegotiation of the marital relationship, and couples who have seemed to be well functioning in the past may differ in their ability to cope with this. Recovering depressed persons become less inhibited and more independent, assertive, and demanding, and this can be misunderstood or negatively received by spouses and prove to be a source of friction and conflict. Furthermore, the reaction of spouses may make it difficult for depressed persons to pace the resumption of previous role responsibilities, or the depressed persons' experimentation with new ways of handling disagreement and hostility may make it difficult for spouses to remain supportive.

Discussions of marital interaction in depression are incomplete without an acknowledgment that wives are more likely to be depressed than husbands. The evidence is that this may be due in part to men's accruing benefits from marriage that women do not rather than to marriage's being inherently depressing for women (Coyne & Gotlib, 1985). However, it is also the case that a variety of sociocultural and economic influences put women at a disadvantage in efforts to renegotiate their marital relationships in times of stress or dissatisfaction. In conducting marital therapy for depression, the therapist is often self-consciously or naively assisting a woman to continue, by other means, a renegotiation of her relationship that has somehow

become thwarted or stalemated. The key to facilitating the husband's participation is to recognize that the hope of reducing the difficulties of living with
a depressed wife may be his principal reason for considering changes in the
relationship that he would otherwise not deem necessary or useful.

THE RATIONALE FOR WORKING
WITH EACH PARTNER SEPARATELY

As noted earlier, it cannot be assumed that both depressed persons and their
spouses have a commitment to therapy or the continuation of the marriage,
or that they agree upon therapeutic goals. We must therefore be careful not
to require that in order to participate in therapy, the couple show a level of
agreement and cooperation the lack of which may have been a major reason
for their seeking therapy. The depressed persons and their spouses are both
more likely to benefit from therapy if they feel that the therapist grasps their
unique perspectives and that they are working toward a personally relevant
goal, with progress that can be marked with observable accomplishments.
Given the couple's initial differences, these conditions may be more readily
established in working with the individual members of the couple separately; much of strategic marital therapy is conducted in this manner.

Conjoint sessions are often regarded as the *sine qua non* of marital
therapy. However, a systems perspective does not require that both partners
be present at all times in therapeutic sessions. Indeed, such a perspective
encourages consideration of how strategic changes in a subsystem (one
member of the couple) can produce changes in the patterning of the whole
couple system—particularly how a motivated spouse can influence the less
motivated spouse and the quality of their relationship.

Even if each spouse is interviewed separately, the approach remains
distinct from a traditional arrangement in which each spouse might receive
individual therapy. Particular attention is given to how the behaviors of
both the depressed person and the partner are aspects of a recursive pattern
involving the other—the locus of the problem lies within neither person but
in what they are doing together. Further, goals and interventions are ecological, in that an effort is made to take into account how each spouse is likely
to react and what new problems and possibilities this will pose.

One important reason for interviewing each spouse separately is that it
allows a frank discussion of that person's commitment to the continuation
of the marriage. In the absence of this, therapists sometimes belatedly
discover that they are doing predivorce counseling when they were about to
congratulate themselves on the successful treatment of a depressed person.
By the time that therapy is sought, marital satisfaction is likely to be low,
and one or both partners may be considering separation or divorce or may
have initiated an affair.

If one or both partners express pessimism about the future of the relationship, the therapist may acknowledge that this is understandable but suggest that treatment is more likely to make a difference if termination of the marriage is not an immediate threat. The therapist requests a moratorium on separation that is longer than the expected duration of treatment. If one spouse cannot accept this, the therapist may inquire how he or she expects therapy to be personally beneficial. If a commitment is obtained from one but not the other spouse, the therapist may express an interest in working with the more committed spouse. In such an instance, the therapist may caution that therapy often involves making important decisions and that if one partner in a relationship does not participate in some way, the decisions that are made may not reflect that person's interests. Generally speaking, the strategic therapist is careful not to express a stronger commitment to either the preservation of the marriage or the usefulness of therapy than that expressed by the spouse being interviewed.

Thus, in these initial meetings with each spouse, the therapist is making a tentative decision about how much attention to devote to each of them. The assumption is that the most efficient use of subsequent sessions is to spend them with a person able to say in some form, "There are some circumstances that are troubling to me; I know that I am not handling them in the best way, and I am potentially open to what you have to say." This may be both spouses or only one. If one spouse remains vague or fails to give an indication of such dissatisfaction or openness, the therapist may express appreciation for that person's willingness to come to the session but indicate an interest in spending the next few sessions with the other spouse. The reluctant spouse may simply be asked to assume the role of observer and be prepared that circumstances may have to get a bit worse in order to get better.

Once these preliminary issues are resolved, a further rationale for interviewing the spouses separately is that it facilitates the gathering of detailed information about how—from each spouse's perspective—problems are occurring in everyday life and how the couple is attempting to solve them. This information is a prerequisite to any reframings or homework assignments. Interviewed together, the couple will often lapse into their characteristic pattern of outbursts and accusations, or alternatively, inhibition and withdrawal, and this interferes with the therapist's ability to obtain a picture of what happens outside of therapy. Such a pattern of interaction is, of course, relevant to therapy, but a brief report of its occurrence is as useful as a drawn-out enactment of it in the therapy room. Furthermore, there is a concern that conflict enacted in the session may reflect the artificiality of the setting and, in particular, the presence of the therapist as a possible ally, referee, or commentator. Such exchanges not only may be unrepresentative of what occurs outside of therapy but may leave the couple less prepared to undertake any initiative for change.

Finally, depressed persons tend to behave less dysfunctionally in the absence of their spouses (Hinchcliffe, Hooper, & Roberts, 1978), and both partners are likely to be less defensive and more flexible and compromising. They will often privately agree to initiate small positive changes that they would reject as unacceptable if they were in the presence of the other. Interviewed together, they may face difficult choices between agreeing to a positive change and resisting the appearance of having made a concession to a hostile and coercive spouse. Further, the opportunity to discuss plans for change with only the therapist is particularly important where there is some risk of failure and therefore the possibility of validating the spouse's accusations of incompetence. The key issues are whether disclosure of a plan for change will induce a debilitating preoccupation with the threat of failure and whether it is less likely that one spouse will fault the failure of the other's efforts if it is not apparent that an effort was made.

INITIAL INTERVIEWING

The use of extratherapy task assignments in strategic therapy has probably attracted more attention to the model than the distinctive style of interviewing that sets the groundwork for them. Yet, in many instances, the delivery of the assignment is secondary to what has been accomplished in the interview. In conducting the interview, the therapist is doing more than just passively absorbing information. By the phrasing of questions and responses to couple's answers, the therapist is simultaneously structuring the couple's framing or definition of their problems, preparing them for reframes, and defining the therapeutic relationship. The interventions that can be designed by the therapist and the extent to which they can be made palatable to the couple may depend upon how these intermediate steps are accomplished.

No matter which spouse is being interviewed, a basic plan structures the initial gathering of information. The therapist seeks to obtain a definition of what the person sees as the problem, how it is a problem, and how it interferes with daily life. Because of the emphasis in strategic therapy on redirecting the couple's problem-maintaining coping efforts, particular attention is given to how each spouse has attempted to solve the problem as he or she sees it. It is also important to determine each spouse's understanding of why therapy has been sought now rather than previously or later. Often there has been a stalemate, an ultimatum, or an incident that one or both spouses see as particularly revealing about their predicament, and strategic planning should take this into account. Finally, an attempt is also made to formulate some concrete, minimal goal for treatment with answers to the question, "What would it take to indicate to you that you were on the right path, even if you were not out of the woods?" Alternatively, it might be suggested, "There is a lot of difficulty and uncertainty in your life, and we cannot expect to take care of it all. Is there one problem such that if we were able to make some small progress in dealing with it, you would feel a bit more able to cope with everything else?"

From the start, the therapist makes repeated reference to the time-limited nature of therapy and utilizes this to prompt each spouse to think in terms of small, observable changes and to share in the responsibility for demonstrating that therapy is not a waste of time:

Therapist: I would like to think that what we are going to do here will make a difference, but we cannot be sure. I don't want it to be a waste of your time, and so maybe we should plan to assess our efforts in five sessions and decide whether we have got enough evidence that we are getting somewhere to justify continuing. What would be a sign to you that we were getting somewhere?

The sign that is negotiated may be the goal of therapy or simply an indentifiable step toward it. What is important is that continuation of therapy be justified by progress, not the lack of it. With a positive assessment of progress, a new target can be identified for the next five sessions.

The therapist obtains the particulars of the couple's everyday life, highlighting the specific exchanges that are seen as problematic, as well as the couple's problem-maintaining solutions and the spouses' relevant positions vis-à-vis each other and the problem. An effort is made to move from abstract definitions of the problem in terms of communication, emotional expressiveness, or whatever to incidents that illustrate these problems and exactly how they are distressing. The therapist guides this process by requesting examples, indicating confusion when complaints are left abstract, or suggesting that therapy would proceed better if the therapist could visualize the occurrence of a problematic situation.

During the interview, the therapist is routinely planting possibilities for subsequent reframings and task assignments. For instance, a depressed patient might repeatedly complain about her spouse's being uncommunicative and unemotional. Casually, the therapist might agree that the spouse is defensive. When this has been accepted, the therapist might propose that the defensiveness indicates vulnerability. With agreement on this point, the therapist is in a better position to suggest supportive strategies appropriate for dealing with someone who is vulnerable rather than someone who is simply withholding. Similarly, a spouse may complain about a depressed person's stubbornness and resistance to influence, and the therapist might agree that the depressed person is too proud to accept helpful advice, even when it would be beneficial. If this is accepted, the therapist might suggest that such pride is often the last refuge of self-respect, and that if someone were to be persistent enough to overcome that pride, it would also be that patient's self-respect that was defeated. The spouse is thus prepared for interventions that are more nurturing than coercive.

The conducting of the interview is also the principal medium by which the therapist defines the nature of his or her relationship to the couple. One working goal is that the couple come to see that therapy is low key and free of the coercion that may characterize their own relationship. Another is that the therapist succeed in establishing and maintaining an appropriately balanced attitude of dead serious play (Haley, 1963). The therapist must bring to the triad of the couple plus therapist a sense of humor and distance that the couple themselves may have lost in their emotional overinvolvement in their struggles. The therapist laughs with the couple but is careful never to convey a sense of laughing at them or of disrespecting their efforts, even when they do so themselves. Furthermore, the therapist makes it clear that the ability to maintain such a balanced, playful perspective is not the result of some moral superiority but the result of the therapist's not having been absorbed in the couple's struggle.

INITIAL INTERVENTIONS

The couple will not always be able to provide clear, informative descriptions of problematic interactions in their everyday life, despite the repeated efforts of the therapist. This provides the opportunity for a problem prescription in the guise of an effort to obtain further information. For instance,

Therapist: I am sorry. You have been patient with my incessant questions, but I just don't understand how your arguments escalate the way that they obviously do. Furthermore, each of you presents your spouse in a way that suggests someone who is too reasonable to get involved in such a no-win encounter. You could save me a lot of time and questions if you could have an argument in which you each got the other to be less reasonable and were both able to report on it. Could you two collaborate in having such an argument and report back to me? Allow yourself some time and you might even pick Tuesday if that's an evening that you have free. . . . I know that this is an odd request, and it would be a sacrifice to therapy for you to comply. If you do decide to go ahead and do it, you ought to reward each other by doing something special afterwards.

Such an assignment may well provide useful information. More important, however, it reframes any argument that occurs in response to it. Namely, the spontaneity and the negativity of the exchange are reduced because it is a response to a request for a helpful initiative. Also, each spouse has a new incentive to resist the provocations of the other and not behave in a way that will be embarrassing to report. The assignment has the potential for precipitating at least a small shift in the way both spouses become engrossed in disagreements that they insist they are attempting to avoid.

Another rather standard assignment is given in the guise of a check on the couple's sensitivity to each other and ability to notice subtle changes. They are asked to do one unannounced thing for the pleasure of the other and one thing that is for themselves or self-indulgent. They are further instructed that in the next session they will separately be quizzed as to what they have done and what they believe the other has done. However, no feedback about the correctness of their guesses will be given, and they are not to discuss the assignment. Again, the assignment may well produce useful information; it is revealing what each partner does and what each guesses the other has done. Even a failure to do the assignment is informative about the willingness of the spouse or couple to comply with subsequent, more demanding task assignments. However, the task has other objectives. It encourages small initiatives and puts each spouse in a position where there will be a loss of face if he or she fails to notice the positive efforts of the other; a climate of positive ambiguity may be created. It also inducts the couple into the basic structure of therapy: Namely, they will provide information to the therapist about their everyday life, receive assignments, attempt small changes, and report back to the therapist. The task is benign, and it encourages resourcefulness, sensitivity to the partner, and individual choice. It can also be a more general metaphor for what will be asked of the couple—that they do things for each other, but not without choice and not to the neglect of their own interests.

SPECIFIC AGENDA AND FOCUSED INTERVENTIONS

The strategic perspective assumes that what the depressed person and the spouse are doing to solve their problems is interdependent and concatenated. Yet, for the purposes of discussion, this can be punctuated in terms of three sets of agendas and foci for intervention: the depressed person, the response of the spouse, and the marriage. This punctuation is, of course, arbitrary, and changes in one area tend to have direct implications for the others. The choice of which area is to be targeted is a pragmatic one, and it depends primarily upon the opportunities provided by the couple and the preferences of the therapist. Frequently, the therapist starts by probing all three fronts and then pursues most vigorously the areas that seem most amenable to change.

Working with Depressed Persons

In eliciting descriptions of depressed persons' problems, the therapist is careful to communicate an awareness that things are indeed difficult and that they have good reason to be depressed or else they would not be. The most basic rule in working with depressed persons is never to dispute their right and privilege to be depressed. When depressed persons seem particularly sensitive about accusations—perhaps from spouses—that they are getting something out of being depressed, the therapist might comment that one would lose a depression if one were happy with it. At some point, it is generally useful to turn the discussion to the topic of why, given that so much is wrong, someone should not be even more depressed. In this way, many depressed persons are better able to identify their resources that if directly asked to do so.

As problem and goal definitions are constructed, depressed persons should be made to feel that they are facing manageable difficulties. One of the therapist's working goals is to assist them in partitioning and framing coping tasks so that any necessity for change is viewed in terms of small steps that they feel empowered to undertake. Generally, an effort is made to construct task assignments so that they are likely to do more than they have agreed to do. For example, a woman indicated that she felt isolated from other women and that there was no good reason for her failing to get together with some woman friends on her days off from work while the children were in school. Although it was not targeted in the therapy sessions, she twice stated that she would do something about this, but twice did not follow through. The therapist and the woman reviewed all that was involved in her getting together with her friends and everything that made it difficult. The woman was asked to procrastinate for a week while she determined how she would deal with all the obstacles that might arise. During the week, she should call one of the friends, but if the matter of getting together came up, she should be deliberately vague and noncommittal about when this could happen. That night she called two of her friends and arranged a women's night out, something that she had previously stated was out of the question.

Just as important as efforts to frame small coping tasks are steps to dissuade depressed persons from taking responsibility for solving problems that are intractable or even maintained by their coping efforts. A depressed man, for example, reported that when his wife unexpectedly began talking vaguely about leaving him, he became solicitous to the point that he alienated her even further. By his own account, he was now pleading with her in a pathetic fashion. Yet, she would not commit herself either to leaving or to staying, and she refused to come to therapy with him. The therapist suggested that it was not clear what would change her mind, but whether they ultimately stayed together or not, his cause was best served by looking after himself. If there was a future to the relationship, he would deal better with it if he did not feel so desperate. If there was no future, learning how to thrive anyway would be the best revenge. The man was also asked whether he would be able to afford two sessions per week if things were to continue to deteriorate. When he replied that he would, the therapist suggested that he might consider not waiting until things got that bad to begin taking care of himself. He was requested to spend at least half the cost of a session on himself per week, doing something he would not otherwise do. His first tasks in dealing with his wife were to be limited to "carrying himself as if he were an interesting person" without attempting to persuade her of this and to observe how she communicated without attempting to influence her.

Depressed persons are frequently avoidant and indecisive, and they can find ample evidence that they are irresponsible and incompetent. Yet, such an unsuccessful style of coping is often maintained by high standards and by a definition of the task at hand that makes any accomplishment seem insufficient and any effort seem futile. The therapist may utilize opportunities to reframe such apparent "irresponsibility" as the result of a willingness to accept too much responsibility. Thus, when a suicidal woman complained that she deserved to die because she had been irresponsible and had disappointed her husband, children, and employer, the therapist commented that suicide was the only exit she knew from the Superwoman role:

Therapist: Contrary to what Barry Goldwater thinks, extremism in pursuit of virtue is a goddamn vice. Other people would probably accept their limitations or make excuses for themselves, but you do not allow yourself that and so depression and attempting suicide is your out. Being depressed at least slows you down. Yet, the problem with depression is that it sometimes lifts when you need it the most and you are again burdened with the sense that you can and should be able to do everything.

The therapist requested and received an antisuicide agreement, but then stated that although it was helpful to him, it was not enough to get her through the week. The therapist further suggested that she take a brief leave from her stressful job. She protested that to do so would be irresponsible. The therapist agreed that someone, particularly Superwoman, might see it that way, but that dead people make bad employees. Finally, a request was made that the woman develop a plan for how she would restrain herself for more than the week if her depression did not hold. Except for some minimal efforts to deal with the children, she was to let her problems be. By the end of the session, the woman expressed genuine relief, and the therapist cautioned her that that would make the agreement to restrain herself harder to keep. The therapist's last comment in the session was: "And I'm not going to tell you to have a good week. . . . That would be a setup. You would only have to work harder to keep yourself down." Within a few weeks she was back at work, but not without some restructuring to everyone's responsibilities at home.

Although adapted to the particulars of this woman's situation, such *restraining* maneuvers are typical of strategic therapy. First, there is a positive reframing of the patients' involvement in their predicaments. Second, going beyond suggestions about how patients might structure their coping tasks to allow themselves to proceed slowly and in small steps, strategic therapists suggest that being depressed has its obvious drawbacks, but that it can serve to restrain someone from trying too hard when resources are depleted or situations are overwhelming. Incongruous comments such as "Depression is like a leaky vacation cottage, and you never know when you are going to be evicted" may bolster this point of view. Additionally, depressed persons may be asked to construct weekly "slough off" lists of important tasks that need to be done but that taken together are likely to prove overwhelming. A set number of these tasks is then selected by the patient to be left undone during the week. Reports of the tasks successfully being left undone are then to be greeted by the therapist as a difficult achievement, and reports that they were completed despite the assignment are to be dismissed with some variation of "No one is perfect."

The rationale for such interventions is that depressed persons are often able to infuse their feelings of sadness with feelings of badness and incompetence and otherwise maintain their dysphoria by taking on too much, failing, or becoming avoidant of trying, and thus validating their negative view of themselves. Further, they are often more likely to discover and utilize their resources if they are restrained from attempting too much rather than prodded to take on what they see as overwhelming.

Discussions of demands and fears of failure often implicate the spouses as the source of demands, or at least as observers and critical commentators. This may lead to opportunities for the therapist to highlight the drawbacks of improvement and to provide depressed persons with a rationale for disengaging from spouses' demands and criticisms and for not struggling so hard to change. Thus, when a depressed patient is recounting her spouse's stringent criticism, a therapist may comment that the husband seems convinced that she can do nothing right and that this has not made it easy for her to prove him wrong. The therapist might then suggest that her husband would be surprised if she pulled herself together and that he might be utterly unprepared for her being competent and independent. Would he feel unneeded and be forced to face his own inadequacies? To bolster this argument, the therapist might inquire if her husband has been inept in dealing with her, and if so, has he been too defensive to admit this? The gist of this line of interviewing is that it should prepare the patient to feel empowered to deal with her partner as someone with limitations and to accept a framing of depression as an active way of protecting the spouse. Frequently, patients are told some variation of the following: "When someone is unbecoming a patient, he or she may have to be especially patient and charitable toward the people around him or her. Others often don't cope well, and they may even be at their worst. No one is perfect. It would be unfair to ask you to be a saint on top of everything else, but please be easy on your partner."

Given this context, when depressed persons produce accounts of incidents that can be construed in terms of spouses reacting negatively to assertiveness or independence, the therapist may suggest that depression is an understandable, but costly, way of protecting spouses: "Depression is a way of shooting yourself in the leg so that you don't worry your spouse about your wandering off." Having identified actions or negative thoughts that depressed persons see as maintaining their plight, the therapist may suggest that one possibility is temporarily doing more of the same as a sacrifice to the spouse and marriage. However, because this is now a chore rather than an affliction, depressed persons should schedule self-rewards: "If you are not paid, you are unlikely to stay on the job." Further, depressed patients may be asked not to flaunt any improvement that they may feel but to do something during the week that would surprise and please the spouse, and to hide it from him or her. Depending on the context, this assignment may be reiterated at the end of the session in the presence of the spouse, but with no explanation and with a request that there be no further discussion of it.

As previously noted, depressed persons are frequently having difficulty renegotiating their relationship with their spouses. At least part of their problem often stems from their inability to take a stand with the spouse, whether because of indecisiveness, inhibition, or simple fear. It is sometimes useful to commit depressed persons to take a stand regardless of whether they deem it appropriate to the particular situation. For example, a depressed housewife complained that her husband was often late coming home from work without notice. Aside from the inconvenience, it represented to her two things. First, he was not taking a stand in dealing with his supervisor when he could, and therefore she couldn't respect him. Second, he was making her life unpredictable, and she had to bear the major responsibility for adapting to *his* problem. In initial discussions of what she might do, she would vacillate between being angry and feeling sorry for him in a way that blocked a commitment to action. For his part, the husband was passive and anxious in sessions, and while he was cognizant of the difficulties that he posed for her, he was equally noncommittal. The therapist suggested to him that things were confusing but that there might be something positive stirring with his wife. Further, if she started feeling better, she might act to protect her more positive mood, and then he might wish she was not so up. The man protested that this was not true and that he was prepared for the necessity for change. The therapist thanked him and stated that for now his job would be to wait until such change came about.

The therapist declined to deal with the problem for a few sessions, stating that it was premature until the woman began insisting otherwise. The therapist then suggested that she should not have to take care of her husband and that he should learn to better attend to her needs. When she agreed, the therapist asked if she was willing to help her husband. Only after obtaining an agreement from her that she would do the assignment would he provide the details of it. He asked her to wait until her husband was late more than 1 hour (a frequent occurrence). For the next night, she was either to get a babysitter or to prepare the children to go out to eat one-half hour after the time that the couple had previously agreed that the husband should be home. Whether or not the husband was home to go with her, she could plan on leaving at the set time. There should be no notes because he already knew what time dinner should be, and her only explanation would be that they were both under stress and needed a break. After she did this three times, the husband asked that he be seen, and work began on both his difficulties at work and their difficulties being clear with each other.

Many depressed persons are initially simply too inhibited to complete such an assignment. For them, the first step must be *in vivo* thought experiments in which they imagine an absurd act of assertion, noncompliance, or rebellion. Thus a woman was asked to prepare a meal of leftovers and place it on the stove as usual. She was then asked to turn the burner on high and to imagine the food becoming a stinking, charred mass. In the fantasy, she was to present the husband with this and state, "Dear, somehow our dinner was ruined, and I'm sorry, but you must take us out to eat." She was then to turn the burner down before the meal was actually spoiled, and, in order to alleviate her guilt for such bad thoughts, be particularly cheerful, acquiescent and attentive when she greeted her husband. The key features of such assignments is that they are absurd and safely in the imagination, and yet they make explicit patients' existing decisions to avoid confrontation, even to their detriment. Frequently, such assignments are followed quickly by spontaneous assertive actions. Further, in the wake of such assignments, straightforward assignments to be assertive become more palatable.

Working with the Spouse

As can be inferred from the preceding section, it is assumed that siding with spouses in efforts to prod the depressed persons into action is unlikely to prove useful. At the same time, therapists should be careful not to side with depressed persons and confuse their framing of their predicament with that of their spouses. Namely, it is important not to ignore spouses' clear statements that there is nothing wrong with their marriages except their partner's depression, if that is their position. In such cases, the focus of therapy with the spouse may become framed in terms of how he or she is dealing with the difficulties that the depressed partner presents to the relationship. Similarly, just because a depressed person complains about a spouse being uncommunicative, the therapist should not take it for granted that the spouse also sees it as a problem. It is probably true that many spouses have defected from therapy when therapists have joined depressed partners in trying to wring an emotional response from them, particularly an allegedly masked sadness or depression.

In general, therapists should make an effort to grasp and acknowledge whatever frustrations, sacrifices, and disappointments may color a spouse's reactions to the depressed person and to the tasks of therapy. In attempting to cope with the depressed partner, the spouse may have stifled complaints, faced what is seen as unjustified hostility and criticism, and made numerous unappreciated concessions. The therapist should be sensitive to these issues from the outset. Further, it is important not to rely too heavily on a spouse's goodwill, altruism, or stated willingness to undertake unilateral change, especially when he or she seems demoralized or outright angry at the depressed person. Wherever possible, the appeal for particular task assignments or therapeutic goals should be based on an identification of the spouse's self-interest.

Early in contacts with a spouse, the therapist should assess the extent to which his or her position can best be summarized as one of underinvolvement or overinvolvement with the distress of the depressed partner. A working assumption of strategic therapy is that the interests of both partners will best be served if the spouse is able to maintain a moderate level of involvement, neither hostilely withdrawing nor becoming overinvolved in efforts to help that are well meant but likely to prove self-defeating and demoralizing to both partners. In providing reframes, setting goals, and assigning tasks, the therapist should attend to the more general goal of assisting the spouse in achieving this moderate level of involvement.

Elsewhere (Coyne, Wortman, & Lehman, in press), my colleagues and I have described the process by which the initial positive commitment, support, and encouragement of spouses may deteriorate to coercion, characterological attack, and rejection. When possible, the therapist should link the occurrence of such miscarried helping to the positive intentions from which it springs. The basic theme is that people would not get trapped into such destructive interactions if they were not so committed to making a difference. When interactions have deteriorated to the point that such positive reframes are no longer possible, the therapist may comment instead on how one must have a tremendous investment in someone to allow that person to get him or her so upset. The fundamental strategy is to connote positively the spouse's efforts and then encourage a de-escalation and a refocus on what the spouse can do to take care of himself or herself:

Therapist: While I can appreciate what you are trying to do, it seems like the more you try, the worse it gets. Maybe it is just a matter of timing. . . . I am concerned that you'll wear yourself out and not be available when your partner needs you most. What can you do to take care of yourself, maybe allow yourself some rest and relaxation before plunging back into the struggle?

Often, spouses have been too absorbed in struggles with their depressed partners to look after their own needs. They are likely to be angry about having made this sacrifice, and it may seem all the more imperative for them to get an immediate change. At least some of their negative affect and unhelpful demands on their partners may be reduced if the therapist legitimizes their needs and wants, particularly as expressed in activities that do not involve the depressed partners. The therapist might even suggest that for the benefit of the depressed person, the spouse do something special for himself or herself on a schedule, whether or not he or she feels such efforts are needed.

The therapist may also take advantage of moments of heightened frustration to commit the spouse to a strategy of backing off. For instance, if the spouse complains that he or she is impotent to effect a change, the therapist might suggest tactfully that one cannot be impotent unless one tries. The therapist might also inquire if the spouse has ever had a roommate (or co-worker), and if so, did the roommate ever get depressed? If the spouse agrees that whether the roommate was in a depressed mood did not matter greatly, the therapist might suggest that the roommate nonetheless recovered, and propose an assignment in which the spouse is asked to treat the depressed partner as either a roommate or a spouse on alternate days and then observe the differential effects. If a spouse reports getting fed up with the depressed person and storming off, the therapist might prescribe that the spouse again get some time away by midweek, suggesting that getting angry again may be what is required to do so.

When the therapist provides a positive reframing for a spouse's behavior and encourages a relinquishing of any excessive responsibility for how the depressed partner feels, the spouse is more likely to adopt more humane interpretations of his or her partner's behavior and reduce demands for immediate change. Often, the therapist will provide a positive reframing to a spouse's behavior and, when this has been accepted, suggest that it similarly applies to the depressed partner. For instance, the therapist may lament with spouses how their efforts merely to defend their own behavior were treated as hostile criticism, how any overture they make is likely to be misunderstood, and how helpless that makes them feel. The therapist is then in a position to suggest that the depressed partners may be demoralized for the same reasons. Incidents that can be construed as involving issues of pride, shame, or the risks of admitting mistakes lend themselves particularly well to such strategies.

With some spouses, the issue is not reducing an emotional overinvolvement that has proven burdensome for both partners or has turned to hostile rejection. Rather, they have removed themselves from the relationship in a way that denies the depressed partners any intimacy or support. In such cases, the therapist may agree with the spouse that it is important to protect himself or herself from the futility of being overinvolved, but may suggest at the same time that his or her distance may maintain the aversiveness of the depressed person. Small moves may then be suggested that are likely to be beneficial to the depressed partner, even while allowing the spouse to maintain at least some sense of not being engulfed.

Working with the Couple

Interventions that target the couple as a unit are generally delivered at the end of the session, and they tend to hold more promise when they build upon what has occurred in the segments with the individual partners. Thus the therapist might comment metaphorically to each person separately, and when this has been accepted, provide a couples-oriented intervention that capitalizes on this:

Therapist: When you are staying in a motel, one has to worry less about the garbage spilling out of the trash can and the dirty towels on the floor, and even the ugly color of the wallpaper, because you know that you will be leaving soon and the maid will come. In your own house it would be different—you live there. You two have decided to stay in the relationship, but you treat it more like a motel room than a home.

At the closing of the session, the therapist might then give them an assignment: Each of them should—without calling attention to what they are doing—pick up one dirty towel and report back to the therapist what this has involved for each of them.

Before asking anything of the couple as a unit, the therapist is careful to acknowledge the problems in the relationship and warn that many of the things that they attempt to do for each other will backfire, go unrecognized, or be misunderstood. Only later will they be able to appreciate the helpfulness of what each is about to do now. Rather than pushing for change, the strategic therapist generally suggests proceeding slowly and cautiously. An effort is made to frame the immediate future explicitly as a time of change, one aspect of which is that they may need to tolerate what they would not want to be a long-term feature of the relationship. Furthermore, there will be a certain quality of noncontingency, in that any rewards for their efforts are not likely to be immediately forthcoming, and there may be real benefits later for not reacting to the partner's negative behavior now. The period may also be framed as a time for indelicacy, with a greater need to be direct and to encourage each other to be direct by not attempting to read the other's mind or fathom how he or she really feels.

There may be specific noxious behaviors that have been salient in the couple's aversive exchanges, perhaps "constructive criticism," depressive complaints about the relationship, idle threats to leave, or unfavorable references to in-laws. Rather than taking sides, the therapist might secure agreement that in calm moments each would accept that one could engage in the aversive behavior less often and that the other could be less sensitive. Scheduled playful enactments of the behavior may then be prescribed in a way that allows for one partner to lose interest in performing the behavior and the other to be less sensitive to it.

Although a resolution of specific problems is sometimes possible and desirable, the therapist should be careful not to pursue an accumulation of minor complaints that are best left to being dissolved with a more general improvement in the marriage rather than being solved. There is sometimes the risk of the therapist adopting an overeager, active problem-solving stance that enourages the couple to be passive, help rejecting, and complaining. The preference is for the therapist to be restrained and even temporizing. Rather than stepping in as a referee, the therapist may dampen the negativity of the couple's exchanges with positive reframing and prescriptions that introduce playful, and even absurd elements.

In obtaining reports of recurring arguments, the therapist should identify what each spouse sees as the most negative aspects of them—perhaps their unpredictability or suddenness, their intensity, their lack of resolution, or the sense of distance that they leave—and what small changes might remove or reduce these elements. Positive reframings of recurrent arguments should be tied to the couple's reports of their details and be compatible with each partner's language and position. That the couple persist in such a pattern may be reframed as evidence of their passion, commitment, romanticism, or refusal to accept a more banal existence. The spilling of accumulated frustrations into an argument may be construed as evidence of the protectiveness that preceded it. Arguments and withdrawal after a period of apparent progress may be reframed as a miscarried effort to get close or a defense against "precipitous intimacy": "At this point, you two porcupines are going to get stuck on each other's quills if you try to snuggle up."

Specific extratherapy assignments may be used to transform recurring arguments into more infrequent or benign occurrences. The paradigmatic transformation by reframing is a couple's framing an interaction as a threatening argument then reframing it as playful. As depicted in Bateson's (1955) classic analysis, play differs from serious activity in its exaggeration or stylization, disruption of key sequences, timing repetitiveness, or limits on how engrossed paticipants become. Thus, the following assignment was given to a couple in whose relationship the wife's overanxiousness and social ineptness were maintained by her husband's monitoring and hypercriticalness: They were to go to a fine restaurant, she was to create a deliberate *faux pas*, and he was to overreact in an exaggerated way. The rationale that was given to the couple was that like weeds, negative spontaneity choked out the occurrence of spontaneous positive exchanges, and the assignment might at least "pull some weeds." (For an extended discussion of this assignment, see Coyne, 1986b.) Other reframes may introduce elements of pretense, ritual, ceremony, or contest.

Different strategies are required with couples for whom the problem is not overt conflict but inhibition and suppression of disagreement. The therapist may praise their mutual protectiveness and respect their willingness to make sacrifices for their marriage, and yet suggest that at some point soon they may feel comfortable enough to encourage each other to disagree. In such a couple, a husband described overreacting when he misunderstood some minimal efforts by his depressed wife to initiate some independent activities. The therapist praised his willingness to encourage her to assert herself similarly. Precisely because he had overreacted, he had given her the opportunity to feel that she was unambiguously right and to put aside her own ambivalence and speak her mind. Even if not particularly pleasant, the overreaction was a gift, and the next week they should exchange gifts by each overreacting at least once. The couple was cautioned that because they were not accustomed to doing such things, they should expect each other to be awkward and perhaps in need of later feedback and coaching. Further, because this was an odd and difficult assignment, they should reward each other by doing something special at another time during the week. Thus the overall strategy is to accept and positively connote reticence and yet to schedule departures from this pattern and praise them as achievements.

POSTSCRIPT: PARADOX, DEPENDENCE ON MARRIAGE, AND DIVORCE AS A SOLUTION

The rationale for the playfulness, deliberate ambiguity, and unconventional tactics of strategic marital therapy for depression lies in some paradoxes of both depression and maladjusted marriages. Therapists are probably more likely to make a positive difference with depressed persons if they accept that depressed persons are powerful in the aversiveness of their powerlessness; that one sure way to remain miserable is to try too hard to be happy; that a certain modicum of comfort may be found in the familiar certainty of depressed persons' discomfort; and that whatever advantages there are to recovery, it is also likely to present new problems.

Therapists are better equipped to deal with the marital issues of depressed persons if they appreciate that these relationships may provide more if each partner depends on them less. Many of the interventions are aimed at covertly assisting both partners to be a bit more self-sufficient or to look elsewhere for the satisfaction of some of their wants and needs. This may be construed as an adaptation to the hopefully temporary limitations of the marital relationship or as a more permanent arrangement. Also, each partner may be more likely to have a positive influence on the other if he or she does not try so hard to exert such influence and does not depend upon having an impact. In some cases, it may even be that change is possible *only* if a commitment to changing the other partner is relinquished.

Finally, preservation of, and positive change in, these relationships may be more obtainable if the couple and the therapist can at least consider the possibility of divorce as a solution. Too often, therapists rigidly and uncritically view divorce as an inherently negative outcome. Although it is also probably true that some therapists are too quick and glib in promoting divorce as the solution to what appears to be a depressing marriage, the more usual problem is that therapists view it as a personal failure, akin to a depressed patient's committing suicide. Anxious to prevent it, they deprive the couple of the opportunity to discover that divorce is an option, even if a costly one, and that their efforts to achieve a better relationship do not have to be so desperate and therefore so self-defeating.

In discussing the possibility of divorce, certain considerations are useful. First, depressed persons are more likely than nondepressed persons to wish that they had never gotten married, yet despite their problems, the majority of them (76%) and their spouses (70%) state that they would marry the same person if they had their life to live over (Merikangas, Prusoff, Kupfer, & Frank, 1985). Therapists should consider whether they are merely alienating these couples by seeming to be sold on an option that they have ruled out. It may even be, as Hinchcliffe, Hooper, Roberts, and Vaughan (1975) suggest, that the persons (i.e., depressed women) who benefit least from conventional marital roles are sometimes most committed to them. However, other statistics can be cited, and I often share them with the couples I treat. Being satisfactorily married may have advantages over being divorced, but the consequences of chronic marital difficulties for physical health and psychological well-being may be more serious than those of divorce (Coyne & DeLongis, 1986; Gove, Hughes, & Style, 1983). Without a change in their marital situation, the prognosis for depressed persons with marital problems is not good (Rousanville *et al.*, 1979). Further, among those whose marital difficulties antedate the onset of symptoms, the outcome of those who divorce may resemble that of women in good marriages (Rutter & Quinton, 1984).

REFERENCES

Bateson, G. (1955). A theory of play and fantasy. A.P.A. *Psychiatric Research Reports, 2*, 177–193.

Beckman, E. E., & Leber, W. R. (1985). The comparative efficacy of psychotherapy and pharmacotherapy. In E. E. Beckman & W. R. Leber (Eds.), *Handbook of depression* (pp. 316–342). Homewood, IL: Dorsey Press.

Birchnell, J., & Kennard, J. (1983). Does marital maladjustment lead to mental illness? *Social Psychiatry, 18*, 79–88.

Briscoe, C. W., & Smith, J. B. (1973). Depression and marital turmoil. *Archives of General Psychiatry, 29,* 811–817.

Coyne, J. C. (1976). Depression and the response of others. *Journal of Abnormal Psychology, 85,* 186–193.

Coyne, J. C. (1985). Toward a theory of frames and reframing: The social nature of frames. *Journal of Marital and Family Therapy, 11,* 337–344.

Coyne, J. C. (1986a). Ambiguities and controversies: An introduction. In J. C. Coyne (Ed.), *Essential papers on depression* (pp. 1–22). New York: New York University Press.

Coyne, J. C. (1986b). The significance of the interview in strategic therapy. *Journal of Strategic and Systemic Therapies, 5,* pp. 63–70.

Coyne, J. C., & DeLongis, A. M. (1986). Getting beyond social support: The role of social relationships in adaptational outcomes. *Journal of Consulting and Clinical Psychology, 54,* 454–460.

Coyne, J. C., & Gotlib, I. H. (1985). *Depression and parenting: An integrative review.* Unpublished manuscript.

Coyne, J. C., Kahn, J., & Gotlib, I. H. (1987). Depression. In T. Jacob (Ed.), *Family interaction and psychotherapy* (pp. 509–534). New York: Plenum.

Coyne, J. C., Kessler, R. C., Tal, M., Turnbull, J. Wortman, C., & Greden, J. (1987). Living with a depressed person: Burden and psychological distress. *Journal of Consulting and Clinical Psychology, 55,* 347–352.

Coyne, J. C., Wortman, C., & Lehman, D. (in press). The other side of support: Emotional overinvolvement and miscarried helping. In B. Gottlieb (Ed.), *Social Support: Formats, processes, and effects.* New York: Sage.

DeLongis, A. M., Coyne, J. C., Dakof, G., Folkman, S., & Lazarus, R. S. (1982). Daily hassles, uplifts, and the prediction of health states. *Health Psychology, 1,* 119–136.

DiMascio, A., Weissman, M. M., Prusoff, B. A., Neu, C., Zwilling, M., & Klerman, G. L. (1979). Differential symptom reduction by drugs and psychotherapy in acute depression. *Archives of General Psychiatry, 36,* 1450–1456.

Dolan, R. J., Calloway, S. P., Fonagy, P., De Souza, F. V. A., & Wakeling, A. (1985). Life events, depression, and hypothalamic–pituitary–adrenal axis function. *British Journal of Psychiatry, 147,* 429–433.

Gove, W., Hughes, M., & Style, C. B. (1983). Does marriage have positive effects on the psychological well-being of the individual? *Journal of Health and Social Behavior, 24,* 122–131.

Haley, J. (1963). *Strategies of psychotherapy.* New York: Grune & Stratton.

Hinchcliffe, M., Hooper, D., & Roberts, F. J. (1978). *The melancholy marriage.* New York: Wiley.

Hinchcliffe, M., Hopper, D., Roberts, F. J., & Vaughan, P. W. (1975). A study of the interaction between depressed patients and their spouses. *British Journal of Psychiatry, 126,* 164–176.

Hooley, J. M., Orley, J., & Teasdale, J. D. (1986). Levels of expressed emotion and relapse in depressed patients. *British Journal of Psychiatry, 148,* 642–647.

Kahn, J., Coyne, J. C., & Margolin, G. (1985). Depression and marital conflict: The social construction of despair. *Journal of Social and Personal Relationships, 2,* 447–462.

Keller, M. B., Klerman, G. L., Lavori, P. W., Coryell, W., Endicott, J., & Taylor, J. (1984). Long-term outcome of episodes of major depression: Clinical and public health significance. *Journal of the American Medical Association, 252,* 788–792.

Kovacs, M., Rush, A. J., Beck, A. T., & Hollon, S. (1981). Depressed outpatients treated with cognitive therapy or pharmacotherapy. *Archives of General Psychiatry, 38,* 33–39.

Leff, M., Roach, J., & Bunney, L. E. (1970). Environmental factors preceding the onset of severe depression. *Psychiatry, 33,* 298–311.

Lowry, M. R. (1985). *Major depression: Prevention and treatment.* St. Louis: Warren Green.

McLean, P. D. (1976). Therapeutic decision-making in the behavioral treatment of depression. In P. Davidson (Ed.), *Behavioral management of anxiety, depression, and pain.* New York: Brunner/Mazel.

McLean, P. D., & Hakstian, A. R. (1979). Clinical depression: Comparative efficacy of outpatient treatment. *Journal of Consulting and Clinical Psychology, 47,* 818–836.

Merikangas, K. R., Prusoff, B. A., Kupfer, D. J., & Frank, E. (1985). Marital adjustment in major depression. *Journal of Affective Disorders, 9,* 5–11.

Noll, K. M., Davis, J. M., & DeLeon-Jones, F. (1985). Medication and somatic therapies in the treatment of depression. In E. E. Beckman & W. R. Leber (Eds.), *Handbook of depression* (pp. 220–315). Homewood, IL: Dorsey Press.

O'Connell, R. A., Mayo, J. A., Eng, J. S., Jones, J. S., & Gabel, R. H. (1985). Social support and long-term lithium outcome. *British Journal of Psychiatry, 147,* 272–275.

Rousanville, B. J., Weissman, M. W., Prusoff, B. A., & Heraey-Baron, R. L. (1979). Marital disputes and treatment outcome in depressed women. *Comprehensive Psychiatry, 20,* 483–490.

Rush, A. J. (1982). Diagnosing depression. In A. J. Rush (Ed.), *Short-term psychotherapies for depression: Behavioral, interpersonal, cognitive, and psychodynamic approaches* (pp. 1–17). New York: Guilford Press.

Rush, A. J., Beck, A. T., Kovacs, M., & Hollon, S. (1977). Comparative efficacy of cognitive therapy and imipramine in the treatment of depressed outpatients. *Cognitive Therapy and Research, 1,* 17–37.

Rutter, M., & Quinton, D. (1984). Parental psychiatric disorder: Effects on children. *Psychological Medicine, 14,* 891–898.

Watzlawick, P., Weakland, J., & Fisch, R. (1974). *Change: Principles of problem formation and problem resolution.* New York: W. W. Norton.

Weissman, M. M., Prusoff, B. A., DiMascio, A., Neu, C., Gorklaney, M., & Klerman, G. L. (1979). The efficacy of drugs and psychotherapy in the treatment of acute depressive episodes. *American Journal of Psychiatry, 136,* 555–558.

Winokur, G. (1986). Controversies in depression, or do clinicians know something after all? In J. C. Coyne (Ed.), *Essential papers on depression.* New York: New York University Press.

PART THREE

THERAPEUTIC STRATEGIES WITH FAMILIES

One of the most challenging aspects of the diagnosis and treatment of affective (mood) disorders derives from the variation across the clinical subtypes of affective illness. In Chapter 5, Ian Falloon and colleagues describe a behavioral family treatment approach, including psychoeducation and communication and problem-solving skills, for families with an affectively disturbed member. This approach has previously been successful in assisting families with a schizophrenic member.

In Chapter 6, the Cornell University Medical College family therapy group describes an inpatient family intervention that was implemented in a clinical trial with affectively disordered patients and their families. Case histories are used to translate quantitative data into clinically meaningful descriptions of treatment outcomes and to illustrate the heterogeneity of clinical problems and strategies for treatment of families with an affectively ill family member.

Epstein and colleagues (Chapter 7) address the issue of family heterogeneity, proposing a clear and comprehensive model for the assessment of family functioning, and a typology for classification of families with an affectively ill member. They also present treatment strategies designed to address dysfunctional patterns of family interaction. Although the patients are relatively homogeneous in terms of affective diagnosis, these investigators have found that problem areas are heterogeneous and that family strengths and weaknesses are diverse. Epstein and colleagues recommend the use of a self-report measure of family functioning to aid in the identification of family problems, strengths, and dysfunctional patterns of family interaction. Use of such structured family assessment instruments can not only aid in treatment planning but guide intervention strategies and assessment of treatment response.

The chapter by Davenport and Adland (Chapter 8) is unique in its exclusive focus on family intervention in manic eposides. Their family treatment vignettes illustrate the chronic, severe, and disruptive course of mania, and highlight, in a way that other chapters do not, the impact on the children of a parent suffering from the affective disorder. The multifaceted family intervention is at once practical and realistic in its goals to assist the family in coping with a chronic condition.

In Chapter 9, Targum presents the less often discussed topic of genetic counseling in the treatment of affective disorders. In a sense, this type of intervention represents a highly refined and specific variant of psychoeducation, enabled by an expanding base of empirical knowledge and technical expertise. Targum outlines the elements of a genetic counseling approach and provides a review of the relevant information on depression.

Melvin Lansky (Chapter 10) offers rich clinical descriptions of family intervention as an effective "vehicle" in the delivery of treatment for affective disorders. He discusses general issues related to the use of family treatments in combination with medication, electroconvulsive therapy, hospitalization, and individual or group therapies, and specific problems or situations (e.g., suicide and concomitant personality disorder) that may call for specific applications of family therapy.

5

Behavioral Family Therapy

IAN R. H. FALLOON
VICTOR HOLE
LESLEY MULROY
LYNNE J. NORRIS
TERENCE PEMBLETON

Behavioral formulations of the psychogenesis of affective disorders have been restricted mainly to depressive conditions. Operant reinforcement and cognitive processes have been invoked to explain the characteristic changes in thinking and behavior that are displayed by a depressed individual. Ferster (1965) and Seligman (1975) employed animal experiments to support their theories of depressive syndromes. Changes in reinforcement patterns that result in an overall reduction in positive reinforcement for adaptive behavior were shown to induce maladaptive passivity in animals, even in the presence of aversive stimuli. Seligman coined the term "learned helplessness" to describe this phenomenon, which appeared to parallel the way in which depressed individuals appear to perceive themselves as unwitting victims of an unpleasant environment that they are unable to modify. This perceived hopelessness is considered a key feature of Beck's theory, which stresses the negative cognitions that distort the interpersonal responses of the depressed person.

Some theorists have observed the effects of social interaction between families and friends and the depressed person (Burgess, 1969; Lewinsohn, Weinstein, & Shaw, 1969; Liberman & Raskin, 1971). The expression of warmth, sympathy, and concern toward the depressed person when he or she is exhibiting depressive behavior tends to reinforce this behavior. On the other hand, relatives often fail to reward constructive or neutral behavior when this is emitted. It is all too easy for families to focus attention almost exclusively on the depressive behavior, which appears as a "despairing cry for love" (Abraham, 1953) or as an expression of infantile helplessness (Klein, 1948). Family members who receive minimal positive responses from the depressed person are prone to become demoralized and hopeless themselves. These negative interpersonal response patterns tend to maintain depressive behavior within the family unit.

These formulations have led to the development of two main behavioral strategies for the treatment of depression. The first aims to increase both the constructive behavior emitted by the depressed person and the frequency of positive reinforcement provided for this behavior by the patient and his or her close associates (Falloon, 1975; Lewinsohn *et al.*, 1969; Liberman & Raskin, 1971). This may be accompanied by efforts to discourage the patient and relatives from giving undue attention to nonconstructive depressive behaviors. The second major strategy is to attempt to modify repetitive negative thought patterns through cognitive restructuring techniques (Beck, Rush, Shaw, & Emery, 1979). Distorted, unrealistic, and exaggerated worrying is replaced by constructive problem solving and the achievement of specific relevant goals.

All of these approaches have targeted the depressed individual for primary intervention, although family members have usually been involved in the overall management plan, albeit in a somewhat peripheral fashion. However, recent findings that suggest that family response patterns may have a central role in the pathogenesis of depressive disorders have led to a review of the significance of family interventions in the management of affective disorders.

STRESS, VULNERABILITY, AND FAMILY COPING BEHAVIOR

The association between environmental stressors and mood disturbance, predominantly anxiety and depression, has a long history. Recently, this association has been supported by several excellent research endeavors. George Brown and his colleagues in London (Brown & Harris, 1978) have provided compelling evidence that a combination of environmental stress factors and psychosocial vulnerability tends to enhance a person's risk of succumbing to a depressive disorder. The stress factors tended to be life events that were perceived as threatening by the subject and that tended to be unresolved within a week, as well as enduring stresses such as persistent financial hardship or inadequate housing. The vulnerability factors that were most significant were a lack of employment, having three or more children under 14 living at home, loss of a mother before the age of 11 by death or separation, and the absence of a close, confiding relationship.

Brown and Harris (1978) concluded that the combined effects of major life stress and vulnerability were potentially able to induce a depressive disorder, albeit usually mild, in otherwise healthy persons. The onset of these disorders was quite protracted, usually developing over months rather than weeks. This contrasts with the manner in which manic episodes tend to be triggered within weeks of a major life event (Ambelas, 1987).

The protection offered by a close, confiding relationship is of particular interest when considering the role of the family unit in the management of affective disturbances. Although Brown's research offers little detail as to how the confiding relationship may operate in preventing depressive episodes, another series of studies helps to elucidate this issue. It is of interest to note that Brown himself provided the initial impetus to this work though his studies of family factors and schizophrenia (Brown, Birley, & Wing, 1972). Several studies have examined the impact of family behavior on the course of depressive (Hooley, Orley, & Teasdale, 1986; Vaughn & Leff, 1976) and bipolar manic–depressive disorders (Miklowitz, Goldstein, Nuechterlein, Snyder, & Doane, 1986). All of these studies have demonstrated a link between low levels of family criticism directed toward the index patient and a reduction in the frequency of major affective episodes. High levels of criticism and hostility toward the patient appear to be markers of inefficient coping behavior in the family unit.

It is apparent that when a person who is vulnerable to episodes of affective disturbance has regular contact with one or more persons who can assist in the resolution of significant life problems, his or her risk of major episodes may be reduced. A confiding relationship is one in which problems can be readily communicated and constructive plans for coping with them developed. High levels of criticism are unhelpful, as, too, are overinvolved, intrusive behaviors, such as persistently solving the problem for the patient. The role of effective problem-solving functions has been supported by recent studies of the interaction between index patients and family members when discussing problem issues (Hooley & Hahlweg, 1986; Miklowitz *et al.*, 1986).

Thus it may be concluded that interventions that aim to enhance the efficiency of family problem-solving behavior may facilitate the management of affective disorders by rapid resolution of the stress of major life events and by assisting the affectively disturbed member in coping with enduring life stressors, including those associated with ongoing difficulties in family relationships.

The development of behavioral family therapy strategies for the management of major affective disturbances in members of the community is under way in the Buckingham Mental Health Service Project in Buckingham, England. This is a comprehensive service that seeks to facilitate home-based management of all mental disorders, with the aim of minimizing the clinical and social morbidity they cause, both for caregivers and for sufferers. The methods employed in the project will be outlined in the remainder of this chapter.

BEHAVIORAL FAMILY INTERVENTION STRATEGIES: AN OVERVIEW

The core ingredient of behavior therapy methods is a detailed and continual assessment of specific presenting problems. Within this empirical framework, a broad range of treatment strategies are applied in a systematic fashion. Rather than assuming that affective disorders such as depression or mania are unitary disturbances of function, the behavior therapist views these disorders as a series of associated behaviors that tend to vary from patient to patient, and in the same patient from hour to hour (Lewis, 1934). These behaviors can be categorized in the following four groups:

1. Motor and verbal output changes: retardation, restlessness
2. Unrealistic self-evaluative statements: self-reproach, unworthiness, hopelessness, bodily changes (depression); or exaggerated self-worth, health, and happiness (mania)
3. Anxiety behavior: tension, fear, obsessions, and compulsions
4. Somatic complaints: changes in sleep, appetite, and sexual desire; weight change, bowel disturbance

The behavior therapist specifies each behavior and then targets an intervention to counter that behavior. The four categories are associated with different behavioral approaches. Activity schedules have been employed successfully with motor and verbal changes (Lewinsohn, Biglan, & Zeiss, 1975). Cognitive restructuring is employed with distorted self-statements (Beck *et al.*, 1979). Anxiety management is effective with anxiety behavior (Marks, 1976). Drug therapies are effective in alleviating somatic complaints (Kessler, 1978).

Family-based intervention in the management of acute affective episodes is essentially delivered by co-therapists, family members, and professionals who assist the index patient to employ the strategies that counter the specific behavior disturbances. When high levels of family tension are evident or when stresses that may have contributed to the affective episode remain, additional stress management strategies may be applied within the family. Education about the nature of the affective disorder and its effective management is an important component of the family-based approach.

Once the acute episode has remitted, family-based stress management, combined with continued drug therapy, forms the basis of an approach to preventing future recurrences. A small percentage of cases show depressive or manic behaviors that persist despite intensive drug and psychosocial intervention. Family management is employed to assist the patient and the family in coping with these problems and in leading relatively unrestricted lives even when recovery is incomplete.

BEHAVIORAL ANALYSIS OF
AFFECTIVE DISTURBANCE
IN THE FAMILY

The baseline assessment of family functioning and the continual review that is conducted as part of every session constitute the framework upon which behavioral intervention strategies are constructed. The initial behavioral analysis may involve hours of painstaking individual and conjoint interviews as well as systematic observation. Where a major affective disturbance is present in one or more family members, other stressful family problems are often evident. Each of these presenting problems, including those associated with the key symptoms of the index patient, is explored in the assessment process. The therapist attempts to obtain the following:

1. *A therapeutic alliance with all family members.* The presenting problems are used as a starting point for the analysis of the functioning of the family as a problem-solving unit. Each component of the system (individual, dyad, triad, etc.) is explored in order to discover its strengths and weaknesses in relationship to the specific problems. At its most straightforward level, this consists of defining the specific contingencies that surround a problem behavior—for example, what precedes a family row or increases agitated behavior, and what the usual consequences are of that behavior. By interviewing each family member individually, the therapist gains a picture of the setting of the presenting problem that is broader than the consensus view provided by a family group. Generalizations tend to be avoided. However, reports of problem behavior are often distorted by the search for simple causal relationships, so that at this stage, the therapist can derive only a series of hypotheses to be confirmed in subsequent observation of the actual behavioral sequences.

2. *Detailed information about each family member's observations, thoughts, and feelings regarding the presenting problems.* This includes the level of understanding of the nature and treatment of the affective disorder.

3. *Information about each family member's interaction within the family system*; his or her attitudes, feelings, and behavior toward the other family members; and his or her support for efforts to resolve the presenting problem.

4. *Information about each family member's functioning* in settings outside the family unit; his or her personal assets and deficits that might be relevant to problem resolution.

Ideally, observations of the family's functioning are conducted in the setting where the presenting problems arise, usually at home. Such naturalistic observations are invaluable, but they may be too costly for routine practice. Alternatives include having the family tape-record interactions at targeted times, time sampling interactions by use of tape recordings with automated time switches, re-enactment of problem situations by family members, or having family discussions about "hot issues." Nevertheless, at least one home visit is an essential part of the behavioral assessment, and it usually provides the therapist with an abundance of valuable information seldom accessible in clinic-based assessments.

The behavioral family therapist is interested not merely in pinpointing the setting in which problem behavior is most likely to arise but also in uncovering the family's past and current efforts to cope with the behavior. It usually emerges that any problem is present only a small proportion of the time and arises only on some of the occasions when it might be expected. Even the most depressed person has extensive periods when his or her main symptoms are not observed. From another viewpoint, most behavior observed in families is positive or neutral (i.e., nonproblematic), and for the most part, families have already learned strategies for coping with the major problems. Thus the therapist is interested in uncovering the contingencies that exist when the problem is quiescent, as well as those that exist when the problem is present but producing minimal distress. It is assumed that the family generally has developed patterns to cope with the problem but that these coping efforts are only partially effective, often because family members are inconsistent in applying them or do not persist in using them, thereby failing to derive the full benefits that are possible. Where such effective strategies can be pinpointed, the therapist is left with the relatively straightforward task of assisting the family in enhancing the efficacy of their preexisting interaction patterns. Such a targeted intervention may take a mere session or two, but the behavioral analysis that precedes it may be a much longer process.

Affective disorders wreak havoc in the everyday routine of family living. A survey of the current activities of each family member is contrasted with that member's desired activity patterns. Family members are invited to describe their most frequent activities, as well as the people with whom they have the most contact, the places where they spend the most time, and the objects that they most often use. Discrepancies between current and expected activity levels help the therapist pinpoint key areas of dissatisfaction, which may assist him or her in defining specific goals related to each family member's quality of life.

In addition to listing activities that induce pleasing responses, family members are asked to discuss aversive situations. Unpleasant situations that tend to be avoided may vary from those involving simple phobias to various family interactions, such as arguments or discussions about finances or sexual concerns. Feelings of rejection, isolation, frustration, coercion, lack of support, mistrust, and intrusiveness may be discussed in this context. Family members are asked to provide clear examples of interactions where they experience these negative feelings.

This survey of reinforcing activities and aversive situations often provides a fascinating picture of the manner in which families' everyday activities intertwine in patterns of mutual reinforcement—positively in happy families, and negatively in distressed families, where confrontation, coercion, or marked avoidance of intimacy may predominate. Interviews in which family members report on daily activities are notoriously unreliable, particularly with patients undergoing episodes of major affective disorders. To obtain a more precise assessment of family activity, it may be necessary to invite family members to complete daily activity schedules.

A final use of the reinforcement survey involves the selection of positive reinforcers that may be employed in the promotion of specific behavior change during the intervention phase. Activities, places, people, and objects that are deemed highly desirable can be employed to mediate change when used as specific rewards for performance of targeted behaviors.

At the completion of the behavioral analysis, the therapist will be able to specify the short-term life goals of each family member and the conflicts and problems that may need to be resolved in order to achieve these goals. Such problems may include the symptoms of the affective disorder and the relationship difficulties that appear to impede problem resolution within the family unit.

FUNCTIONAL ANALYSIS: A BEHAVIORAL SYSTEM

The behavioral analysis provides a clear basis for identifying a list of potential intervention targets. However, such a list does not tell us where to begin. The behavioral family therapist aims to pinpoint the key deficits within the family group that once resolved, will lead to maximal change. It is assumed that the patterns of family behavior that are observed at any point will represent the optimal response of every family member to the resolution of the existing problem. Even when chaotic, distressing responses are observed, every family member is attempting to resolve the problem (or achieve the goal) in the manner he or she considers most rewarding (or least distressing), given all of the constraints imposed by the biopsychosocial system at that time.

Rather than attempting to impose his or her own optimal solutions to a problem, the behavioral family therapist aims to employ minimal intervention—intervention that will build upon existing family assets. For example, where one family member is observed to be able to get a depressed person to assist with household chores, the therapist examines that member's behavior closely and pinpoints the specific effective strategies that he or she employs. A note is made that effective strategies are already present within the family unit and that the skilled member may be used to train others in the intervention plan.

The functional analysis involves exploration of the family system from a behavioral perspective, so that a long list of potential targets for intervention can be reduced to one or two specific issues that can be addressed in a straightforward manner. These issues are not restricted to purely psychosocial parameters but may include biological variables such as changes in hormonal systems that may trigger or maintain an affective disturbance, or the specific benefits of drug therapies. If the latter are observed to produce significant relief of specific symptoms in an efficient manner, they are strongly advocated, despite evidence that family patterns of behavior may appear to have contributed to the onset or maintenance of the episode.

Thus a purely pragmatic approach is employed, one that endeavors to facilitate effective problem resolution and goal achievement for every family member in the most efficient manner. Of course, this includes efforts to ensure that similar problems do not recur in the future. In most cases of major affective disorders, interventions are targeted to multiple systems: drugs to correct biological deficiencies, psychological interventions to correct cognitive–behavioral problems, family interventions to enhance family problem-solving functions, and social interventions to deal with stresses related to finances, work, and friendship.

CASE EXAMPLE: JANE

An example of this approach involved Jane, a depressed woman, who had recently resigned from her job as a social worker after the threat of an assault by a client's husband. Her problem was made worse by an exacerbation of her long-standing fear of crowds. This caused her to become housebound, to withdraw from social activities she found very rewarding, and to place increasing demands upon her husband for friendship. The accidental death of her daughter 5 years earlier had not been discussed with her husband. This had created persistent tension between them that limited the emotional support he could give his wife at this time. He tended to take over her role as homemaker, leaving her with limited rewarding daily activities. In addition, she was experiencing the effects of the hormonal changes associated with menopause. Her family doctor had given her a course of antidepressants that she had not completed because of unpleasant side effects.

The behavioral family therapist postulated that Jane had become persistently depressed not as a result of biological, psychological, or social factors— despite the presence of abundant problems in these areas—but primarily because of the breakdown in her intimate communication with her husband, which had effectively precluded her obtaining support to resolve the stressors she had experienced at work and at home, and her symptoms of anxiety. Under the treatment plan that was devised, the first step was to reestablish the intimate communication of feelings, needs, and wishes between husband and wife, initially to address the specific problem of Jane's anxiety symptoms, and then to facilitate open discussion about their daughter's death.

At the completion of the functional analysis, the behavioral family therapist is able to draw up an initial intervention program with one or two clearly defined therapy goals, and a systematic treatment plan targeted to these goals. A time frame is defined, and a contract for a specific number of sessions is agreed upon with the family. Continual measures of progress toward the goals are defined in order to guide the therapist from session to session, and a date is set for a detailed review at the end of the contracted sessions. After this review, goals and intervention plans may be modified or changed, and a contract for further therapy developed.

BEHAVIORAL FAMILY INTERVENTION DURING ACUTE AFFECTIVE EPISODES

For acute episodes of major affective disorders, it is common practice to treat patients in a hospital. The role of caregiving is transferred from the family to nursing and medical staffs on a hospital ward. However, with the trend toward community care of persons with mental disorders, families are generally expected to provide more extensive care at home. Family management of severe acute episodes of depression or mania involves training family members in many of the skills employed by excellent nurses. At all times, the management plan is based upon the behavioral assessment of family functioning, although it is usually necessary to begin the initial intervention strategies before comprehensive family assessment has been conducted. However, when the therapist is able to operate from a community-based service, cases tend to be detected before an episode is fully developed, so that a more extensive assessment may be feasible.

The minimal assessment involves a problem-oriented appraisal of the major symptoms of the disorder in the index patient; the factors that appear to reduce, and those that appear to exacerbate, the severity of these symptoms; the coping behaviors of family members; their levels of distress associated with the index patient's disorder, as well as other stressors; and the problem-solving skills of the family unit. If the family appears able and willing to continue caring for the index patient, training in management skills is begun without delay. If the family does not appear capable of providing the management required, even with considerable assistance from the therapy team, alternative care (e.g., hospital, day hospital, residential care) is arranged.

The acute phase of family management includes (1) education about the disorder, (2) family stress management, and (3) specific strategies for symptom management.

1. *Education about depressive or manic episodes.* The patient and family receive one or more sessions aimed at enhancing their understanding of the nature of the major affective disorder from which the patient is

suffering. This includes discussion about the range of symptoms, diagnosis, and theories of etiology. A biopsychosocial perspective is employed that considers genetic, biological, cognitive–behavioral, and sociological factors. This model is used to provide a rationale for an integrated approach to management. A longitudinal perspective is emphasized, with methods to ensure effective rehabilitation and the prevention of recurrent episodes. The education focuses on the active contributions that the index patient and family members can make to the long-term outcome of the disorder. Specially prepared handouts are provided and further educational input is provided whenever it is indicated during the intervention program.

2. *Family stress management.* Crucial to the success of family management of acute episodes is the ability of the family to cope with the added stress that the disorder places upon the household. Families are taught a six-step problem-solving approach, which involves pinpointing stressful problems, brainstorming potential solutions, evaluating and choosing the best alternative, and planning and reviewing efforts to implement that solution. When stress is high, families are encouraged to conduct problem-solving discussions at least once a day. When symptoms are severe, a therapist may be present to convene these discussions. However, unless stress is overwhelming, the therapist adopts the role of coach to the family, assisting the members in employing the structured approach efficiently in seeking their own solutions and devising their own plans.

3. *Specific strategies for symptom management.* The key symptoms (problems) of the affective disorder are pinpointed by the therapist, patient, and family. A behavioral analysis of each problem is conducted, and a specific intervention strategy planned, using the family problem-solving structure. However, in these instances, the therapist adopts a participant role in the discussion, assisting the family in employing validated strategies for symptom resolution. Examples of such strategies include the use of activity schedules and operant reinforcement to promote constructive activity; cognitive restructuring to promote realistic self-evaluative statements; anxiety management strategies for phobic, obsessional, and panic symptoms; relaxation strategies (psychological or pharmacological) for muscle tension and insomnia; tricyclic drugs for anorexia, weight loss, loss of sexual desire, and retardation; and tranquilizing drugs for agitation, pressure of thought, and hyperactivity.

Whenever possible, the specific effects of each intervention are assessed by introducing the interventions one at a time and measuring specific changes in the targeted problem behavior in a multiple-baseline design. This process assists in the continuing functional analysis of the disorder. For example, when generalized improvement occurs following the introduction of an antidepressant drug directed primarily at severe anorexia, it may be postulated that a primary disorder of biological systems existed. When a cognitive–behavioral strategy produces similar changes, it would tend to support the existence of a predominantly psychosocial deficit. However, the conclusions of such speculation should be viewed with caution in light of our very limited understanding of the origins of affective disorders.

The severity of the disorder in the index patient and the management skills of the family members will determine the level of input from the therapy team. This will vary from sessions held once a week to work with the patient and family two or three times daily. These sessions are conducted in the family home and involve practical training in specific skills, with instructions, demonstrations, guided practice, and supportive coaching. Emphasis is placed upon shaping the preexisting skills of family members and self-help strategies for patients. Patients and family members keep records of the problem behaviors and intervention strategies.

CASE EXAMPLE: SYLVIA M

Sylvia was a 59-year-old woman who lived with her retired husband, Alan. She was a very active member of the small village community in which she had been born. Over a period of several months, she had gradually lost interest in her social activities and had experienced difficulties in concentrating and with sleep and appetite. She became filled with thoughts of unworthiness and self-reproach and felt that she should be punished for her misdeeds. She was unable to manage the home and unable to sit still, pacing restlessly around the house.

Her husband was very supportive and had taken over the household management. When it was evident that Sylvia's behavior was too much of a burden for Alan, he sought the assistance of their family doctor, who immediately consulted with the mental health service. Sylvia was assessed as suffering from a depressive disorder, and an initial program was begun that involved activity scheduling for motor restlessness and an antidepressant drug for sleep and appetite disturbance. The patient, her husband, and a daughter who lived nearby participated in two sessions of education about depressive disorders. After 4 weeks, neither the drug nor the behavioral intervention had shown any significant impact on the problems, and Alan was unable to cope with Sylvia's periods of extreme agitation. A hospital admission was arranged.

After 5 months of hospital management, including an extensive search for neuroendocrine abnormality and the use of various drugs, activity programs, and two courses of electroconvulsive therapy, her condition remained unmodified. Her husband was eager to have her returned to his care, and a 4-week period of family management was contracted. For 5 days per week, 2 hours of therapy in the morning and 2 hours in the afternoon were provided by a team of trained therapists. Three problems were targeted, and specific strategies were devised for alleviating them, as follows:

1. *Agitated, restless behavior.* The therapist established a goal for Sylvia of spending 20 minutes continuously engaged in a constructive activ-

ity. They coached Alan and his daughter to help Sylvia engage in low-stress activities that she formerly enjoyed, such as knitting, baking cookies and cakes, and strolling in the village. Alan was shown how to prompt her to attend to the task at hand when she showed signs of restlessness and to provide positive reinforcement for all her efforts.

2. *Unrealistic, negative self-statements.* The therapist established a goal of minimizing the frequency of Sylvia's repetitive, spontaneous statements of unworthiness and self-reproach. Alan tended to respond to these unrealistic statements by telling Sylvia that they were untrue, that she had always been a good wife and mother. He was taught either to ignore these statements or to introduce a different topic of conversation through a comment or a question. Therapists demonstrated the effectiveness of this strategy in reducing Sylvia's negative self-statements and in increasing her everyday conversation.

3. *Alan's stress.* It was observed that Alan became burnt out at times. On these occasions, he would become tearful and distressed. This tended to upset Sylvia, who became agitated and increased her negative self-statements. Alan was taught to employ structured problem solving when he was aware that he was becoming overwhelmed and to plan to have friends, relatives, or therapists give him a break from Sylvia's care on a regular basis.

Daily assessment of these goals was conducted on systematic scales by Alan and the therapists. After 2 weeks, little change had been noted in Sylvia's agitated behavior. A small dose of thioridazine was prescribed for the morning and the evening. After 4 weeks, ratings of agitated behavior had improved by 50% on an 8-point scale. Constructive activity had increased to targeted levels. Appetite and sleep had returned to normal. Alan was reporting feeling more able to cope and was beginning to pursue his own activities and interests.

The frequency of Sylvia's negative self-statements showed little reduction after 4 weeks. It was observed that Alan was visiting friends and relatives but had great difficulty not responding to these remarks. However, Alan now experienced less distress when Sylvia made negative statements about herself, despite having great difficulty preventing himself from reassuring her. Further coaching was provided, not only for Alan but also for their daughter and several other relatives and visiting friends. A cognitive approach was not feasible in this case because Sylvia continued to have difficulty concentrating in complex discussions.

Once the acute episode had been resolved, further behavioral analysis was conducted and the emphasis shifted to preventing future exacerbations of the disorder. The intensive therapeutic input was gradually reduced as further improvement occurred. Subsequent goals for Sylvia included increasing homemaker activity and reestablishing social behavior outside the home. Alan continued to develop his own interests and activities as the need for his caregiving role declined. Further education that was provided about the nature of depressive disorders stressed recognition of the early warning signs of an exacerbation and the importance of immediately reporting these signs to the mental health professionals so that intensive management could be provided with minimal delay.

This case study illustrates the strategy of home-based family intervention with a severe episode of an affective disorder that was unresponsive to good hospital-based management. Such cases are relatively rare, and they require the cooperation of very supportive relatives who are prepared to take the role of co-therapists. A more typical case of acute disturbance, such as that of the social worker, Jane (described earlier), can be treated in a much less intensive manner. Nevertheless, the close collaboration with key relatives enables specific strategies to be employed on a day-to-day basis, thereby greatly increasing the efficiency of the therapy.

PREVENTION OF EPISODES OF MAJOR AFFECTIVE DISORDERS

Once the acute episode of depression or mania has remitted, attention switches to strategies that may help reduce the risk of recurrence. Prophylactic drug therapy involving continuation of low doses of antidepressants (for depressive disorders) or lithium therapy (for bipolar disorders) has been well established. The effectiveness of drug prophylaxis is limited, however, by several factors, perhaps the most important being the patient's ability to adhere to the prescribed regimen. Antidepressants and lithium are characterized by a broad range of unpleasant side effects that discourage long-term compliance. An important aspect of family management is the further education of patients and their families regarding the prophylactic benefits of these drugs, strategies for coping with their side effects, and methods of maintaining high levels of compliance.

However, even when excellent drug taking is maintained, the prophylaxis provided is restricted. Recurrent episodes remain common in a large proportion of cases. Evidence that environmental stress may contribute to episodes has led to the application of behavioral family therapy strategies to the prevention of episodes of affective disorders. The methods are identical to those that have shown promise in preventing recurrent episodes of schizophrenia (Falloon, Boyd, & McGill, 1984). In addition to family education, families are assisted in improving their problem-solving functions so that they may better cope with a wide range of intrafamilial and extrafamilial stresses. Stress is not avoided; rather, the family unit collaborates to deal with stress in a highly efficient manner. This entails regular family discussions, effective interpersonal communication, and a structured approach that facilitates problem resolution. A behavioral analysis that focuses upon the family problem-solving functions provides the framework for this approach.

CASE EXAMPLE: COLLEEN AND ANDREW L

Colleen was a 39-year-old housewife, married to Andrew, a 40-year-old systems analyst. They had a 19-year-old son, David, who had just begun studying economics at a university in Scotland. Colleen was referred for management of a chronic bipolar disorder following discharge from a hospital after partial remission of a severe manic episode had been achieved. She was receiving large doses of fluphenazine decanoate and lithium carbonate.

During the past 20 years, Colleen had had at least seven severe episodes of mania and numerous, less disturbing depressive episodes. These episodes lasted from 6 months to 2 years, and during the most recent 5 years, she had spent less than 24 months out of the hospital. Indeed, the only period of long-term stability in her disorder had occurred when she and her husband has spent 3 years in the United States. During that time, she remained very well. It was noted that this was the only time she had established a circle of supportive friends and had felt free of significant stresses. Her husband's job led to frequent moves, which appeared to trigger episodes.

Colleen and Andrew were well informed about the nature of her disorder and had learned to detect the earliest signs of a recurrence. Andrew noticed her becoming tense, anxious, and irritable. However, they often experienced difficulties getting effective medical assistance at this stage. Andrew had great difficulty coping with Colleen's outbursts of aggression and spending sprees. He tried to play along with her high spirits, to reason with her in a calm manner, or to minimize contact with her during manic episodes. None of these strategies seemed to help, and they both agreed that their lives now almost completely centered around the disorder. Both had a wide range of interests but had been unable to pursue them for several years.

Colleen defined her short-term goal as taking over the household management again, that is, planning meals, cooking, and cleaning. Andrew targeted two goals: learning to cope more effectively with Colleen's episodes so that she could stay at home, and taking a short trip abroad on a work assignment. Their problem-solving and communication skills were observed to be good, although they seldom sat down and discussed problems.

The therapist initially contracted for ten home-based sessions, to include education that stressed the drug and psychological strategies used in the management of manic episodes, communication training that focused on increasing the direct expression of everyday positive and negative feelings, and the establishment of regular structured problem-solving discussions.

The education sessions enabled Colleen to understand the rationale for long-term drug prophylaxis and to accept that although her weight gain may have been induced by the drugs, weight loss could be accomplished only by a program of sensible dieting and exercise. Andrew learned that it would be helpful for him to persist with his calm approach to Colleen during her manic states and to avoid confrontation. The importance of making assertive requests for help at the earliest sign of an episode was stressed. Their family practitioner was given a list of Colleen's early warning signs, with instructions to contact the mental health service whenever these signs became apparent.

Several sessions were devoted to improving communication skills. The skills for which training was received included mutually expressing positive feelings in an appropriate manner for everyday pleasing behavior, making requests for behavior change in a nondemanding manner, expressing displeasure in a manner that is likely to lead to constructive problem resolution, and listening in an attentive, empathic way that assists in pinpointing and defining problems or goals. Each session was conducted in a workshop fashion, with guide sheets, therapist demonstrations, behavior rehearsal of brief interaction sequences, and between-session practice assignments.

The couple quickly achieved competence in these communication skills and were able to incorporate them into their marital interaction. Andrew no longer worried that he could not express any negative feelings toward Colleen lest he upset her and trigger an episode. Colleen felt less inhibited in expressing her positive feelings and affection toward Andrew.

They quickly adopted the six-step problem-solving approach and conducted weekly discussions during which Colleen planned her household chores for the week and they both planned activities together. After ten sessions, they were able to demonstrate excellent communication and problem-solving skills and were coping with everyday stresses in a highly efficient manner. The therapist reduced the frequency of sessions, but in view of the severity of Colleen's disorder, continued to provide monthly sessions for 2 years. The couple continued to convene regular problem-solving discussions. Colleen had taken over the household management fully, had established a network of friends, and had taken up several hobbies. She had coped with several very stressful situations, including three occasions when Andrew had made business trips abroad, and an operation that Andrew had had to remove a thyroid tumor, which was found to be benign. Throughout this 2-year period, she had remained free of all symptoms. She continued to take lithium carbonate with excellent compliance, and the fluphenazine decanoate had been reduced to a low dose.

Andrew was more settled in his work and was less concerned about making trips abroad. He was now able to pursue his hobbies with enthusiasm and to enjoy a satisfying social life with his wife.

Although it is not possible to attribute the improvement in the course of this woman's disorder to the family management approach, similar benefits have been observed in a series of cases in which we have employed similar methods. Not in all cases have patients remained free of recurrent episodes, but even where further episodes have emerged, a combination of early intervention and drug and psychosocial approaches has enabled the patients and families to cope with each successive episode in a more effective manner, with progressively less distress to patients and relatives alike.

CONCLUSION

The efficacy of behavioral family therapy in the management of major affective disorders has not been subjected to rigorous scientific evaluation. In combining it with other behavioral strategies and pharmacotherapy, we have observed added benefits. The observation that family collaboration enhances the management of acute mental disorders has been made in hospital-based studies (Gould & Glick, 1977). The most striking benefits have been noted in the long-term management of affective disorders, where the family approach has been associated with considerable improvements in the stability of several cases where recurrent episodes were frequent and drug prophylaxis was relatively ineffective. In addition, we have noted that early detection of the symptoms of major depressive or manic episodes has enabled immediate and intensive drug and family therapy to modify the severity of these episodes.

Controlled studies of these methods are needed in order to examine these clinical impressions in detail. A study of the incidence and prevalence of major affective disorders in an epidemiologically defined population in Buckingham is currently in progress. A family-based management approach is employed in treating all patients with mental disorders who come to the primary health care service. Preliminary findings suggest that the frequency of episodes of major affective disorders is declining. We suspect that these benefits may have derived, at least in part, from the behavioral family therapy methods we have employed.

REFERENCES

Abraham, K. (1953). Notes on the psychoanalytical investigation and treatment of manic-depressive insanity and allied conditions. In D. Bryan & A. Strachey (Trans.),*Selected papers on psychoanalysis*. New York: Basic Books.

Ambelas, A. (1987). Life events and mania—A special relationship? *British Journal of Psychiatry, 15*, 235–240.

Beck, A. T., Rush, A. J., Shaw, B. F., & Emery, G. (1979). *Cognitive therapy of depression*. New York: Guilford Press.

Brown, G. W., Birley, J. L. T., & Wing, J. K. (1972). Influence of family life on the course of schizophrenic disorders: A replication. *British Journal of Psychiatry, 121*, 241–258.

Brown, G. W., & Harris, T. O. (1978). *Social origins of depression*. London: Tavistock.

Burgess, E. P. (1969). The modification of depressive behaviours. In R. Rubin & C. M. Franks (Eds.), *Advances in behavior therapy*. New York: Academic Press.

Falloon, I. R. H. (1975). The therapy of depression: A behavioral approach. *Psychotherapy and Psychosomatics, 25*, 69-75.

Falloon, I. R. H., Boyd, J. L., & McGill, C. W., (1984). *Family care of schizophrenia.* New York: Guilford Press.

Ferster, C. B., (1965). Classification of behavioral psychotherapy. In L. Krasner & G. Ullmann (Eds.), *Research in behavior modification.* New York: Holt, Rinehart & Winston.

Gould, E., & Glick, I. D. (1977). The effects of family presence and brief family intervention on global outcome for hospitalized schizophrenic patients. *Family Process, 4*, 503-510.

Hooley, J. M., & Hahlweg, K. (1986). The marriages and interaction patterns of depressed patients and their spouses. Comparing high and low EE dyads. In M. J. Goldstein, I. Hand, & K. Hahlweg (Eds.), *Treatment of schizophrenia: Family assessment and intervention.* Berlin: Springer-Verlag.

Hooley, J. M., Orley, J., & Teasdale, J. T. (1986). Levels of expressed emotion and relapse in depressed patients. *British Journal of Psychiatry, 148*, 642-647.

Kessler, K. A. (1978). Tricyclic antidepressants: Mode of action and clinical use. In M. A. Lipton, A. DiMascio, & K. F. Killam (Eds.), *Psychopharmacology: A generation of progress.* New York: Raven Press.

Klein, M. (1948). *Contributions to psychoanalysis, 1921-1945.* London: Hogarth Press.

Lewinsohn, P. M., Biglan, A., & Zeiss, A. M. (1975). Behavioral treatment of depression. In P. O. Davidson (Ed.), *The behavioral management of anxiety, depression and pain.* New York: Brunner/Mazel.

Lewinsohn, P. M., Weinstein, M. S., & Shaw, D. A. (1969). Depression: A clinical research approach. In R. Rubin & C. M. Franks (Eds.), *Advances in behavior therapy.* New York: Academic Press.

Lewis, A. (1934). Melancholia: Clinical survey of depressive states. *Journal of Mental Science, 80*, 277-378.

Liberman, R. P., & Raskin, D. E. (1971). Depression: A behavioral formulation. *Archives of General Psychiatry, 24*, 515-523.

Marks, I. M. (1976). The current status of behavioral psychotherapy: Theory and practice. *American Journal of Psychiatry, 133*, 253-261.

Miklowitz, D. J., Goldstein, M. J., Nuechterlein, K. H., Snyder, K. S., & Doane, J. A. (1986). Expressed emotion, affective style, lithium compliance and relapse in recent-onset mania. *Psychopharmacology Bulletin, 22*, 628-632.

Seligman, M. E. P. (1975). *Helplessness: On depression, development, and death.* San Francisco: W. H. Freeman.

Vaughn, C. E., & Leff, J. P. (1976). The influence of family and social factors on the course of psychiatric illness: A comparison of schizophrenic and depressed neurotic patients. *British Journal of Psychiatry, 129*, 125-137.

6

Inpatient Family Intervention

JOHN F. CLARKIN
GRETCHEN L. HAAS
IRA D. GLICK

Two major hallmarks of state-of-the-art psychotherapy research are the definition of a model of the target disorder/pathology and the use of a manualized therapy that attempts to alter the specifics of the condition. In the study reported here, we constructed an inpatient family intervention package focused on two specific aspects of a particular psychiatric population: the occasion of hospitalization of a family member, and family education and coping with a specific disorder, namely, an affective disorder.

Surprisingly, the utilization of family intervention in inpatient settings has expanded exponentially, although controlled clinical research in this area is almost nonexistent. Until now, there had been no single controlled study of family intervention on an inpatient service. Influenced by the prior research on outpatient family intervention with schizophrenics and affectively disordered patients as well as by our own clinical observations, we decided to implement the study of a manualized family intervention for affective disorders. Our approach was most influenced by the specific, practical family intervention utilized with schizophrenics and their families on an outpatient basis by Goldstein and colleagues (Goldstein, Rodnick, Evans, May, & Steinberg, 1978).

Hospitalization of a family member is a crucial event in many ways. The family is in distress and can use assistance in coping with the stressful situation. A hospitalization dramatizes the severity of the mental disorder in the identified patient, thus potentially eroding any existing denial around the difficulty. As a corollary, faced with the severity of the condition, the family is potentially open to treatment in a new way. Contact with members of the mental health profession during the hospitalization enables the family and the patient to form what may be lasting impressions of the nature of the disorder, of mental health professionals and how they work, and of how helpful treatment can be, and expectations regarding the possible benefits of such assistance in the future.

The development of our brief family intervention was informed by the nature of affective disorders in several ways. It was designed to provide information to the patient and the family—information specific to the type of disorder (i.e., bipolar or unipolar). As the literature on affective disorders suggests, these families often have marital and family conflict that would make the task of coping with the patient's illness more difficult. Depressed patients feel particularly vulnerable to family and marital stressors, and marital friction is the most common event reported during the 6 months prior to the onset of depressive symptoms (Paykel *et al.*, 1969). Marital and family conflict is high in both depressive (e.g., Weissman & Paykel, 1974) and bipolar (Davenport & Adland, Chapter 8, this volume) samples. In addition, there is often the complicating influence of chronic personality disorders among the affectively ill. In one study, it was noted that the prevalence rate of personality disorder was 23% among bipolar patients and 37% to 53% among depressed patients (Charney, Nelson, & Quinlan, 1981).

The literature on expressed emotion (EE) clearly indicates that the family can have significant impact on the course of schizophrenic and affective illness (e.g., Vaughn, Snyder, Jones, Freeman, & Falloon, 1984). Moreover, research on family treatments for schizophrenia has shown that certain deleterious family factors (hostility, overinvolvement) can be changed with family intervention, thereby improving the course of recovery (Falloon *et al.*, 1982; Leff, Kuipers, Berkowitz, Eberlein-Vries, & Sturgeon, 1982). The literature on EE and affective illness is less extensive but growing. What data there are (Hooley, 1986) suggest that among those depressed patients who are married, those with high EE spouses show a pattern of hostile and non-self-disclosing communication.

SPECIFIC HYPOTHESES OF OUR STUDY

Given the association between family environmental stress and affective disorder, coupled with the growing evidence that family intervention can be helpful in the course of a major psychiatric condition such as schizophrenia, we hypothesized that a brief inpatient family intervention (IFI) would be clinically useful for serious affective disorders. Hypotheses were formulated concerning the mechanism of action and the role of specific mediating and final goals of intervention as outlined in Figure 6.1. The accomplishment of the specific targeted treatment goals of IFI was expected to lead to improved family attitudes toward the patient and toward the use of mental health services in the future. In addition, it was hypothesized that positive family attitudes toward treatment would promote (be associated with) patient compliance with aftercare treatment—both pharmacological and psychosocial. Furthermore, we hypothesized that successful achievement of

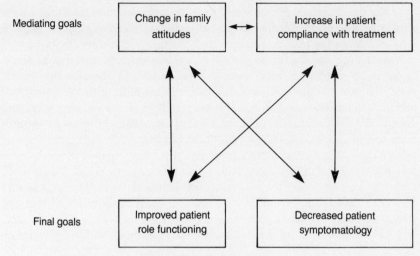

Figure 6.1. Goals of IFI.

these *mediating* goals of IFI would be instrumental in achieving the *final* goals: improved patient role functioning and decreased symptomatology.

It should be emphasized that our goals for IFI were quite modest, since we were using a brief family intervention, limited to the hospitalization phase, with no control over outpatient follow-up. In addition, we were dealing with patients whose affective pathology was in the most severe range, severe enough to occasion a psychiatric hospitalization. This affective pathology was probably caused in varying degrees by biological factors not under the direct influence of family intervention.

PATIENTS AND THEIR FAMILIES

Subjects in this investigation were 50 patients with DSM-III major affective disorders who were consecutively admitted to the hospital and screened for admission to the study using the following criteria: (1) recent admission (within 1 week of admission to the unit), (2) a minimum age of 18, (3) availability of family or significant others for family intervention, and (4) an anticipated length of stay sufficient for a minimum of six sessions of family intervention.

As a group, the 21 bipolar patients were predominantly white (81%) and female (67%). The mean age was 32, and two thirds of the cases were between the ages of 18 and 47. Marital status was quite varied, with 48% single, 43% married, and 9% divorced, separated, or widowed. Of these 21 patients, 48% had no previous hospitalizations, and 33% had no previous episodes of illness. There was a more seriously ill subgroup (14%) with three or more previous hospitalizations, and 19% with three or more previous bipolar episodes.

The 29 unipolar patients were predominantly white (62%), with almost equal distribution of males (45%) and females (55%). The mean age was 38, with two thirds of the patients between the ages of 26 and 50. In terms of marital status, 48% of the patients were single, 31% married, and 21% divorced or separated. A total of 62% of the patients had no previous hospitalizations, and 48% had no previous episodes. In contrast, 14% had experienced three or more previous hospitalizations and three or more previous episodes.

TREATMENT ASSIGNMENT

Within the first week of admission to the hospital, all patients (and families) who satisfied the selection criteria and consented to participate in the study were randomly assigned to one of two treatment conditions: multimodal hospital treatment *with* IFI or multimodal hospital treatment *without* IFI (the "comparison treatment" condition).

Of the 21 bipolar patients, 12 received IFI and 9 received the comparison treatment. Among the 29 unipolar patients, 17 were randomized to IFI and 12 received comparison treatment.

The standard hospital treatment included medication when indicated, individual sessions with a primary therapist, and group and milieu treatment.

DESCRIPTION OF IFI

Inpatient family intervention is a brief psychoeducational and problem-focused family treatment structured to assist the patient and his or her family in coping with the patient's hospitalization. We will describe here some of the assumptions, goals, and strategies of this intervention.

We call our approach "family intervention" rather than "family therapy" because the latter term has some connotations that are not applicable to work in an inpatient setting. In family therapy, it is usually assumed that the "patient" is the family, and that the problem does not reside in one individual but in the interaction patterns of the family as an interpersonal system. Family therapy theorists place a strong emphasis on "circular causality," that is, the hypothesis that the repetitive interactions among individuals in the family group cause and reinforce the psychiatric problems that come to our attention. Although there may be many problems that can be viewed usefully from this perspective, we suspect that severe affective psychopathology that requires psychiatric hospitalization cannot be so explained *in toto*.

WORKING MODEL OF AFFECTIVE DISORDERS

Our first basic assumption is that *the affective episode is not caused solely by family environment or family communication problems.* We operate with the understanding that although greatly influenced by psychosocial factors, these disorders are partly biological in nature. Thus we do not assume that the manic or depressive symptoms are under total control of the repetitive family interaction patterns. Furthermore, it is quite misleading, we believe, to infer that the family interaction patterns seen at the time of the hospitalization are typical or that such patterns of interaction caused or even maintained the symptomatic behavior in the identified patient. We operate with the view that the family is doing what it perceives as necessary for coping with the situation. This assumption assists the clinician in establishing an alliance with the family by reducing attitudes of blame toward them.

Second, *we assume that psychoeducation, that is, the provision of information about the affective disorder, will enable the family to use its own strengths in coping with the condition.* It is often the case that the information provided is not readily accepted or digested by the family. Rather, the process of providing information itself can be instrumental in building a therapeutic alliance with the family and in working through basic maladaptive attitudes toward the disturbed family member. This process can also promote more effective utilization of the mental health treatment system.

Third, *we assume that the crisis period of hospitalization is not the time to discuss at length, or to rehash, long-standing family and marital conflicts.* Such conflicts may or may not be related to the affective episode, and therefore focusing on these is not a first priority. The timing and sequencing of intervention is most important here. The first task is for the clinician to assume an active role in directing the dialogue so that the family does not become distracted by intense emotional turmoil or attend to long-standing family conflict or blame for the patient's episode. The task is to deal with the issues and matters at hand. This entails asking (and discussing) several key questions: What immediate crises might have preceded the hospitalization? What is the nature and prognosis of the affective disorder, and what treatment will be needed upon discharge from the hospital?

TREATMENT GOALS AND
THERAPEUTIC STRATEGIES OF IFI

Six immediate treatment goals define and guide delivery of IFI: (1) helping the patient and family to accept the reality of the affective disorder and to develop an understanding of the current episode, (2) identifying possible precipitating stresses relevant to the current episode, (3) identifying likely future stresses both within and outside the family, (4) elucidating the family interaction sequences that produce stress on the identified patient, (5) planning strategies to manage or minimize future stresses, and (6) educating the patient and family regarding the nature of the treatment and the need for continued treatment following discharge from the hospital.

The six goals of IFI were to be pursued differentially (in varying degrees of emphasis or not at all), depending upon the existing problems and needs of each family case. The family therapist and the supervisor set the goals for the case at the beginning, and at discharge the family therapist rated the extent to which each goal was achieved.

Based upon the goals of IFI, we delineated strategies and techniques to assist the therapists in achieving these goals. In general, the strategies involve psychoeducation, task-oriented interventions, and problem solving, with little emphasis on psychodynamic or structural family therapy strategies. These latter strategies were seen as too invasive for a brief intervention in the context of hospitalization for a severely debilitating disorder.

ASSESSMENT PROCEDURES

Table 6.1 outlines the goals of family intervention and the instruments utilized to measure them. The extent of accomplishment of the treatment goals of IFI was rated by the family clinician at the completion of family intervention (time of hospital discharge). Family attitudes were measured by the Family Attitude Scale (FAS), a 53-item self-report scale filled out by a significant family member. The scale measures family attitudes toward the patient, willingness to accept professional help, emotional involvement with the patient, perceived family disruption and burden caused by the patient, and family reliance upon social support. (For further description of this scale, see Chapter 2, this volume.) The final mediating goal, patient compliance with aftercare treatment, was measured by a section of the Role

Table 6.1. Assessment of the Goals of IFI

Targeted domain	Instruments	Assessor
Rating at discharge of family's treatment absorption	Family goals in IFI	Family clinician
Clinical ratings of patient status and role functioning	Role Performance and Treatment Scale Global Assessment Scale Psychiatric Evaluation Form	Independent assessor
Family attitudes toward patient and treatment	Family Attitude Scale	Family member

Performance and Treatment Scale (RPTS) that assesses patient compliance with treatment following discharge from the hospital.

The final goals of IFI were improved patient role functioning and a decrease in symptomatology. Role functioning was measured by a composite score derived from items on the Psychiatric Evaluation Form (PEF) and the RPTS. Symptomatology was assessed by a composite score from the Global Assessment Scale (GAS) and the PEF.

Patients and families were assessed at four times: on admission, at discharge, and at 6- and 18-month follow-ups.

RESULTS

Following an average hospital stay of 47.5 days ($SD = 27.7$), results at discharge showed differential effectiveness of IFI, with a positive treatment effect specific to female patients with an affective disorder.

Final Goals and Outcome of IFI

Global Functioning and Symptoms

For the entire group of 50 patients (combining both unipolar and bipolar patients), there were no main (overall) effects of treatment on a composite measure of patient global functioning and symptomatology. However, at 6 months, there was a trend for an interaction effect of treatment and diagnostic subtype ($p < .09$); this reached a level of significance ($p < .05$) at 18 months. Inspection of the mean (average) scores indicated that for bipolars, there was better outcome with IFI, whereas for unipolars, there was better outcome with the comparison treatment.

Role Functioning

Similarly, on a composite measure of patient role functioning, there was no main effect of treatment. Again, there was a significant interaction of treatment with affective disorder subtype at both the 6-month ($p < .02$) and the 18-month follow-up ($p < .001$). Again, the bipolar patients did better with the IFI, and the unipolar patients did better with the comparison treatment.

Mediating Goals of IFI

On the family attitude composite scores, there were no main effects of treatment at either 6 or 18 months. However, there was a treatment-by-subdiagnosis interaction effect on one of the two family composite measures at 6 months—attitude toward the patient/family burden. Families of bipolars treated with IFI showed more positive attitudes and less family burden than did their counterparts treated in the comparison group. Among the unipolar families, the reverse effect was found (consistent with the results for patients)—families treated with the comparison treatment showed more positive attitudes and less burden than did families treated with IFI.

Relationship of Mediating and Final Goals of IFI

For affectively disordered patients treated with IFI, follow-up data revealed a significant positive correlation between overall achievement of the treatment goals of IFI (as rated by the family clinician at discharge) and patient outcome on the global functioning–symptomatology composite measure at 6 months ($r = .39; p < .03$) and the role-functioning composite measure at 18 months ($r = .35; p < .05$).

For the bipolar patients, the ratings of overall achievement of IFI treatment goals correlated significantly with patient outcome on the composite measure of global functioning and symptomatology at 6 months ($r = .60; p < .04$).

For the unipolar patients, ratings of achievement of the treatment goals of IFI did not correlate significantly with patient outcome or family attitudes at either 6- or 18-month follow-ups.

It was also hypothesized that the achievement of the IFI treatment goal of increasing family support for patient posthospitalization treatment compliance would correlate with the patient's actual compliance with posthospitalization treatments. Results supported this hypothesis, indicating a significant positive correlation between achievement of IFI Goal 6 (family support of patient compliance) and follow-up ratings of patient compliance (medication and psychosocial treatments) at 6 months ($r = .60; p < .004$), and a trend for a correlation with medication compliance at 18 months ($r = .34; p < .10$). This correlation was strongest for bipolar patients and their families on a measure of overall treatment compliance at 6 months ($r = .78; p < .006$), a relationship that attenuated at 18 months ($r = .49; p < .09$) and was accompanied by a trend for a correlation with medication compliance ($r = .52; p < .09$) at 18 months. For the unipolar patients and their families, the correlation between achievement of IFI Goal 6 and patient treatment compliance was less strong and less stable, showing a trend ($r = .55; p < .06$) at 6 months.

Treatment Goals of IFI for Bipolar and Unipolar Disorders

Given the differential effectiveness of IFI for bipolars (as compared with unipolars), one might wonder whether the immediate treatment goals of IFI were different for the two affective disorder subgroups. To assess this possibility, we compared goals set for unipolar and bipolar IFI patients with the overall rating of goals achieved as assessed by the family clinician. The relative emphasis placed on the six goals of IFI was essentially the same for the two diagnostic subgroups. In terms of the overall rating of achievement of goals, the bipolar and unipolar IFI groups were not rated significantly differently. In addition, in the judgment of the family clinician involved, the overall ratings of achievement of the family goals were essentially equivalent for the two diagnostic subgroups. On a 5-point rating scale, the bipolar group had a mean rating of 2.69, and the unipolar group, of 2.58. Thus it would appear that differences in outcome at follow-up could not be attributed to differences in either targeting the goals of treatment or achieving these goals as assessed at discharge.

ILLUSTRATIVE CASES

To provide a rich description of the clinical situation for the reader, we have selected to discuss one unipolar and two bipolar cases from the study. To make the cases somewhat representative of the aggregate results as described we have selected two good outcome bipolar cases treated with IFI and a good outcome unipolar case treated without IFI.

CASE EXAMPLE:
BIPOLAR DISORDER TREATED WITH IFI

Mr. M, a 35-year-old married claims adjuster, was functioning well until 10 days prior to his admission to the hospital, when he was informed by his employer that he would be temporarily rotated to another center, which would require a longer commute. He quickly became quite angry and upset about this change and began to think that his supervisors were out to get him. This was the beginning of a number of sleepless nights, during which he would think of ways to "get even." He began to experience an extreme oscillation of moods from crying periods to highs. During the highs, his speech was pressured, he wrote down many ideas, and he called old friends with whom he had not spoken for years. He began to abuse Quaaludes. He complained of tightness in his testicles and had thoughts of mutilating his genitalia. On the day prior to admission, he had to leave work because of uncontrollable shaking. He came to the psychiatric clinic for evaluation on the advice of friends and relatives and was admitted with a diagnosis of bipolar disorder.

Mr. M was a college graduate and a veteran of the Vietnam War. His parents lived many states away. The patient and his spouse of some 8 years lived next door to her parents, with whom they got along well. Mr. M was described by himself and his wife as a meticulous person, always concerned about procedure being carried out "by the book." At times, he experienced some difficulty in dealing with authority figures, questioning their motives and judgment.

The patient was immediately placed on chlorpromazine, and by the second night of hospitalization, he was sleeping more regularly. He was assigned (at random) to IFI. By the third hospital day, his appetite was improved, and he began to show some perspective on his recent bizarre thoughts and behavior. Four days after admission, he was placed on lithium carbonate, the chlorpromazine was reduced, and his mood stabilized and thought disorder disappeared. The IFI sessions were held (seven in all) with patient and spouse and focused on support for the wife during the hospitalization, assessing precipitating stress on the couple, education about the affective disorder, support for aftercare, and assessment of the marital relationship. The couple responded well to the IFI goals and intervention, and at discharge the therapist rated the overall success of these family meetings at "3" (out of a maximum possible "4").

On admission to the hospital, Mr. M had a GAS score of 32, with severe or extreme ratings of speech disorganization, hallucinations, suspicion–persecution, disruption of daily routine and leisure time, and denial of illness on the PEF. Upon discharge 28 days later, his GAS score was 60, with only a moderate rating of agitation and excitement on the PEF. He was discharged to his home, with follow-up medication treatment at a clinic in his area. He did not feel he could afford a private therapist.

At the 6-month follow-up, the patient had a GAS score of 69. He was working full time at the job he had held prior to hospitalization. He reported doing better in setting limits with clients on the job, and though he still had some hostile feelings toward authority figures, they were well modulated. He noted a continuing difficulty in separating himself from the job, and several weeks ago had felt upset and depressed for several days, but this passed. He was happy in his marital relationship and took his medication faithfully, with support for this from his wife.

At the 18-month follow-up, the patient received a GAS score of 70. He was working successfully at the same job, residing with his wife, and actively pursuing hobbies and a social life. He had continued his lithium treatment until 1 month prior to the 18-month follow-up, at which time he decided, against his wife's wishes, to quit the medication and cancel the appointments with his physician. He had become somewhat hypomanic and grandiose, but he denied any major problems.

From prehospitalization through follow-up, this patient's marital status (married) and living situation (with wife) remained stable. His primary role functioning went from an initial negative change (full-time work prior to hospitalization but only part-time functioning at the 6-month follow-up) to a more positive adjustment at the 18-month follow-up.

Mrs. M completed the FAS at admission, at discharge, and at 6 and 18 months. From admission and throughout follow-up, Mrs. M had a positive attitude toward treatment, with an openness to social support. Also during this period, her attitude toward the patient was one of acceptance, with little sense of burden from her husband.

This was a sudden-onset, stress-related bipolar episode that was successfully treated with hospitalization and medication. The patient's marital relationship was good prior to the episode, and his wife was quite supportive of both the patient and his continuing need for medication treatment following hospitalization. The IFI seemed to fit into the context of this supportive relationship and probably enhanced the wife's resolve that her husband continue with treatment.

CASE EXAMPLE: BIPOLAR DISORDER TREATED WITH IFI

This was the third psychiatric hospitalization for a 27-year-old single white female who lived with her mother and two younger sisters. Two months prior to admission, the patient began therapy at a low-cost clinic, was placed on medication, and began working part time as a receptionist–administrator at a retirement home. Two weeks prior to admission, the patient's antidepressant medication was decreased by the clinic and subsequently decreased further by the patient because she felt "elated." The patient began to be irrtitable at home, arguing with her mother and sisters, shopping a lot, getting little sleep, pacing, and talking and laughing to herself. She was brought to the clinic by her mother and a sister who felt they could not control her hypomanic symptoms. She was admitted with a diagnosis of bipolar disorder, manic, with mood congruent psychotic features, plus concomitant alcohol and marijuana abuse.

The patient's father was a heavy drinker (probably an alcoholic) who abandoned the family when the patient was 7 years old. She was a good student through high school. During college years, the patient had a history of drug abuse (heavy marijuana abuse, occasional use of LSD, and use of Quaaludes), moved to three different colleges, and repeatedly became envolved in triangles in which she would vie against another woman for a man's attention and end up isolated and alienated. Five years ago, the mother developed malignant melanoma, and the patient and her sisters left school and went to work in order to support the family. At one point, the patient was managing five different carpet stores. During the past several years, however, her general level of adjustment and work functioning had noticeably decreased. She fell in love with a male friend and proposed marriage to him, even though they had never dated. He rejected her proposal, but for the following 2 years, she obsessively talked of him as if he were going to marry her. At the same time, she became preoccupied with learning about her absent father.

The patient was assigned (at random) to IFI, and there were seven sessions during the hospitalization, all including the mother and one including the two sisters. The focus of IFI was on the relationship between the mother and the patient, the enlistment of family support against the patient's drug abuse, discussion about the mother's illness, and discharge planning.

On admission to the inpatient service, the patient was rated as 33 on the GAS, with "moderate" to "severe" ratings on the PEF on measures of agitation–excitement, belligerence–negativism, denial of illness, and overall severity of illness. Upon discharge, she had a GAS rating of 60.

At the 6-month follow-up assessment, the patient was rated 64 on the GAS, with no symptoms on the PEF beyond the mild range. She had been in a day hospital treatment program throughout most of the follow-up period and was in total compliance with her medication regime. Family treatment occurred once per week with a psychologist at a local clinic. Her mother's illness had progressed, and the patient had taken major responsibility for household chores. She was doing clerical work part time, and managing this successfully. She had dated several men, one regularly, and she had not let any of these relationships get "too serious."

At the 18-month follow-up, the patient received a GAS score of 70, with only mild ratings of agitation–excitement and anxiety on the PEF. She was not abusing alcohol or drugs. She was working full time in an administrative position in a retirement home, and was doing so well she had received a promotion. She was the major homemaker and was handling this well. She continued to comply with her medication regime. Most important, the patient was doing all of this despite the death of her mother several months earlier, the mother toward whom she had felt so attached and dependent. She felt she was still grieving for her mother, and at times felt mildly depressed and guilty. She felt the most pressure from the relationship with her boyfriend, since he was, she said, then pressuring her to marry him.

From prehospitalization through follow-up, this patient's marital status (single) and living situation (with her mother) remained the same over most of this interval. Her primary role functioning improved as she went from part-time work (prehospitalization) to full-time employment by the time of the last follow-up.

On the FAS, the mother and sister indicated an above-average positive attitude toward treatment and openness to social support from admission on to discharge and follow-up. In contrast, the family was below average in their attitude toward the patient and felt much burden at admission and discharge. At the follow-up periods, this attitude toward the patient had reversed.

An interesting sidelight of this case is that the patient can serve as her own "control," contrasting the two previous hospitalizations and their follow-ups with the hospitalization and its aftermath in which she received IFI. After her first hospitalization at age 26, she was discharged with decreased symptoms and referred to individual therapy. She was then readmitted within 5 days, with a resurgence of psychotic thinking and extreme anxiety. She did take her medications upon discharge, but admitted lying about the seriousness of her symptoms upon first discharge. In addition, she was very upset over an appointment mix-up with her new individual therapist in which she could see her for only a few minutes. The mother brought her back to the clinic with complaints of suicidal ideation, and the patient was readmitted to the hospital.

This story is in sharp contrast to the postdischarge process after the target hospitalization some 1 year and 4 months later. during this later hospitalization, the patient, mother, and sisters laid a careful foundation for her discharge, including plans for day hospital treatment and medication. The family's support for a stand against drug and alcohol abuse was also elicited.

It would appear that the IFI treatment was successful in countering the patient's (and possibly the family's) denial of the illness and its seriousness. By focusing on the illness and needed treatment, the patient was successfully inducted into follow-up care that involved medication, day hospital treatment, and then medication only. It may well be that one of the reasons that IFI was apparently successful in countering any denial of illness when it did was because of the prior treatment avoidances and subsequent illness episodes.

CASE EXAMPLE: UNIPOLAR DISORDER TREATED WITHOUT IFI

Mrs. A, a 72-year-old white married woman, was brought to the emergency room by her husband of 46 years because she "won't do anything." During the prior 3 weeks, the patient had begun complaining of weakness and headaches, and had refused to do her usual household chores. In addition, she began to "talk nonsense," in her husband's words, and to complain that her family was against her and that she was making the family sick. Her appetite decreased, she could not concentrate or read, and she occasionally became tearful. She had not expressed suicidal ideation, but at times seemed convinced that she was dead and buried. She was diagnosed as having major affective disorder, depressed type, with no Axis II disorder.

The elderly couple had three daughters, one of whom currently lived with them. There had been no family history of major psychiatric disorder. Prior to the illness episode, the patient, as described by her retired husband had been a cheerful woman whose major focus in life was her family and who typically was concerned about others but was shy and somewhat avoidant of contacts with those outside the family. This patient had had one prior episode of depression at the age of 60, and this was successfully treated with medication.

This patient was randomly assigned to the comparison treatment condition (standard hospital treatment without IFI). After a neurology consultation that revealed no signs of any neurological disorder, the patient was started on a course of six ECT treatments. She responded with dramatic improvement in affect and resolution of psychotic symptoms. Following hospitalization for 35 days, she was discharged to an outpatient psychiatrist, who saw her for medication and support.

On admission to the hospital, Mrs. A had a GAS score of 31, indicating a poor level of overall functioning requiring hospitalization. On the PEF, she was rated as having severe symptoms of agitation, social isolation, belligerence and negativism, and depression, with severe disruption in daily routine. At the time of discharge, some 35 days later, the patient had a GAS score of 75, indicating that she was functioning extremely well and had few obvious symptoms.

At the time of our 6-month follow-up, she had a GAS score of 80 and was complying with follow-up care with a psychiatrist (three visits, with a final one planned). Since discharge, she not only had handled her usual household chores but also had nursed her husband during his 2-month recovery from abdominal surgery. She had resumed her involvement with the family, including visits with daughters who lived nearby. Husband and wife noted that family relations were supportive, and our rater noted that the family reported no identifiable difficulties. At the 18-month follow-up, the patient had a GAS score of 85.

From prehospitalization through the follow-up period, this patient's marital status (married), living situation (with her husband), and primary role functioning remained consistent.

At admission, at discharge, and at 6 months, the patient's spouse had a below-average attitude toward treatment and openness to social support. It was only at 18 months that this attitude became more positive. In his attitude toward the patient, the husband felt a sense of burden at admission, but by discharge and throughout follow-up, he had an above-average positive attitude toward the patient.

In retrospect, this appears to be a case of sudden-onset depression in which biological factors were probably most prominent. The patient had no concomitant personality disorder. The treatment was predominantly biological, and the depressive episode was interrupted and abbreviated with this intervention. The patient returned to a relatively conflict-free and supportive family environment in which husband and daughter lived normal lives.

Also in retrospect, there would appear to have been little need for family intervention. The husband in no way blamed his wife for her condition and saw it as an atypical situation that needed psychiatric intervention. One even gets the impression that psychoeducation about depressive illness was not much needed here. Both husband and wife saw the need for both the hospitalization and the aftercare, and she complied with all treatments. It should be noted, however, that at the time of admission, it is not always clear that a family like this one will be so conflict free and cooperative with treatment. Recall, for example, that this patient came into the hospital saying that her family was against her, and that the husband reported on the FAS that she was a burden. In this case, it was part of a psychotic thinking process. In some cases, however, such symptoms reflect prolonged family conflict.

This case is somewhat unrepresentative because of the advanced age of the affectively disordered patient. We do not have enough data in each of the age ranges to ascertain the effects of age. There is some growing evidence to suggest that late-onset depressions may be more heavily influenced by biological processes (Stoudemire & Blazer, 1985). How this factor might affect the need for family intervention is not clear.

We have the clinical impression, buttressed somewhat by the research results showing that comparison unipolar patients did better without IFI, that in some cases family intervention may actually be disruptive for patients and their families, at least during an illness episode. For example, in this particular case, though it is hard to see how family psychoeducation could have been harmful, questioning the family at length about possible long-standing family conflict, implying that it precipitated the current depressive episode, might have been detrimental.

DISCUSSION OF RESULTS

Inpatient family intervention is a brief intervention with a major focus on psychoeducation for the patient and family who are coping with a diagnosed psychiatric condition. It was anticipated that with affectively disordered patients and their families, IFI would enable family members to decrease their sense of burden in coping with the disorder and would improve their attitudes toward follow-up care for the patient following discharge from the hospital. It was hypothesized that with the accomplishment of these mediating goals of IFI, the patient would have a better outcome, both in terms of fewer and less severe symptoms and in terms of improved role functioning, in the context of better compliance with posthospitalization treatment.

At the point of discharge from the index hospitalization, affectively disordered patients and their families who were treated with IFI were significantly better than patients and families who received a comparison treatment. This positive effect was almost totally accounted for by the improvement of the female patients with affective disorders.

This positive effect on affectively disordered patients without regard to subdiagnosis did not continue into the 6- and 18-month follow-up periods. However, when the results of IFI at follow-up were examined with regard to subdiagnoses, some important differences appeared.

There is evidence in our study that both the mediating and the final goals of IFI were accomplished with the bipolar patients and their families. Bipolar IFI families showed a significantly improved attitude toward the patient and a lowered sense of burden in coping with the illness. Likewise, the final goals of IFI were achieved with the bipolar IFI patients, since they showed significantly reduced symptoms and improved role functioning at follow-up as compared with the non-IFI bipolar patients. In addition, a correlational link was made between the achievement of the mediating goals of IFI and the final goals of patient outcome. Most specifically, there was a significant positive correlation between achieving the goal of improving family attitudes toward treatment compliance during IFI and subsequent treatment compliance by bipolar IFI patients. This linkage of the mediating goals of IFI with the final goals of patient outcome is only correlational and does not prove causality, but it is suggestive and in the hypothesized direction.

In an unexpected but rather interesting contrast, IFI was not effective in achieving either mediating or final goals with the unipolar patients and their families. It was not effective in enhancing family attitudes toward the patient and the burden of illness on a composite score. The achievement of the IFI goals did not correlate with patient outcome or family attitudes on follow-up. And finally, in terms of the final goals of IFI treatment, patients in the comparison group were significantly better on measures of symptomatology and role functioning than were unipolar IFI patients.

Both the success of IFI and the link between the mediating and the final goals of IFI treatment with the bipolar group are encouraging. In contrast, the apparent failure of IFI treatment with the unipolar group is puzzling. There may be something about the unipolar disorder itself that is not being addressed in IFI. On the other hand, rather than the affective disorder diagnosis, there could be important variables correlated with affective disorder subdiagnosis that are interacting with the treatment variable and that could otherwise account for the differential outcome. If so, however, the data in this study are not helpful in clarifying these findings. The bipolar and unipolar groups were not significantly different at baseline on such potentially important variables as socioeconomic status, prior functioning, indices of severity of illness, incidence of severe personality disorder, history of prior treatment compliance, and treatment compliance following hospitalization.

Alternatively, it could be argued that although the general goals of IFI are equally appropriate for both bipolar and unipolar patients, it may have been that in this study the goals were somewhat differentially applied to each of the two diagnostic subgroups, since the clinician determined at her discretion the differential application and weight of the six goals of IFI, depending upon the specifics of the individual patient and family. We assessed this possibility and found that the relative emphasis on each of the goals was roughly equivalent for bipolar and unipolar patients and their families. Also significant was the finding that achievement of the goals—as rated by the family clinicians—was equivalent for the two diagnostic subgroups.

Is IFI efficacious for affectively disordered patients and their families? Our results suggest that this question cannot be answered without reference to the specific subdiagnosis (bipolar or unipolar) of major affective disorder. These results suggest that a brief psychoeducational and problem-solving form of family intervention during hospitalization *is* effective with bipolar disordered patients and their families. In contrast, unipolar patients did significantly better without IFI than with it. The efficacy of IFI for this diagnostic group has not been demonstrated, and there is a need for replication of results for the bipolar patients before firm conclusions can be drawn from this study.

GUIDELINES FOR FUTURE RESEARCH

We hope that the study reported here will lead to further refinements in research on family treatments for affective disorders. In an effort to guide future research efforts, we will briefly discuss problems in the design of our study and methods for improving the design for use in future research studies.

1. *Monitoring of therapeutic intervention.* In this study, we were not able to videotape the entire sample of therapy sessions. This would have been helpful in terms of ensuring both consistency and competency in the delivery of the treatment. We are impressed with the recent literature that suggests substantial variance among individual therapists (e.g., Luborsky *et al.*, 1986) and deficient skills and/or decreased competence on the part of therapists when faced with patients (and, probably more so, families) who are hostile toward the therapist or the therapy itself.

2. *Timing of the family intervention.* We are impressed with clinical accounts suggesting that overstimulation, perhaps as occurs during family sessions in the acute phase of an illness, can be detrimental to patients with serious mental disorders like schizophrenia (see Heinrichs & Carpenter, 1983). We suspect that the same principle applies with other serious Axis I conditions, as, for example, the major affective disorders. In families with a member having a major affective disorder *and* notable family conflict, the issue of *timing* the family intervention around a series of extraillness family issues is extremely important. We have the suspicion, but few data to back it

up, that some families with a unipolar patient did better without IFI *precisely because when the IFI was used, it allowed conflictful material to surface too soon*—before the patient was sufficiently recovered and able to benefit from such intervention.

3. *Assessment of the impact of IFI on the family.* It seems clear that assessment of the progress toward achieving mediating goals of family intervention is, at present, problematic and lacking any well-defined and valid methodology. The typical mediating goals of most family interventions involve some change in family interaction patterns related to problematic or symptomatic situations (e.g., parental reactions to depressive withdrawal). In this study, the identification and measurement of mediating goals included assessment of key family members' attitudes toward the patient, the illness, the family's burden in coping with the illness, and the need for further treatment. We have no direct evidence that these attitudes correlate with key behaviors within or outside of the treatment context. In addition, there are probably other key behaviors of family members that significantly influence the patient and his or her progress—behavioral dimensions that we did not measure in this study. In the future, studies of actual patient family interactions may assist us in both targeting intervention and measuring pretreatment-to-posttreatment changes.

4. *Heterogeneity of the patient sample.* Finally, we are impressed with the heterogeneity of the patients who meet DSM-III criteria for a major affective disorder. To assume that one has a homogeneous sample of patients (and families) by virtue of selection by diagnostic criteria alone is to take a superficial and shortsighted view of the patient and his or her family as well as the complexities of the interaction of patient, family, and therapist. Other important variables may influence or modify patient and family outcome; these include prior treatment compliance, sex of the identified patient, sex of therapist, socioeconomic status, religion, and race. Furthermore, there are probably other suspected and unknown variables that influence receptivity and response to IFI. One of the possibly important, but insufficiently studied, variables is the Axis II personality diagnosis of the identified patient. Unfortunately, we did not have a reliable diagnosis of the Axis II pathology for the patients included in this study. Prior research suggests that an affective disorder group would have a substantial number of individuals with coexisting personality pathology. It is our impression that personality disorders of both the patient and family members heavily influenced the receptivity to, and the issues raised by, the IFI sessions, although these disorders were not directly assessed using measures designed to tap personality *per se.*

5. *The addition of an outpatient treatment phase to IFI.* One can only wonder what would have happened if we could have followed up IFI with some *outpatient* family sessions. In this study, we did not include posthospitalization follow-up therapy sessions, primarily because we were interested

in evaluating the specific effects of an *important* family treatment. Future studies should assess the impact of postdischarge "booster" family intervention sessions that build on a positive response to family work during the inpatient phase and follow through on work that requires a more extended period of time. In the future, it may be possible to differentiate between families needing no further postdischarge intervention and those needing further family intervention because of such factors as family denial of illness or long-standing conflict and lack of support for the patient. The next step in systematic research on IFI would be to test the incremental benefits of continuing such treatment into the posthospitalization recovery phase.

REFERENCES

Charney, D. S., Nelson, C. J., & Quinlan, D. M. (1981). Personality traits and disorder in depression. *American Journal of Psychiatry, 138,* 1601–1604.

Falloon, I. R. H., Boyd, J. L., McGill, C. W., Razani, J., Moss, H., & Gilderman, A. (1982). Family management in the prevention of exacerbations of schizophrenia: A controlled study. *New England Journal of Medicine, 306,* 1437–1440.

Goldstein, M. J., Rodnick, E. H., Evans, J. R., May, P. R. A., & Steinberg, M. R. (1978). Drug and family therapy in the aftercare treatment of acute schizophrenics. *Archives of General Psychiatry, 35,* 1169–1177.

Heinrichs, D., & Carpenter, W. (1983). The coordination of family therapy with other treatment modalities for schizophrenia. In W. McFarlane (Ed.), *Family therapy in schizophrenia* (pp. 267–288). New York: Guilford Press.

Hooley, J. M. (1986). Expressed emotion and depression: Interactions between patients and high versus low EE spouses. *Journal of Abnormal Psychology, 95,* 237–246.

Leff, J. P., Kuipers, L., Berkowitz, R., Eberlein-Vries, R., & Sturgeon, D. (1982). A controlled trial of social intervention in the families of schizophrenic patients. *British Journal of Psychiatry, 141,* 121–134.

Luborsky, L., Crits-Christoph, P., McLellan, A. T., Woody, G., Piper, W., Liberman, B., Imber, S., & Pilkonis, P. (1986). Do therapists vary much in their success? Findings from four outcomes studies. *American Journal of Orthopsychiatry, 56,* 501–512.

Paykel, E. S., Myers, J. K., Dienelt, M. N., Klerman, G. L., Lindethal, J. J., & Pepper, M. P. (1969). Life events and depression: A controlled study. *Archives of General Psychiatry, 21,* 753–760.

Stoudemire, A., & Blazer, D. (1985). Depression in the elderly. In E. E. Beckham & W. R. Leber (Eds.), *Handbook of depression: Treatment, assessment, and research* (pp. 556–586). Homewood, IL: Dorsey Press.

Vaughn, C. E., Snyder, K. S., Jones, S., Freeman, W., & Falloon, I. R. H. (1984). Family factors in schizophrenic relapse: Replication in California of British research on expressed emotion. *Archives of General Psychiatry, 41,* 1169–1177.

Weissman, M. M., & Paykel, E. (1974). *The depressed woman: A study of social relationships.* Chicago: University of Chicago Press.

7

Combined Use of Pharmacological and Family Therapy

NATHAN B. EPSTEIN
GABOR I. KEITNER
DUANE S. BISHOP
IVAN W. MILLER

In this chapter, we shall describe clinical experiences encountered in the course of our research program in studying the application of a combination of standard ward therapy, including the appropriate psychopharmacological agents, and family therapy to cases of major affective disorders, that is, major depression and bipolar disorder. At the time of writing, our experience with major depression was more extensive because of difficulties encountered in recruiting bipolar disorder cases for the research study. Consequently, we have more data on depressive cases than on bipolar disorders.

We will not address the treatment of transient dysphoric states, adjustment disorders, dysthymias, or grief reactions, but will restrict our discussion to the serious cases diagnosed as major depression and bipolar disorder that necessitate hospitalization for the patient. Treatment of the patients and their families begins while the patient is hospitalized and continues on an outpatient basis for as long as is considered necessary.

We begin with a literature review, followed by empirical findings from various studies of families of patients with affective disorders. These studies demonstrate that family functioning may have an impact on the course of depressive illness and that continued problematic family functioning may interfere with the recovery process and even be associated with higher rates of patient relapse. We then present the rationale for our treatment approach, both for the pharmacological aspect and for our problem–centered systems therapy of the family. Some attention is given to the heterogeneity of clinical problems presented by the patients with whom we have worked. Finally, we describe some fascinating phenomena that we uncovered in our clinical work and present a loose grouping of varying responses to therapy that we have observed in our cases.

LITERATURE REVIEW

A recent literature review (Keitner, Baldwin, Epstein, & Bishop, 1985) demonstrates that few definitive findings have been published in the important area of family functioning in the affective disorders. The few better designed studies available suggest that during the acute episode of major depression, female patients report impairment in all social roles. They report decreased verbal and nonverbal communication leading to friction with husbands and children; increased reticence, submissiveness, dependence, guilt, and isolation; and decreased sexual satisfaction. These women describe high levels of tension and self-preoccupation. Their parenting skills seem impaired, leading to behavioral problems in their adolescent children. Their work performance is reported to be impaired, particularly in the home, but less so outside the home. The degree of disturbance experienced during the acute episode is reported to be partly a function of their premorbid adjustment. With resolution of the depressive episode, their social and family functioning approximates, but does not match, that of nondepressed populations.

Depressed male patients are reported to be vulnerable to relapse if their families are characterized by criticism, hostility, overprotection, and overinvolvement. A family that is encouraging and supportive without being stifling seems to protect against relapse.

During the acute episode of bipolar affective disorder, the impact on families is reported to be substantial, with disturbed marital relationships manifested by vague caretaking roles, tenuous loyalties, lessened affection, and disturbed parenting. These parental problems lead to anxiety, tension, and excessive health concerns in their children. For many of the patients who receive and respond well to medical plus psychosocial treatment, the family disturbances appear to subside, and many families report marital satisfaction during remissions that is similar to that in families without an affectively disturbed member.

Despite these reported findings, which seem to be quite consistent, definitive conclusions are difficult to draw because of the significant methodological limitations of the studies on which they are based. These include inadequate diagnostic specificity, use of unvalidated measures, lack of comprehensive assessment of a variety of family variables, lack of objective measures of family functioning, lack of controls for simple negative response, bias in the reporting of depressed patients, and lack of appropriate control groups and/or skill norms.

EMPIRICAL FINDINGS

A recent study by our group (Keitner, Miller, Epstein, & Bishop, 1986) also supports the finding that during the acute phase of a major depressive episode, there are areas of family functioning that are significantly disturbed. The family functioning of 39 patients with major depression and their families was assessed during an acute depressive episode using the Family Assessment Device (FAD; Epstein, Baldwin, & Bishop, 1983; Miller, Epstein, Bishop, & Keitner, 1985), a self-report measure assessing seven dimensions of family functioning of the McMaster model of family functioning (Epstein, Bishop, & Levin, 1978). These scores were compared to those of 22 nonpsychiatric families who also completed the FAD. The results indicated that during the acute episode, depressed families did not differ from nonpsychiatric families in overall family functioning but rather, showed specific dysfunction in the areas of communication, problem solving, and affective responsiveness. However, since these two groups were not matched for demographic characteristics, these differences may have been attributable to other factors.

In a subsequent study (Miller, Kabacoff, Keitner, Epstein, & Bishop, 1986), we compared the family functioning of five groups of psychiatric patients categorized by diagnosis: major depression; bipolar disorder, manic; schizophrenic; adjustment disorder; and alcohol dependence. The FAD was administered to the patients and the families of these patient groups during the first 10 days following hospitalization. An additional sample of 23 families *without* a member with psychiatric disorder was matched to the psychiatric groups on demographic variables. The results of this study indicated that families of patients with major depression had poorer levels of family functioning than did families of the patients in the other psychiatric groups, and that they were significantly worse than nonclinical families in all dimensions of family functioning. Identical results were obtained when controlling for the potential bias by the patient by using only the scores of the nonpatient family members. This study replicated our previous finding of significant dysfunction in families of patients with major depression and suggested that these difficulties are more severe during the acute depressive episode than during acute episodes experienced by patients in the other psychiatric groups examined.

In another analysis, a series of *t* tests was used to compare the mean family FAD scores of 15 families with bipolar patients (scores were obtained during the patients' hospitalization for manic episodes) with the FAD scores of 23 nonclinical control families. Since seven comparisons were conducted, a $p < .01$ significance level was used to control for the experimentwise error rate. These comparisons indicated that the families with a bipolar disordered patient reported significantly poorer functioning than controls on the affective involvement, affective responsiveness, and behavioral control scales. Using health–pathology cutoff scores for the FAD, the bipolar families averaged approximately twice the percentage of unhealthy families that the control group averaged. Families with bipolar patients do exhibit significant disturbances in family functioning, particularly in the areas of affective involvement, affective responsiveness, and behavioral control (Epstein, Miller, Keitner, Bishop, & Kabacoff, 1985).

There is also preliminary evidence that family functioning can affect the course of depressive illness. In their seminal study, Vaughn and Leff (1976) reported that depressed patients whose relatives had an elevated level of critical comments in a structured interview were three times more likely to relapse within the following 9 months than were those depressed patients whose relatives had low levels of critical comments. Rounsaville, Prusoff, and Weissman (1980) investigated the relationship between the course of social adjustment (including marital adjustment and disputes) and depressive illness in women who were receiving maintenance antidepressant drug treatment. Overall, social adjustment during the acute episode did not predict subsequent relapse. However, approximately one half of the depressed women reported significant marital difficulties. Of these women with marital difficulties, those whose marital problems did not improve were significantly more symptomatic after 8 months of maintenance drug treatment than were those women whose marital difficulties had improved.

Our own study (Keitner, Miller, Epstein, Bishop, & Fruzzetti, 1987) on 25 patients with major depression and their families who have met criteria for recovery by 1 year showed that there was a significant improvement in family functioning, particularly in communication, behavior control, and general functioning. However, a comparison of these clinically improved families with a matched sample of nonclinical families showed that even after recovery from depression, the clinical families continued to function at a more unhealthy level than the nonclinical families in all areas but particularly in general functioning, problem solving, and communication.

In another analysis, we divided the same depressed patients into those whose family functioning had improved from their acute episode to recovery versus those whose family functioning had stayed the same or deteriorated after recovery. Overall (using the General Functioning subscale of the FAD), patients with families that showed improvement in family functioning ($n = 20$) recovered more quickly (4.1 months) than patients with families that showed no improvement in family functioning ($n = 8$), who took 8 months to recover. Improved family functioning was thus associated with a shortened depression episode. In summary, there is evidence to suggest that family functioning may have an impact on the course of depressive illness, and that continued problematic family functioning may either impede the recovery process or actually be associated with higher rates of relapse.

There have been almost no studies assessing the effect of family treatment on the course of affective disorders. Glick and his co-workers (1985) have recently reported on the evaluation of inpatient family interaction treatment at discharge and at 6-month follow-up on patients with schizophrenic and affective disorders. They found that for patients with major affective disorders, there was a significant treatment effect on discharge, as measured by the Global Assessment Scale, for those patients who had family therapy in addition to the other treatment modalities utilized in modern inpatient treatment. This effect was diminished at the 6-month follow-up. Interestingly, female patients with affective disorders who were treated with inpatient family therapy did significantly better at discharge and follow-up than did their male counterparts.

Among the preliminary results of our combining family therapy with pharmacological and standard inpatient milieu treatment of patients with bipolar disorders (Epstein *et al.*, 1985), we have data suggesting that family treatment does indeed produce some important effects. Those families who received family therapy reported greater improvement in family functioning than those who did not receive family therapy in conjunction with the other therapies. The effect of these perceived improvements in family functioning on the course of the bipolar illness over time periods longer than 1 year is unknown at this time.

Overall, there does appear to be sufficient evidence to be concerned about the impact of affective disorders on the families of patients, and of the families on the course of the illness, and therefore to include family therapy in the therapeutic repertoire currently available for these conditions.

RATIONALE OF TREATMENT APPROACH

Prior to detailing our clinical experiences in working with families with patients suffering from affective disorders, we wish to present our treatment rationale.

Although we are still far from understanding the etiological basis of the affective disorders, the current evidence implies an etiology in which many factors—biological, psychological, and social—contribute to the illness state. We do not share the belief of some clinicians that biological and psychosocial factors are antithetical, either–or elements that mutually exclude each other as possible etiological factors. On the contrary, we believe that each element contributes in some as yet unknown fashion and in a varying degree to the etiology of these conditions. Neither aspect can be ignored in the treatment and understanding of these disorders.

Pharmacological Approach

Pharmacological treatment has been shown, in numerous studies over the past 20 years, to be most effective in contributing to the alleviation and stabilization of the affective disorders. Such treatment helps not only to reverse the acute phases of the illness but also to prevent, or at least reduce, relapse in these recurring and chronic illnesses.

We use tricyclic antidepressants when the depression is of such severity and duration that it interferes with the person's ability to function or creates a significant risk of suicidal behavior. Features of depression that have been associated with good response to tricyclic antidepressants include insidious onset, weight loss and anorexia, middle and late insomnia, and psychomotor disturbance. Conversely, a poor response to tricyclic antidepressants is associated with hypochondriasis, hysterical traits, and delusions (Bielski & Friedel, 1976). We use monoamine oxidase inhibitors when there is a failure to respond to the tricyclic antidepressants. We use antidepressants during the depressive phase of a bipolar illness, but do so carefully because of their propensity to precipitate manic episodes and increase the rate of cycling of the affective disorder.

No antidepressant on the market has been proven to be better than others. We choose the appropriate antidepressant based on the patient's history of use of a particular drug, on the patient's particular symptoms, and on the desire to avoid different side effects. Amitriptyline, for instance, is quite sedating and therefore most useful with a patient who is experiencing a great deal of anxiety, agitation, and insomnia. Desipramine, on the other hand, being much less sedating and less anticholinergic, would be the drug of choice for a patient whose depression is characterized mainly by hypersomnia, psychomotor retardation, anergia, and anhedonia as well as by more significant cardiovascular abnormalities.

A number of "new" antidepressants (amoxapine, trazodone, maprotiline) have been introduced recently with claims of greater efficacy and fewer side effects. However, none of these new drugs provides significant advantages over established antidepressants in terms of clinical efficacy, speed of onset of therapeutic action, fewer side effects, or increased specificity of action (Ostrow, 1985).

Combining pharmacological treatment with family treatment has had additive effects for both therapeutic modalities. Pharmacological treatment helps to improve the concentration, energy, interest, and motivation of depressed patients, so as to make them more amenable to looking at family issues. Family therapy, on the other hand, has been very helpful in enlisting the family's support for drug management in terms of improving compliance and giving the patient more support during the early phases of pharmacotherapy, when the drug has not had an opportunity to exert its full effect. The more family members understand about the illness, the more they feel a collaborative part of the treatment process, and the more they are likely to support a combined family and pharmacological approach. We discuss basic issues with respect to drug treatment with all family members. We review side effects with them and also discuss the time frame within which symptoms can be expected to begin to remit.

Family Therapy Approach

Our use of family therapy requires a more detailed explanation because its effectiveness has yet to be systematically demonstrated. We do not hold the belief that familial pathology in and of itself can give rise to an affective episode and that the resolution of family pathology will therefore "cure" severely ill affectively disordered patients. We do believe that it is likely that family pathology can operate through some intervening variable or variables to contribute to the development of an affective disorder in patients who are in some way vulnerable to these conditions. Consequently, it is reasonable to assume that relieving some of this family pathology would lessen the vulnerability of such patients.

At the very least, we believe that families of patients can be given a great deal of support by a proper therapeutic approach and in the process can be educated with regard to current knowledge about these disorders, enabling them to understand the conditions better. Such education and support of family members can aid them in being highly supportive of the patient and of the total treatment approach. Studies published over the past few years (Falloon *et al.*, 1982; Leff, Kuipers, Berkowitz, Eberlein-Fries, & Sturgeon, 1984) have demonstrated that such results are forthcoming in the application of family therapy to the treatment of schizophrenic patients and their families. It has been demonstrated that such family involvement is most effective in reducing exacerbation of the schizophrenic illness and readmission to the hospital.

Problem-Centered Systems Therapy of the Family

The family therapy approach utilized by our team is called *problem-centered systems therapy of the family*. This treatment approach was developed by our research group based upon years of clinical research and several "generations" of outcome studies (Epstein & Bishop, 1981). It, in turn, is based upon the McMaster model of family functioning—a conceptual model of family functioning also developed by our group.

In the course of carrying out family functions, families deal with a number of tasks, which we group into three areas: basic tasks, developmental tasks, and hazardous tasks. "Basic tasks" are instrumental in nature and include such fundamental issues as the provision of food and shelter. "Developmental tasks" encompass those family issues that arise with the natural processes of growth, which we differentiate into two sets—those associated with the individual developmental stages that each family member goes through, and those associated with family developmental stages. "Hazardous tasks" include the crises that arise in association with illness, accidents, loss of income, job changes, and moves.

The McMaster model considers family functioning along the following dimensions: problem solving, communication, family roles, affective responsiveness, affective involvement, and behavioral control. "Problem solving" is defined as a family's ability to resolve problems to a level that maintains effective family functioning. A family problem is seen as an issue that threatens the integrity and functional capacity of the family, the solution of which presents difficulty for them. For clinical utility, problems are subdivided into instrumental and affective types. Instrumental problems are the mechanical problems of everyday life, such as finances and housing. Affective problems are those related to feelings.

"Communication" is defined as the way in which the family exchanges information. The focus is solely on verbal exchange. Nonverbal aspects of family communication are tremendously important but are excluded because of the methodological difficulties of collecting and measuring such data. Communication is also subdivided into instrumental and affective areas. In addition, communication is assessed along two other vectors: the clear versus masked continuum and the direct versus indirect continuum. The former focuses on the clarity with which the content of the information is exchanged. Is the message clear or is it camouflaged, muddied, vague, and masked? The latter vector considers whether the message goes to the person for whom it is intended.

"Family roles" are the repetitive patterns of behavior by which individuals fulfill family functions. Family functions are divided into instrumental and affective areas, and also into necessary versus other family functions. In considering the role dimension, two further concepts are considered: role allocation, which incorporates the concepts of the assignment of responsibilities for family functions, and role accountability, which involves the process of a family member being made accountable for the responsibilities that he or she has been allocated.

"Affective responsiveness" is defined as the ability to respond to a range of stimuli with appropriate quality and quantity of feelings. The responses are divided into two classes: welfare feelings, exemplified by affects such as love, tenderness, happiness, and joy, and emergency feelings, exemplified by fear, anger, sadness, disappointment, and depression.

"Affective involvement" is defined as the degree to which the family shows interest in and values the activities and interests of the family members. The focus is on how much, and in what way, family members show an interest and invest themselves in each other.

"Behavior control" is defined as the pattern that the family adopts for handling behavior in three specific situations: physically dangerous situations, situations involving the meeting and expressing of psychobiological needs and drives, and situations involving socializing behavior both inside and outside the family (Epstein, Bishop, & Levin, 1978).

Problem-centered systems therapy of the family focuses on the specific problems of the family, including those problems presented by the family in coming to therapy and those identified during the assessment stage. The model stresses the active collaboration of family members with the therapist at each stage of therapy. The family must agree to work in this collaborative arrangement throughout the therapy process or else there is no therapy; the therapeutic contract is based upon this total mutual commitment. The therapist's ideal role in this model is that of catalyst, clarifier, and facilitator. The family members should actually do most of the therapy work. They are involved openly and directly in identifying, clarifying, and resolving the difficulties and problems of the family. The therapist carefully explains his or her actions to the family every step of the way and makes sure they clearly understand and agree to what he or she is doing. This open approach extends to the family responsibility for its own actions and ensures that the family understands, accepts, and is prepared for each step of the therapeutic process. This therapy model is tailored to a treatment encounter ranging from 6 to 12 sessions stretched over a period of time that varies from weeks to months to years, depending on the issues of each case. The length of the individual sessions may also vary considerably. Early assessment sessions may be longer, whereas the later task-setting sessions may be as short as 15–20 minutes.

The major stages of the treatment are assessment, contracting, treatment, and closure. Each stage contains a sequence of steps, the first of which is always orientation. Orientation to the assessment stage is quite detailed and sets the tone and direction of therapy. All later orientations are much briefer and are used to indicate a change in the focus and task. After general orientation, each step needs to be approached systematically, with a therapist guiding the process. At the conclusion of each stage, the therapist and family need to review and reach agreement on what has been accomplished before moving on to the next stage.

1. *Assessment.* This stage consists of four steps: (1) orientation, (2) data gathering, (c) problem description, and (4) clarifying and agreeing on the problem list. During the assessment stage, we are concerned with orienting the family to the beginning of the treatment process; identifying and detailing the structure, organization, and transactional patterns of the family; and carefully elucidating all the problems that currently exist. The therapist should therefore take as many sessions as necessary for completing a full assessment. During this stage, all necessary investigations are carried out, including full psychological and biological assessments of any or all individual family members as necessary, such as clinical psychiatric evaluations, psychological and neuropsychological testing, EEG and brain imaging, and full physical examination.

2. *Contracting.* The goal here is to prepare a written contract that delineates the mutual expectations, goals, and commitments regarding therapy. The steps in this stage are (1) orientation, (2) outlining options, (3) negotiating expectations, and (4) contract signing. For each option, it is the therapist's responsibility to clarify what his or her function, if any, might

be and to explore the possible consequences of each alternative. Family members are asked to negotiate among themselves what they want from each other, that is, what specific behavioral changes they want to see in each other. Family members are given the major responsibility for defining their expectations, while the therapist's responsibility is in helping each member express his or her expectations in concrete behavioral terms so that progress may be clearly identified and assessed. We then establish a written contract that lists the problems and specifies for each what has been agreed upon as a satisfactory outcome.

3. *Treatment.* This stage consists of four steps: (1) orientation, (2) clarifying priorities, (3) setting tasks, and (4) task evaluation. Priorities are clarified by ordering the problem list according to the family's wishes. Family members negotiate specific tasks that if carried out during the following week, would represent a move in the direction of meeting their expectations. If a task is accomplished, we provide positive reinforcement; if a family fails to complete its task, the original assessment and task negotiations are reviewed.

4. *Closure.* This stage consists of four steps: (1) orientation, (2) summarizing treatment, (3) establishing long-term goals, and (4) follow-up. The family members are asked to summarize what has happened during treatment and what they have learned. They are also asked to discuss and set some long-term goals. When follow-up is arranged, it is scheduled far enough into the future to allow the family a full opportunity to deal with issues as they arise.

This model allows for a well-structured and ordered assessment and evaluation of the family, followed—if agreed upon by the family *and* the therapist—by a carefully defined, clearly spelled out treatment in which the problems of the family are worked on with the aim of achieving effective *solutions.* We believe that families of all patients with affective illnesses should be seen for a family assessment as early in the treatment process as possible. Such an assessment is not to be confused with an interview of the patient's family for the purpose of obtaining further information regarding the illness of the patient, although this is often necessary and helpful. The objective of a family assessment conducted according to the approach spelled out by our therapy model is a full understanding of the family's functioning along a number of dimensions. This knowledge contributes to an understanding of the framework in which the affective episode occurred and the context in which it will be treated.

Not all families require family therapy, since comprehensive assessments often reveal healthy family functioning. Nevertheless, even a healthy family can benefit from education regarding the illness and from a generally collaborative and supportive approach by the treatment team. If family pathology is uncovered in the course of the family assessment, it can be addressed at the appropriate time in the course of the disorder.

HETEROGENEITY OF CLINICAL PROBLEMS

The most salient factor encountered by our group in the course of our clinical experience with this project has been the complex and confusing heterogeneity of clinical problems and issues subsumed under the diagnostic rubric of affective disorders. It is obvious that although DSM-III has been a useful step in the right direction, there are *many* disorders gathered under the diagnostic labels now in existence. Clinically, one finds any number of family problems as well as a variety of individual psychopathology in these patients and families. Currently, there is no research support for the hypothesis that a particular family constellation or interactional style invariably leads to or is associated with affective illness. Factors such as the premorbid functioning of the family, the developmental stage of the family, the health of family members (particularly the presence or absence of psychiatric illness), the family's social and financial situation, and the availability of external supports all bear on a family's level of functioning and on its capacity to deal with crises, including current affective disorder episodes.

Apart from the heterogeneity of factors related to the families of patients, there is marked heterogeneity in patients. One encounters the gamut of individual psychopathology in patients with affective disorders. Notable complicating factors are the issues of concurrent dysthymia and/or character disorders of various types. In many of our clinical encounters with these patients, we have found the major affective disorder component of the illness to respond quickly to therapy, only then to be faced with a concomitant underlying dysthymia and/or severe character disorder that proves most resistant to our treatment endeavors. We shall discuss some examples of this type of case in the next section. All varieties of intrapsychic conflicts may be encountered in these patients in the course of treatment. To complicate matters even further, these varieties of psychopathology may also be encountered in one or more members of the patient's family. It should therefore be obvious that any therapeutic approach adopted in these cases must be broadly based, flexible, and responsively creative in order to deal with all the possible complications of psychopathology.

CLINICAL EXPERIENCES

Prior to describing specific cases, we would like to comment on two related phenomena encountered frequently in intensive work with families of affectively disordered patients. Aspects of these phenomena can be seen in all types of family work with patients having varying illnesses. Affective illness highlights some of these interesting aspects.

Affectively disordered patients frequently complain strongly about various members of their families—often offering many specific examples of gross misbehavior or maltreatment by such family members. Although these statements are sometimes true, they are frequently groundless, with no evidence being found for them after intense and careful work with such families. Furthermore, these complaints often disappear in direct relation to the clearing of the current affective episode of the patient concerned. Many of these patients vehemently deny having made these statements, much less having believed them, once they have recovered from their current episode.

These experiences are fascinating. Sound psychodynamic theory demands that a therapist take into serious consideration these complaints and accusations. Yet, as stated, we often find them groundless following very careful, intensive exploration. At this point, we do not know what to make of these phenomena other than that in some way, they reflect the severe cognitive distortions of these patients. The therapist and treatment team must be very cautious in dealing with these statements: Attention must be paid to them, yet the family must not be wrongly painted by a brush wielded by a severely ill individual whose perceptions and judgment are grossly distorted.

The second phenomenon encountered in our work is that ward and treatment team staff frequently read pathology into the manner in which family members relate to the identified patients. As an example, the team reported that every night when a husband came in to visit his wife, he would sit there and ignore her, and often would talk to other visitors or just sit by himself and read. This example of the husband's behavior was used by several team members to justify their hypotheses that this couple had a basically bad relationship and that the husband's active rejection of his wife was the real cause of her depression. Close examination and follow-up of these "accusations" led to the following information: It was not the husband who rejected the wife while visiting her. She was so depressed that for a long period she could not relate to anybody. She would greet him most perfunctorily on his arrival in the ward to visit and then would withdraw to a corner by herself. He would then be forced to be by himself to read or relate to others on the unit. The wonder was why this devoted and faithful man came to visit his wife night after night following a hard day's work despite such total withdrawal by her. As her depression cleared, she began to relate to him and enjoy his visits, and his perseverance was thusly rewarded. Intense exploration with the couple during the height of her withdrawal from him and after her depression cleared failed to reveal any difficulties in their marital relationship—much to the surprise (and disappointment!) of some of the team members.

A similar phenomenon occurred in another case—that of a woman in her early 40s with a severely malignant, long-standing depression. A number of treatments were tried with very limited success. Whenever her depression lifted slightly, she would be granted her request to go on home visits with her husband. These visits would invariably be followed by a worsening of her depression on the next day. This intensification of the illness began to be viewed by members of the treatment team as an indication of mistreatment by the husband while the wife was home and as clear evidence of a severely disturbed relationship between the couple. Close examination of both members of the couple failed to reveal any evidence for either hypothesis. Nothing much happened at home, and both partners denied any negative feelings or behaviors while on pass. When this patient's depression finally cleared and she went home on pass a number of times prior to discharge, she returned feeling very well, happy, and joyous. The positive feelings carried over between visits. Obviously, what was being observed previously was merely an indication that the patient's illness was still very severe and that she could not yet tolerate the stress of a home visit. It was no reflection on her relationship with her husband.

To repeat: Treatment teams must be most careful to gather clear evidence to justify hypotheses regarding observed behavior. We must not forget that we are dealing with severe illness in which factors other than intrapsychic or interpersonal ones are often operative.

Specific Case Examples

On reviewing our extensive and growing experience with combined family and pharmacological treatment of the affective disorders, an interesting loose grouping of responses to therapy seems to be evident. Although this grouping is by no means firm or clearly defined as yet, we feel our preliminary observations and experiences are interesting enough to report.

Rapid Response to Treatment

A number of cases of depression have shown a remarkably rapid clearing of what appeared to be severe symptoms of depression once the family issues that were problematic were delineated during a comprehensive family assessment and once the family members and the therapist developed a mutually satisfactory treatment contract. The depressive symptomatology has included severely depressed affect, withdrawal from social and occupational activities, loss of weight and appetite, disturbed sleep, and serious suicide attempts.

CASE EXAMPLE

A prime example of this type of case was CQ, a 17-year-old high school junior who was admitted to the hospital following a 4 to 6-month history of depression, heavy drinking, and drug abuse; a series of potentially dangerous car accidents; angry arguments and hostile, unpleasant behavior with parents and sibling; and a suicide attempt.

Family assessment revealed a family unit that had functioned very well until about 1 year prior to the patient's admission to the hospital. At that time, the father had suffered a serious work injury and was forced to stop work and lead the life of a handicapped individual at home. The father had become quite depressed over the past year and had withdrawn from a fairly close, warm, and outgoing relationship with the identified patient. This series of events was accompanied by the death of the paternal grandfather, with whom the patient was very close and of whom he was most fond. These serious losses precipitated a serious depression in this patient, which was expressed primarily by his acting-out behavior. This behavior was responded to angrily by the parents, which produced further hostile behavior in the patient. This pattern of troubled transactions continued until the family assessment during the early part of the patient's hospitalization.

When these elements were teased out during the initial family interview, and when the preexisting healthy connections and relationships were reestablished, the patient's depressive, hostile, sullen behavior dramatically changed to his more usual outgoing, warm, and likeable behavior. Subsequent to several family therapy sessions, the reestablished positive behavior continued at home following the patient's early discharge from the hospital. The family lived some distance from the hospital, and the father found the automobile ride a severe strain on his disabled back. The family members stated that they felt they couldn't put the father through this strain, and they arranged for follow-up treatment at a mental health center in their home community. Apparently, a sound treatment relationship was never really established at this center, and the family drifted out of therapy without notifying us. About 6 months following hospitalization, the patient shot himself in his school classroom. We feel that in the absence of continued satisfactory treatment, the family regressed to its previous depressive patterns.

We have seen quite a few other examples of similar abrupt changes in a patient's depressive symptomatology during the course of the initial comprehensive family assessments. In a number of other cases, the improvement continued for the duration of the treatment and for a considerable length of time following treatment termination. To the best of our knowledge, many of these improvements continue up to the present—a period of 1 to 3 years. Interestingly enough, this type of rapid response was seen across a wide age spread in the identified patients.

Minimal Family Pathology

In some families, there is minimal, if any, family pathology—even during the acute phase of the illness of the identified patient. This phenomenon may occur even in cases where the depression in the patient has been protracted. Our therapeutic approach in these situations is restricted to supporting the family unit and carefully educating its members concerning all aspects of the patient's condition. We clearly emphasize that they are in no way responsible for the illness and indicate in every way we can how much we empathize with their burden of coping with an affectively ill member. We point out how difficult it is to watch loved ones suffer as much as these patients do but yet how supportive their concern and care can be to these patients in the long run. We encourage them to lead as normal a life as possible and not to be overcome with guilt and/or overconcern. This approach has proven most helpful in allowing family members to see themselves as collaborating members of the treatment team. They frequently express their appreciation for being treated as responsible, intelligent individuals and, particularly, for not being patronized or made to feel guilty about contributing to the patient's illness.

In our study of the effectiveness of family therapy in addition to standard pharmacotherapy in treating a bipolar disorder, we have included a specific educational component in the family treatment. For the sake of efficiency and consistency, we have prepared a 30-minute educational videotape of a simulated family session between a psychiatrist and a family with one member having a bipolar disorder. Reviewed in the tape are major issues concerning the signs and symptoms, causes, course, treatments, and common family problems connected with bipolar disorders. Major content areas are emphasized with slides and voice-over edited into the film. The videotape focuses on practical issues and provides specific answers to questions commonly asked about bipolar illness. The videotape is shown by the family therapist, who is available to answer questions concerning the information presented. We have also used the videotape with families not included in the treatment study, as a means of providing them with some basic information prior to our initial family meetings. Most families have found the information to be very helpful and seemed to be much better prepared to discuss specific and meaningful issues with their therapist in the family assessment and treatment sessions.

Broader Family Pathology

We have seen a variety of cases where a wide spectrum of family pathology is present, yet the patients and the family as a whole respond very well to the combination of pharmacological and family therapy. In these patients, proper pharmacological treatment is seen to definitely improve the affective episode, and while this is occurring, the patient and family are working on their family problems in the ongoing family therapy.

CASE EXAMPLE

An example of this situation was a 16-year-old boy (NQ) who was severely depressed and was admitted following serious suicidal threats and at least one serious attempt. He was living at home with his widowed mother, who was a health care professional. His father, the mother's first husband, had died when the patient was 3 years old, and the patient had no real recollection of him. The mother remarried several years later, and with this second husband, the patient developed a warm and positive relationship. Unfortunately, this man died suddenly about 1 year prior to the patient's admission to the hospital. Both of the mother's husbands were alcoholics—a fact unknown to the patient. The mother had actively contrived to conceal from the patient the facts concerning the alcoholism of her second husband. The patient was too young to be aware of the alcoholism of his biological father.

The mother's stage management of the illness of her second husband was indicative of her overall behavior in general and of her behavior in relation to her son in particular. She was a strong, competent individual, with a great deal of ego strength, yet had great difficulty in establishing warm, intimate, sharing relationships. She was primarily a "caregiver" who had difficulties with other aspects of the marital and parenting roles. The patient felt alienated and distant from his mother. He found it difficult, if not impossible, to really talk to her—a fact that surprised her no end when it was revealed during the family assessment. The boy was lonely and isolated, and he became seriously depressed. It became obvious, on further history taking, that his biological father's alcoholism was a manifestation of a probable affective disorder, from which our patient was obviously suffering in the form of overt depression rather than being covered over by alcoholism or drug abuse, which was probably absent because of the patient's young age.

The family therapy focused on the serious problems in the relationship between the patient and his mother. As the patient's depression eased as a result of the drug therapy, he was able to work positively in the family therapy and took the lead in many aspects of the treatment situation. It was much easier for him to effect change than it was for his mother, because she had developed a much more rigidly fixed characterological pattern. Nevertheless, she worked at it assiduously, and both were able to respond positively to therapy. They had maintained the improvement at the time of a postdischarge follow-up about 1 year later.

We have encountered a number of cases similar to this one, where the identified patient improved once on medication, and the patient and family simultaneously worked effectively and with considerable success during the ongoing family therapy.

Freeing the Family of Severely Depressed Patients

This last group of patients was the most difficult of all, yet in some ways, perhaps the most interesting. These patients were admitted with a wide range of very severe depressive symptomatology, often following serious suicide attempts. It proved difficult to engage these patients in any type of therapy, and once involved in family therapy plus antidepressant drug treatment, the depressive symptomatology disappeared only to reveal severe underlying character pathology and/or severe dysthymia—which in turn proved impervious to further therapeutic efforts. It is almost as if these people refused, at any cost, to give up their remaining pathology, even though they were suffering intensely and were causing much suffering on the part of everyone involved with them. Frequently, they sabotaged further therapeutic work and fled therapy, only to reappear in the emergency room following further suicidal attempts. In our experience, family therapy in these cases often may have a beneficial result insofar as it helps other family members to free themselves from the pathological web of involvements previously woven within the family by all members around the pathological behavior of the identified patient. This freeing often reduces the secondary gain and pathological power previously granted to the identified patient and ameliorates his or her pathological behavior to some degree.

CASE EXAMPLE

An example of this type of case was DN, a young married woman in her late 20s, who was admitted to the hospital in a severe depression following some recent suicide attempts and threats. She was depressed and anorectic, had lost much weight over a long period of time, had much difficulty sleeping, and could no longer continue in her job or look after her children. Her husband was most concerned about her behavior and was terrified she would carry through on her threats to kill herself. On the ward, she behaved in a highly misanthropic fashion—surly, hostile, barking at anyone who tried to make contact with her. She resisted any kind of therapy for some time, stating that she wanted to die anyway, so why bother. After some days of persistent confrontation, she grudgingly agreed to give family therapy and drug treatment a try. After several weeks of antidepressant therapy, her overt depressive symptoms diminished considerably. However, she still manifested underlying severe character pathology. She refused to work on changing these behaviors, which included her need to avoid close contact with anyone (including her husband and colleagues at work), her need to hang on to unusual eating and sleeping habits, her refusal to gain weight, and her refusal to develop more pleasant patterns of social relatedness and a less bitter and hostile approach to life in general.

During the work of family therapy in this case, the husband made remarkable—and to us, highly unexpected—behavioral changes. Prior to the beginning of family therapy, the husband had been highly resistant to getting involved in the treatment situation, even more so than his wife. His attitude to the treatment team was an unspoken "This is not my problem— she's the sick one—fix her up and don't blame me." He was overprotective toward his wife, and because he was so terrified by her suicidal threats and suicide potential, he was consequently easily and often manipulated by her. He saw himself as her protector and at the onset of hospitalization "defended" her from the therapy team.

When we prevailed upon him to join his wife in the family assessment, his behavior changed remarkably. It seemed that for the first time he realized that he was not to blame for his wife's severe illness and highly unpleasant behavior. He began to understand that we were not out to put him down but were merely trying to enlist him as a collaborator in a very difficult and complex process that was very important to his wife.

As a result of the therapy, he was able to free himself from being a prisoner to his wife's hostile, depressive behavior. He was able to avoid being "sucked in" to do battle with her; he could stand up to her with dignity and self-respect and could walk away from useless, mutually destructive encounters. He quickly learned that life thereby was much more pleasant for him: Once his wife realized that he would not be seduced into battle, she frequently gave up trying to get him involved in her pathology and began to treat him with more respect.

When this level of function was reached in the therapy, the wife stated very clearly that she would refuse to participate in any further therapy. The therapist revealed the options open to the husband when faced with this ultimatum from her. The husband chose to stay with her under his new rules of operation and to develop a life of his own in addition to his relationship with her. He was able to enjoy their children more and to involve himself in satisfying activities outside the home with friends. He cared for his wife despite her serious pathology and was able to tolerate her then somewhat lower level of hostility and general misanthropy. He was encouraged to contact the therapist for further help at any time. Posttermination follow-up about 1 year later found the couple functioning at the level achieved at discharge. The husband was still quite satisfied with the outcome, and the identified patient was continuing in her sullen, dysthymic fashion but was making no more suicidal threats or gestures; they were getting along at this level.

In many other cases of this general type, treatment was ended similarly, that is, with a somewhat limited result. In some cases, the results were null. These patients continued to reappear at the hospital following further suicide attempts or threats, or with just plain, simple severe depression—only to repeat the process over again.

One of the interesting aspects of these cases is that the severe, overt "depressive" symptomatology is that which is most responsive to therapy. It is the underlying character pathology and/or dysthymia that resists all the weapons available in our present therapeutic armamentarium. This area is one in which further research is sorely needed.

CONCLUSION

The combination of pharmacotherapy and family therapy that we have used in our research program has provided us with interesting results and a rich panoply of clinical findings. As we continue these studies, we hope to learn more about such elements as the cost-effectiveness of our therapeutic endeavors and to tease out more factors involved in the clinical complexities that we have attempted to provide a glimpse of in this chapter.

REFERENCES

Bielski, R. J., & Friedel, R. O. (1976). Prediction of tricyclic antidepressant response. *Archives of General Psychiatry, 33,* 1479–1489.

Epstein, N. B., Baldwin, L. M., & Bishop, D. S. (1983). The McMaster Family Assessment Device. *Journal of Marital and Family Therapy, 9,* 171–180.

Epstein, N. B., & Bishop, D. S. (1981) Problem-centered systems therapy of the family. In A. Gurman & D. Kniskern (Eds.), *Handbook of family therapy* (pp. 444–482). New York: Brunner/Mazel.

Epstein, N. B., Bishop, D. S., & Levin, S. (1978). The McMaster model of family functioning. *Journal of Marriage and Family Counseling, 4,* 19–31.

Epstein, N. B., Miller, I. W., Keitner, G. I., Bishop, D. S., & Kabacoff, R. I. (1985, May). *Family dysfunction in bipolar disorder: Description and pilot treatment study.* Paper presented at the meeting of the American Psychiatric Association, Dallas.

Falloon, I., Boyd, J. L., McGill, C. W., Razani, J., Moss, H. B., & Gilderman, A. M. (1982). Family management in the prevention of exacerbations of schizophrenia. *The New England Journal of Medicine, 306,* 1437–1440.

Glick, I. D., Clarkin, J. F., Spencer, J. H., Haas, G. L., Lewis, A. B., Peyser, J., DeMone, N., Good-Ellis, M., Harris, E., & Lestelle, V. (1985). A controlled evaluation of inpatient family intervention—I. Preliminary results of the six-month follow-up. *Archives of General Psychiatry, 42,* 882–886.

Keitner, G. I., Baldwin, L. M., Epstein, N. B., & Bishop, D. S. (1985). Family functioning in patients with affective disorders: A review. *International Journal of Family Psychiatry, 6,* 405–437.

Keitner, G. I., Miller, I. W., Epstein, N. B., & Bishop, D. S. (1986). The functioning of families in patients with major depression. *International Journal of Family Psychiatry, 7,* 11–16.

Keitner, G. I., Miller, I. W., Epstein, N. B., Bishop, D. S., & Fruzzetti, A. (1987). *Family functioning and the course of major depression.* Manuscript submitted for publication. *Comprehensive Psychiatry, 78,* 54–64.

Leff, J., Kuipers, L., Berkowitz, R., Eberlein-Fries, R., & Sturgeon, D. (1984). Psychosocial relevance and benefit of neuroleptic maintenance: Experience in the United Kingdom. *Journal of Clinical Psychiatry: Sec. 2, 45,* 43–48.

Miller, I. W., Epstein, N. B., Bishop, D. S., & Keitner, G. I. (1985). The McMaster Family Assessment Device: Reliability and validity. *Journal of Marital and Family Therapy, 11,* 345–356.

Miller, I. W., Kabacoff, R. I., Keitner, G. I., Epstein, N. B., & Bishop, D. S. (1986). Family functioning in the families of psychiatric patients. *Comprehensive Psychiatry, 27,* 302–312.

Ostrow, D. (1985). The new generation antidepressants: Promising innovations or disappointments? *Journal of Clinical Psychiatry: Sec. 2, 46,* 25–30.

Rounsaville, B. J., Prusoff, B. A., & Weissman, M. M. (1980). The course of marital disputes in depressed women: a 48-month follow-up study. *Comprehensive Psychiatry, 21*, 111–118.

Vaughn, C. E., & Leff, J. P. (1976). The influence of family and social factors on the course of psychiatric illness. A comparison of schizophrenic and depressed neurotic patients. *British Journal of Psychiatry, 129*, 125–137.

8

Management of Manic Episodes

YOLANDE B. DAVENPORT
MARVIN L. ADLAND

INTRODUCTION

In April 1984, members of the panel of the National Institute of Mental Health/National Institutes of Health (NIMH/NIH) Consensus Development Conference on Mood Disorders: Pharmacological Prevention of Recurrences, held on the NIH campus in Bethesda, Maryland, concluded that recurrent mood disorders, or affective illnesses, are associated with high prevalence and serious consequences and remain both underdiagnosed and undertreated in the nation's population. They noted that patients who have had a manic episode, or both a hypomanic and a depressive episode, are at a particularly high risk for recurrence. Further, they reported findings from a summary of 14 follow-up studies of bipolar disorder that recurrences among patients maintained 1 year on lithium carbonate were reduced by 50% and were less severe in intensity when compared to recurrences among patients on placebo. In addition to stressing the efficacy of lithium treatment for the majority of diagnosed bipolar patients, it is most significant that this important report also acknowledged the usefulness of psychotherapy in conjunction with pharmacotherapy to reduce disruptions in occupational and marital and family life associated with bipolar illness (NIMH/NIH, 1985).

Bipolar illness is generally acknowledged to have strong genetic and biological components. It is known to occur in families, and its presence in one or more members of a family often has a catastrophic and lasting impact upon the entire family. Since the advent of lithium carbonate and other antimanic and antidepressant drugs to treat the psychosis and to control the extreme mood swings of the illness, pharmacotherapy alone has been the treatment most often prescribed for the management of this chronic familial disorder. A conceptual treatment model developed that focused on the biology and biochemistry of the identified patient, with relief of symptomatic disturbance through medication as the primary goal. This approach tended to subordinate the existence of external or psychosocial factors that may influence the illness course or even trigger a genetic predisposition. It also failed to consider that the specific psychopathological and maladaptive character traits associated with a severe mood disorder and present even during euthymic phases have a part in the suffering and distress of patients and families, a part that remains totally untouched by the introduction of medication.

In the predrug era, the intrapsychic state and interpersonal interactions, as well as the family constellation, of the bipolar manic–depressive patient were of interest to psychoanalytic investigators. Because of the recurrent, cyclothymic factors related to the course of their illness, specifically the rapid appearance and escalation of florid symptoms and the difficulties experienced by the bipolar patient in forming a therapeutic alliance, these investigators were often unsuccessful in their psychoanalytic treatment endeavors. Long-term hospitalization was frequently the outcome. It is ironic, then, that with their mood episodes better controlled with medication, enabling them to be more accessible to psychotherapy, bipolar patients currently remain largely remote from a treatment approach that might alter and enhance their lives.

Bipolar patients are difficult to treat. Many patients, including those for whom medication has been prescribed, deny that they have an illness. Some acknowledge only the biochemistry of the illness, which can be "cured with a magic pill." Many patients refuse to comply with a prescribed medication regime, and the unfortunate consequences associated with a possible episode recurrence evoke anxiety and stress. The extreme highs are often characterized by outrageous, alienating, destructive behavior. The depressive episodes, characterized by marked dependence and often accompanied by suicidal ideation, gestures, and attempts, are stressful for patient, family, and therapist. It is not surprising that many clinicians have limited themselves exclusively to prescribing and monitoring medication in treating the bipolar patient.

In previous studies, we reported psychodynamic features of multigenerational bipolar families, presenting specific themes and behavioral patterns found cross-generationally among the families studied, regardless of individual family characteristics. We hypothesized that these maladaptive patterns transmitted within the family system of the potential manic–depressive patient may interact with genetic vulnerability and have some part in the cultural transmission of the illness (Davenport, Adland, Gold, & Goodwin, 1979). In a continuation of this work, we have also explored the contributions of the family system of the manic–depressive patient from the perspective of early child-rearing practices in families with a manic–depressive parent (Davenport, Zahn-Waxler, Adland, & Mayfield, 1984). In conjunction with the use of lithium carbonate for the patient, we have long advocated the inclusion of the spouse and family in the psychotherapeutic work

(Davenport, Ebert, Adland, & Goodwin, 1977). In this chapter, we will describe the effects of family treatment of the manic–depressive bipolar patient and suggest strategies and methods for intervention.

BIPOLAR ILLNESS AND ITS SYMPTOMATOLOGY

Mental illnesses characterized by severe disturbances of mood have been known since biblical times. However, it was not until the early 20th century that Kraepelin (1913/1921) systematically described manic–depressive disorder as a separate entity, distinguishing it from schizophrenia. Kraepelin noted then that manic–depressive psychosis had a good prognosis and that the disease was probably the result of a genetic deficit. This prognosis may have been viewed as relative compared to the chronicity and intensity of disturbance experienced by the chronic schizophrenic, for patients with manic–depressive illness, even unmedicated, may have periods of remission between recurring episodes. More recent studies, however, suggest that the course of bipolar manic–depressive illness is associated with a high degree of psychiatric and social morbidity. It is estimated that though the number of recurrences may vary among individuals, 70% to 90% of all bipolar patients will experience a median of 11 episodes during their lifetimes. Recent estimates are that diagnosed bipolar disorder is prevalent in at least 1% of the population in this country at any given time, or approximately 4 million people.

In fact, this may be a low estimate, since the presence of hypomanic symptoms between episodes of morbid depression have not always been recognized. Many patients emerging from a period of deep depression are unable to recognize the feelings of extravagant elation that may follow as other than normal good feelings. A spouse or family member, well aware that such feelings seem exaggerated and are predictive of troublesome behavior, may fail to fully recognize or report the hypomanic symptoms. Symptoms associated with the onset of a major depression may go undetected as well, until dysfunction can no longer be denied.

To understand how bipolar illness can affect and disrupt the lives of patients and families, it is necessary to define it and its symptomatology. Most adults have experienced periods of depression and of elation that can be considered normal and appropriate situational reactions. For example, the depression that may follow a death, divorce, job loss, and so forth, and the joy and high spirits associated with a happy event, such as a wedding, promotion, or birth of a child are examples of this. Such feelings tend not to be pervasive and are self-limiting. But when the depression or hypomanic moods are associated with disabling symptoms that persist over a defined period and interfere with normal life functioning, treatment may be necessary. Without treatment, episodes will recur, leading inevitably to a downward progression in economic, social, psychological, and occupational position.

The revised third edition of the *Diagnostic and Statistical Manual of Mental Disorders* of the American Psychiatric Association (1987), or DSM-III-R, has divided the mood disorders into bipolar disorder and depressive disorders. Bipolar disorders are further divided into mixed, manic, and depressive disorders. For the depressive phase in bipolar disorder, the following criteria, according to DSM-III-R, must be met: First, a dysphoric mood must be present, characterized by loss of interest in all common activities and by feelings of sadness, depression, and irritability. Second, at least five of the following symptoms must have been experienced daily over a period of 2 weeks: increased or decreased appetite; sleep disturbances—insomnia or hypersomnia; psychomotor agitation or retardation; loss of interest in activities, including decreased sexual interest; loss of energy and fatigue; feelings of shame, guilt, and unworthiness; difficulties in thinking and concentrating; indecisiveness; suicidal thoughts and ideation. Neither preoccupation with a mood-incongruent delusion or hallucination, nor bizarre behavior has dominated the clinical picture when the affective syndrome has remitted, or was present prior to its development.

The criteria for mania, acording to DSM-III-R, include the presence of a high, expansive, or irritable mood of persistant duration. At least three of the following symptoms must be present for a period of 1 week, or four symptoms if the mood is only irritable: increased social and sexual activity, talkativeness, flight of ideas, grandiosity and inflated self-esteem, decreased need for sleep, distractibility, and excessive involvement in pleasurable activities associated with poor judgment. Neither preoccupation with a mood-incongruent delusion or hallucination nor bizarre behavior dominates the clinical picture when an affective syndrome is not present, that is, before it developed or after it has remitted. The diagnosis of bipolar disorder is not used when the main diagnosis is schizophrenia, dementia, or some organic mental disturbance with mania. In mania, if there are delusions, they are mostly mood congruent.

Bipolar disorder has an earlier average age of onset, generally before the age of 30, in contrast to unipolar disorder, where average age of onset is in the middle or late 30s. There appears to be no correlation between bipolar disorder and marital status; bipolar disorder appears more often in persons of higher socioeconomic class who have high educational and social achievement levels; and the prevalence rates between men and women appear to be approximately the same. Although the interrelationship between alcoholism and affective disorders is not well understood, alcoholism is often associated with mania. It has been suggested that many bipolar patients may use alcohol in their efforts to medicate an oncoming episode. Loss of employment, bankruptcy, high divorce rates, and financial ruin are also associated with manic behavior, and this, in turn, may lead to social isolation, shame, and humiliation for the patient and family.

Unfortunately, many hypomanic patients appear to feel extremely well, at least in the initial phases of an episode. The high spirits and energy, increased libidinal drive, and creativity typical of hypomania in the early phases of the illness often create an attractive aura for the family. Spouse and family members may also be caught up in this phase, a period that may, in time, become frightening to them. Specific behavior not in itself extreme may, over time, become an important clue for the family of an oncoming manic episode. One spouse informed us that before his wife's diagnosis was finally made, he would join her in Saturday morning shopping sprees across the city where they live, gleefully stopping at every street-corner stand to purchase illuminated paintings. His rationale, until the enormity of their purchases impressed him, was that he participated because he "feared her tastes were too tacky." Some patients repeat the same behavior with the onset of each new episode. One spouse reported that she would always know when her husband was becoming hypomanic because, unable to sleep, he would arise at 3 or 4 A.M. to make lengthy long-distance telephone calls "to save money." Many bipolar patients experience "mini-episodes" of depression and mania, even though they are taking medication and appear to be symptom free. Such episodes are generally manageable outside of the hospital, but they remain worrisome and may ultimately be destructive to the marital relationship. Some patients and families are sufficiently alert to early prodromal symptoms of depression or mania to be able to report them. In such instances, medication may be adjusted and hospitalization averted.

In a study in which they analyzed the progression of symptoms during the course of a manic episode in 20 hospitalized bipolar patients, Carlson and Goodwin (1973) provide an excellent account of three stages of mania. They describe the euphoria that seems to predominate in the initial stage of the patients' illness with increased psychomotor activity, including increased initiation and rate of speech and increased physical activity. The patients they describe were expansive, grandiose, overconfident, sexually preoccupied, and, though coherent, sometimes tangential. They had an increased interest in religion; inappropriate spending of money and increased smoking, telephone use, and letter writing were also observed. When the patient's many demands were not immediately satisfied, the mood would become one of irritability. These patients, though hospitalized, were not considered grossly out of control, and the behavioral symptoms described are, in fact, similar to those of bipolar patients who may remain in the community.

In the second stage, pressured speech and psychomotor activity increased further. Although the mood was predominantly euphoric, increased dysphoria and depression were noted. Irritability increased to open hostility and anger, and the accompanying behavior was frequently explosive and assaultive. Cognitive disorganization also increased, and racing thoughts progressed to flight of ideas. Earlier paranoid and grandiose thinking were now apparent as frank delusions.

The third stage, seen in 70% of the patients these investigators studied, was characterized by a panic-stricken, desperate, hopeless state, accompanied by frenzied and frequently bizarre psychotic activity. Incoherence and loosening of associations were observed, as were bizarre delusions. Ideas of reference, hallucinations, and disorientation as to time and place were present in this stage. Third-stage patients require hospitalization and are generally in seclusion.

The patients in this study were hospitalized in a research setting where it was possible to study the course of mania prior to the institution of drug treatment. All of the patients eventually received lithium carbonate treatment; some of the stage-three, or more disturbed, patients were treated with phenothiazines as well, and all responded positively to medication.

It is our impression that only a few clinicians other than those practicing in hospitals have experience with the more severely disturbed manic patient. However, prior to hospital admission, families are subjected to angry, assaultive, bizarre, and destructive behavior often relieved only by the arrival of the police or other help. Because they have lived through the experience, family members are usually able to provide an accurate first-hand account of events preceding an episode.

For example, the onset of Mrs. Smith's manic–depressive illness occurred at age 28. A highly competent attorney with no history of previous mood disturbance, she was married and the mother of one child. Both her father and a paternal uncle had been hospitalized for depression, and a maternal aunt had committed suicide. Mrs. Smith had participated actively in an important election campaign, working long hours, making speeches, and seeming to enjoy the rigors of political life. In retrospect, it appeared that she had not been sleeping; was both hyperactive and hypertalkative; had created a scene in her office, loudly insulting everyone in sight, which was uncharacteristic of her usual behavior; was expressing grandiose thoughts about her own fitness to become governor of her state; and for two successive nights before her hospital admission had not slept and had failed to come home because she was "too busy." She was taken to a hospital by the police and admitted for treatment of her manic episode after disrobing in a public park where she had been scheduled to speak for her candidate. She was treated with lithium carbonate, with symptom remission occurring in 20 days.

Later, in a conjoint therapy session, her husband asked in a subdued manner if she could remember what had happened and how she had felt during the episode. Her response was, "I can't remember being there. It's like amnesia. It's only after others keep telling me that I did something that I could remember being there. It's like being dead." Although she knew she had been manic, on a conscious level she appeared unable to realize that she had been inappropriate and unpleasant. When asked how she was currently feeling, she referred to the presence of dysphoric feelings and to her sensations in seclusion as the mania subsided.

Mrs. Smith: It's like being born every time I wake up. It's like coming out of the womb. I have my own personal checklist. First I check my senses, I open my eyes and see, but I don't know what I'm looking at, so I smell to see if I'm breathing, and listen to hear. And I go through the senses. Once I'm aware that I'm alive and not dead, I can begin to talk to others. It's only then do I find out where I am and what day it is. As they gave me more information, I slowly put the pieces together. Every day I wake up and go through this process and it gets easier and easier until I'm normal. As normal as I am today.

Another example of the onset of a manic episode in a hitherto undiagnosed patient occurred when Mr. Jones, 38 years old, was admitted to the hospital in restraints, having been brought from the high school where he was teaching. He had arrived at the school before classes, angry and upset, claiming that he had "lost his car." His mood escalated during the morning. He became hypertalkative, loud, and obscene, attracting the attention of the principal, who thought Mr. Jones was intoxicated. The hospital admission history provided by Mrs. Jones revealed that her husband had experienced several episodes of severe depression in the past. Most recently, he had been preoccupied with concerns that he would not be promoted to head of his department. At home, he had been autocratic, domineering, and threatening to his children. Mrs. Jones had resorted to sending the younger children to neighbors, while the older children crept into the house through windows to sleep, to avoid their father who had taken over the main floor of the home. Mr. Jones also had a positive multigenerational family history for affective disorder, including a grandmother who had died after 25 years in a mental hospital.

Depressive episodes, which are features of bipolar disorder, can also have a lasting impact for patient and family. Depression is a ubiquitous disorder with far-reaching effects. The onset of a clinical depression is generally more insidious then hypomania, but when untreated, a single episode can last an average of 1 year. Feelings of helplessness, worthlessness, guilt, anxiety, irritability, and lethargy are often experienced and are accompanied by behavioral changes. Frequent weeping, slowed speech and movement, agitation, inability to accomplish simple daily tasks (even those involving self-care), diminution or cessation of interest in previously pleasurable activities, impairment of occupational functioning, and suicidal gestures and attempts may have as devastating an impact upon the quality of life for patient and family as manic episodes. Studies at NIMH of lithium carbonate, the drug of choice in the treatment of bipolar disorder, have demonstrated its effectiveness in the treatment of depressive episodes, especially for bipolar patients. When pharmacological treatment is successful, however, the emotional and social problems of having had an episode of either depression or mania nonetheless remain for most patients and their families long after the episode has ended.

Studies of the manic–depressive patient conducted prior to the availability of effective medications consisted of descriptions of the intrapsychic dynamics and character structure of the bipolar patient that were intended to enable clinicians to understand pathogenesis and prescribe psychoanalytic treatment approaches. Now that pharmacotherapeutic interventions are available, these early investigations tend to be disregarded by many clinicians. However, it is our contention that more than drug treatment alone is needed for managing the intrapsychic and intrapersonal distress of the patient and for reducing the burden and impact that this illness has upon marriage and family. As suggested earlier, even with the best of current pharmacological treatments, bipolar patients remain at risk for recurrence and disruptions in their occupational, family, and social lives. In addition, approximately 20% of all diagnosed patients are nonresponsive to pharmacotherapy; some patients discontinue their medications; and others appear to break through medication, experiencing mild to severe mood episodes.

REVIEW OF THE LITERATURE

Freud (1917/1950) and Abraham (1924/1949) were among early psychoanalytic investigators who examined the family constellation of the bipolar patient and described the interpersonal interactions among its members. The early mother–child relationship, in which individuation and loss are first experienced and mastered, was viewed by them as a defective nurturing experience, with loss of narcissistic input and rage at the lost object central to their formulations regarding the continuing problems of the potential bipolar patient.

Jacobson (1956) also described an infantile narcissistic dependency on the lost object as central to the ego defect and interpersonal difficulties of the adult bipolar patient that were brought to the patient's marital relationship. Cohen, Baker, Cohen, Fromm-Reichmann, and Weigert (1954) focused on the early cultural environment and childhood events in the life of the bipolar patient, citing an unusual consistency in conforming to rigid family rules as an explanation of both the abnormal character formation of the patient and the repetitive recurrence of the disorder in families. Bipolar families were depicted as placing a high premium upon conformity in order to raise family social and economic status. Children were described as being pressed into service by the mothers to achieve prestige for the family, while fathers in these families were described as weak, though lovable. In addition to the thrust toward conventionality, they also saw hypomanic patients as possessing a certain social facility, able to provide an appearance of closeness by their liveliness, talkativeness, and social aggressiveness, an aggressiveness they perceived as being motivated not by hostility but by need, emptiness, and dependency. These patients were further described as being able to form only one, or a few, close dependent relationships, seeming to see others as either good or bad, with no allowance for human frailty (Cohen, *et al.*, 1954). Gibson (1958), in a continuation of this work pertaining to the family background and early life experience of the manic-depressive patient, described four characteristics of the manic–depressive character structure: (1) difficulty in dealing with feelings of envy and competition, (2) strong dependency drives, (3) the use of denial as a defense, and (4) a value system based on social conventionality.

Janowsky, Leff, and Epstein (1970) described the interpersonal maneuvers of the acutely manic patient in an article aptly entitled "Playing the Manic Game." They described their clinical experience in treating 15 acutely manic patients in a hospital setting. They observed how often the manic patient alienates family, friends, and therapists, and cited the following five types of activity in which the manic patient engages in order to induce discomfort in others: (1) manipulation of the self-esteem of others; (2) perceptiveness to vulnerability and conflict, which enables them to sense, reveal, and exploit areas of covert sensitivity in others; (3) projection of responsibility, or the ability to shift responsibility in such a way that others become responsible for their actions; (4) progressive limit testing, or "upping the ante," described as a phenomenon whereby the manic extends the limits imposed on him or her; and (5) alienating family members, a process by which the manic distances himself or herself from the family. They viewed the presence of these characteristics in the patients they studied as hallmarks of the interpersonal activity of the bipolar manic patient. In addition, these authors provided us with a classic description of manic and hypomanic behavior, contributing an important link in our understanding of how these patients can create such havoc in their significant relationships (Janowsky *et al.*, 1970). However, rather than the manic's having some clairvoyant or exceptional ability to discern weaknesses in others as they suggested, it may be that in actuality, the manic does not have greater perceptiveness but, as part of the expression of his or her illness, lacks inhibitions. Other people, in fact, may see as the manic sees, but have learned to exercise appropriate control and withhold comment.

Fitzgerald (1972) is among the few early investigators of drug and psychotherapy interaction who described issues related to treating the bipolar manic patient with lithium in combination with family therapy. He saw the manic episode as part of a behavioral pattern within manic–depressive psychoses that along with the chronic disorder, created emotional, social, legal, and psychological disturbance in the patient and those around him or her. For long-term prophylaxis, he advocated the use of medication along with "vigilance, individual and family therapy." However, in the years since his article was published, most clinicians have continued to rely on medication alone in treating the bipolar patient acutely, prophylactically, and in remission.

FAMILY ISSUES IN THE TREATMENT
OF BIPOLAR PATIENTS

In this section, we summarize our studies with collaborators at NIMH in which psychodynamic features of manic–depressive families and treatment issues were examined.

Initially, the interpersonal relationships of the married bipolar patient and spouse were studied, and the complex themes and features significant in the marital relationship were reported (Ablon, Davenport, Gershon, & Adland, 1975). During the course of multiple-family group therapy with married couples with a manic–depressive spouse, major themes related to their difficulties with loss and grief consistently emerged. Among these themes were (1) fears of recurrence of illness in spite of medication (2) the sense of helplessness in marriages that lacked ego boundaries, (3) the need to control all affect and defend against closeness, (4) the use of denial to manage hostility and anxiety, and (5) themes related to parental loss and failure to grieve (Ablon *et al.*, 1975).

Predominant interactional patterns found among bipolar families in which the illness had occurred in more than two generations also were studied, and the following additional characteristics identified: (1) unrealistic standards of conformity and self-expectation among all families' members; (2) displacement of parental feelings of low self-esteem onto the parents' own children; and (3) the tendency for members of the families to remain bound together and isolated in a closed system with little socialization outside the family network, limiting the opportunity for the introduction of new and different responses. We noted that these characteristics were not unique— that they could be found in many family constellations—but that their existence congruent with episodic illness in the bipolar family tended to perpetuate the self-defeating behavior, chaos, and disorganization observed. We suggested that the parents' inability to attend to their own wants and needs and the continual repression of grief and of the awareness of feelings were transmitted to the children born into these families. The relationship that formed between the married partners because of their own early life experiences led them to behavior that supports the denial of feelings. On the other hand, as part of a circular mechanism, the continual repression of rage, grief, and affection, even during well stages, reinforces the sense that the expression of feelings is not safe. Ultimately, the repression results in a chronic state of turmoil with destructive features, a condition that becomes the binding stable force in the bipolar family dynamic. In spite of medication, many bipolar couples and families continue to lead their lives as if there is nothing but the despair of depression or the euphoria of mania. There is no "grey area." The expression of affect or feeling remains unsafe, and within the bipolar family system, there seems to be a continuous collusion in the denial of feelings. Consequently, the appropriate communication of feelings is likely to be experienced as a loss of control that could be destructive to intimate relationships. The defensive maneuvering to avoid confrontation with conflict observed in the bipolar marital dyad is an unwillingness to replicate feelings of rage and grief over earlier unresolved parental losses and disappointments (Davenport *et al.*, 1979).

Manic–depressive families maintain close ties with their members, and the family unit continues to provide the major interactional experience for children born into such families. When seven infants were born at approximately the same time to couples with at least one parent in treatment at NIMH for bipolar disorder, we had an opportunity to test our hypotheses regarding the significance of psychocultural and psychodynamic factors in the familial occurrence and perpetuation of the disorder. When mothers from bipolar families participated with their offspring in a structured laboratory playroom paradigm, we found that by 18 months, children of bipolar parents showed less overt emotional response to temporary loss and separation from their mothers than did normal children. Mothers from bipolar families also showed fewer positive feelings toward their children and were significantly less active in interactions with them than normal control mothers. By 2 years of age, children with a bipolar parent had difficulty sharing with friends and handling hostility, and they exhibited measurable patterns of aggression. There were consistent differences in the bipolar and normal control children, and the social and emotional problems of the bipolar children appeared comparable to the interpersonal problems of their parents. Developmental deficits and mood disturbance constitute a major part of the pathology found in bipolar families, features that require a major psychotherapeutic treatment effort (Davenport *et al.*, 1984).

THE BIPOLAR FAMILY AS PATIENT

Historically, family therapy developed primarily as an effort to study and understand the function of the family in relation to the etiology of schizophrenia in order to provide treatment. In his excellent review of the family therapy field, Lansky (1981) noted that these early investigations "yielded no convincing evidence that family processes in and of themselves can cause schizophrenia" (p. 6). If family therapy was intended to alter pathological family systems sufficiently to reverse the schizophrenic process, in reality it served primarily to "modify the course of the disease rather than affect a cure" (p. 6).

The development, beginning in the early 1950s, of effective psychotropic drugs to treat many of the psychotic disorders previously considered untreatable, helped to forge a split between practitioners of biological psychiatry and the family therapy movement. The medical model, with its emphasis on diagnosis, phenomenology, and the treatment of the individual patient removed the onus of blame from the family but also led to the practice of excluding the family from the treatment. On the other hand, family therapists, tending to withdraw from treatment of the more severe disturbances or psychopathologies, focused on the development of theories of family systems and techniques to the exclusion of the need for diagnosis and pharmacotherapeutic treatment of the individual patient. As Lansky noted, psychoanalysis also evolved during this period, and concepts of object relations, projective identification, splitting, the psychology of the self, mirroring, and idealizing transferences were elaborated upon and added to a growing armamentarium of psychoanalytic insights in an effort to assist mental health professionals in understanding the intrapsychic and interpersonal experiences of the individual. However, it is our contention that the manner in which mental disturbance can so control and isolate bipolar patients and their families requires that clinicians understand the interdependence and utilitarianism of both the medical model and the family systems model.

We have alluded earlier in this chapter to our understanding of specific psychopathology found in the bipolar family system and to our treatment efforts combining pharmacotherapy and psychotherapy. In considering the treatment of the bipolar family, questions inevitably arise regarding indications for family therapy as well as for individual, couples, and group therapy. Is it possible to treat the hypomanic patient, and if so, at what stage in the cyclical process is treatment best begun? What evidence is there that psychotherapeutic treatment has an effect on outcome for patient and family? To address, first, the issue of the effectiveness of adjunctive psychotherapy, a comparative study was made of the outcomes of 65 married bipolar patients who had been hospitalized at NIMH for an acute manic episode and later discharged on lithium (Davenport *et al.*, 1977). At follow-up, which occurred from 2 to 10 years after discharge, it was found that 18 patients had experienced rehospitalization for an episode recurrence (some had independently discontinued medication), 14 patients were divorced, 2 were separated, and 3 had committed suicide. However, 12 patients who had been treated in a multiple-family therapy modality conjointly with their spouses had experienced no rehospitalizations or marital disruptions and were having a more benign posthospitalization course as measured by work status, social functioning, family functioning, and mental status. We found that involvement of the spouse in the psychotherapy counteracted the efforts of patients to distort, deny, and leave treatment; that fears regarding the genetic component of the illness could be addressed; that earlier drug and psychotherapeutic interventions occurred when a family member was present to warn of oncoming signs of episode recurrence; that the multiple-family group therapy modality supported the thrust toward socially desirable behavior (including medication adherence), and that anxiety-provoking transference issues, especially those of intimacy and closeness, could be more easily regulated than in a traditional dyadic therapy setting.

In a subsequent study of adherence to a prophylactic regime in which the medication-taking and appointment-keeping behaviors of 48 bipolar patients treated in two lithium clinics were assessed, a significant correlation between nonadherence and poor outcome was found (Connelly, Davenport, & Nurnberger, 1982). Patients who had been seen in one of the clinics in which family therapy was a conjunctive modality had a significantly better rate of adherence to their drug regime, and continuity of care was associated with appointment-keeping adherence. Although these were small samples in which premorbid or pretreatment differences were not accounted for, statistically the results tend to support the usefulness of conjunctive psychotherapy in which patient and family can be engaged.

At what stage is it possible to initiate family therapy if the patient is manic, hypomanic, or acutely depressed? Productive family work can begin as part of obtaining the history, identifying family interactional and interpersonal problems, and reviewing with them the diagnosis and probable course of the disorder. Sadly, there are yet families who traverse doctors offices and family agencies describing the ongoing chaos and despair in their homes without receiving recognition that the behavior they are describing may be symptomatic of a bipolar disorder. Denial on the part of the patient and often the family is also an impediment to early recognition and treatment. However, once the diagnosis has been established, and patient, family, and therapist, are willing to deal with it, we believe the work can begin. It has been our experience that families are willing to be involved and to become a part of the treatment process. Family members can provide the clinician with valuable information, and their involvement gives them an opportunity to learn about the illness in a systematic manner and to reduce individual anxiety through questions and resultant discussion. Interpretation, intervention, and reeducation designed to change maladaptive defenses, improve communication patterns, and introduce constructive coping mechanisms are the goals if the family psychopathology is to be altered.

On a few occasions, we have held conjoint sessions with patients and their spouses in the patients' seclusion rooms in order to continue therapeutic work already begun. We have also escorted seclusion-room patients to the family therapy room and have witnessed their ability to behave appropriately in the company of spouse and children. We have also participated in family sessions in which the patient was in an acute depressive phase and have been surprised to note that it is possible for the withdrawn, seemingly mute patient to rouse and respond with feeling at times when something of a provocative nature has been said by another family member. Most hospitals today have some understanding of the desirability of avoiding total isolation of the psychotic patient, and many are experimenting with Dutch doors outside the seclusion room or with double doors that provide access space between seclusion room and corridor, where patient and a staff member or a family member may sit together. A certain tenacity on the part of the therapist, concern and consideration, and perhaps an intuitive understanding of how much the patient, family members, and the therapist can bear will dictate therapeutic efforts with the acutely ill patient.

What is gained by such intervention? Perhaps little apparent insight into psychic structure at such times, but availability and persistence are key words in both short- and long-term treatment. These qualities in the therapist are essential for the treatment to succeed, and differ from those that were generally experienced by these patients in their early lives. More often, they have experienced rejection and isolation as responses to their expression of feeling. This is why the continuity and availability expressed through regularly scheduled and maintained meetings causes many patients to remark to their families and therapists that the conjoint family meetings were the most important happening in their hospitalization because they learned that they were not alone. We have treated bipolar patients for many years and believe that the continuity and trust established during the early acute and difficult phases of an episode, before medication was started or before it began to have an effect, enabled many patients to continue to take their medication and to come with their families after discharge to outpatient sessions.

Family members, particularly in the initial sessions, gain an understanding of the basic symptomatology of the disorder, so that the patient no longer appears as bestial or noncaring but instead as suffering from a specific disorder. We have often included in sessions children as young as 6 years of age. Throughout the course of parental illness, they may have suffered from the unavailability of a parent, along with inconsistency in nurturance. They may not understand the reasons for the distress experienced, but they can talk about it, and seem to gain strength and support from the total family sessions: Childrens' fantasies, especially regarding causality, are often worse than the reality. Family members, as well, have an opportunity to discuss the impact of the manic or depressed behavior on their lives, in a less harsh and judgmental environment. A spouse who can describe the vicissitudes that result from a patient's writing of bad checks may not always find that future behavior is necessarily modified by the open expression of anger but will at least learn in the family session to control the bank account and the use of credit cards by the patient with less guilt feeling. We have found that family therapy work with the bipolar patient provides a framework for assessing intrafamilial interactions and for intervening, so that communication skills among family members can be improved and conflict solving can be learned. When the marital partners are seen alone, sexual problems can be addressed, negative feelings and anger expressed, and new techniques of adaptation learned. Family sessions are generally very lively when the patient is hypomanic, and sometimes it appears that the therapist's function is to contain the discussion providing boundaries and controls. But the euphoric behavior, the distortions and exaggerations, in time become grist for the therapeutic mill.

Because children are so important and so intimately involved in the life of the bipolar family, we have suggested that modifications in child rearing may be possible through interventions emphasizing the following ideas in the family therapy: (1) that at successive developmental stages, a variety of behaviors by the child may be age appropriate; (2) that the expression of feelings, whether grief, anger, or affection, is acceptable; (3) that loss and change occurs in the early mother–infant relationship and throughout life; (4) that in order to accomplish this, there must be a capability for mourning and resolution; (5) that conflict and differences are not inherently destructive; (6) that limit setting is a parental responsibility, reflecting parental concern, that helps children learn to control impulsive feelings and to mourn; (7) that dependence is a perfectly appropriate human experience, but that excessive and rigid family interdependence hinders maturation and healthy development; and (8) that observing and participating in experiences with other families can produce growth and strength (Davenport *et al.*, 1984).

CASE PRESENTATIONS

THE CASE OF MRS. JONES

Mrs. Jones is a 50-year-old married mother of 8 offspring whose first psychiatric disturbance occurred 8 years ago. A depressive episode characterized by profound lethargy, weeping and sadness, inability to complete minimal household tasks, and eventual withdrawal to bed led to outpatient treatment with tricyclic antidepressants for a period of 2 years, with little change. The depression had occurred in proximity to the marriage of her oldest child and only daughter. A full-blown episode of mania led to an extended hospitalization, which lasted 1 year. During that time, she was treated unsuccessfully with various antidepressants, including monoamine oxidase inhibitors and carbamazepine as well as lithium carbonate. Since discharge from the hospital, she has continued to cycle unrelentingly, with periods of hypomania lasting 2 weeks and alternating with similar-length periods of severe depression. Currently, she is on a regime of low doses of lithium and carbamazepine, which has altered the severity of the episodes slightly but has not changed the frequency.

The history obtained from Mr. Jones presented a premorbid picture of an energetic and intellectual woman who was resourceful and well liked in the community where the family lived. Both her deceased father, who committed suicide when the patient was 16 years old, and her paternal grandfather had histories of pronounced mood swings and are assumed to have had bipolar illness. The paternal grandfather lived in the family home until his death, and the patient vividly recalls the profound effect this model of depression and hypomania had upon her childhood.

At the time family therapy began, the older Jones children had assumed responsibility for cooking the meals, managing the shopping and the laundry, and generally attending to the needs of the two younger children so that they were properly dressed and sent off to school. During the first four family sessions, all of the children were present. They discussed the resentments they felt when their mother's mood switched from depression to hypomania, especially how they resented her attempts in the first few days of mood elevation to reestablish her standards and control. They felt that she was oblivious to what was actually happening in the family and explained that her unavailability during a depression, when they had to be responsible, was experienced as an abandonment. In this family, however, it became clear that in spite of resenting their mother's seeking to reclaim control during the first hypomanic days, the children nonetheless preferred her to be hypomanic, when fantasies could be acted out, no limits were set, and the children were swept along in the infectious high spirits of the patient.

During hypomanic periods, Mr. Jones perceived his wife as untrustworthy, a spendthrift, and neglectful of him and the children. Mr. Jones also seemed to prefer the hypomanic phase, which is unusual since many bipolar spouses prefer the period when the patient is depressed and less active. Although he resented the patient's threats of divorce that invariably occurred during her hypomanias and that were linked to her lack of access to money and credit cards which he controlled, Mr. Jones also experienced comfort and gratification from the high energy level and the excitement of the hypomanic phase. He was pleased by the increase in sexual activity and excited, as well, by the patient's many plans and ideas, which, though sometimes bizarre, were perceived as sound and reasonable enough to be tolerable.

During the year the patient was in the hospital, the family was seen weekly. After that, Mr. Jones and the children came in only when there was a marital or family-focused problem or when they felt a need for support during a particularly trying episode. Mrs. Jones continued as an outpatient in individual therapy for many years. Over time, sessions focused on the despair she felt about her remorseless illness, her losses, and her sense of being a "useless" person. In individual sessions, she was able to articulate conflictual and ambivalent feelings, areas that became available because of the family work. During "good" periods, she would talk about the possibilities that she could reintegrate and become a functioning person again. With two exceptions, she remained out of the hospital. One of them entailed a brief stay when she was admitted for reevaluation of her medication. The other occasion, which was also brief, occurred when the therapist who had treated the patient and her family throughout this period announced her departure from the area. Shortly afterward, the patient had an episode in which she smashed and destroyed objects in her house, and the therapist was summoned in the middle of the night. The patient insisted that the destructiveness had nothing to do with the coming loss of the therapist—that it merely represented anger felt toward Mr. Jones, who happened to be away on a business trip. Needless to say, this painful incident was also invaluable in the psychotherapy in working through the termination.

This may not be a vignette that portrays success, because the patient continues to have cycles and remains severely impaired by her illness. However, the marriage is intact; the children are coping relatively successfully in high school and college, and have dealt well with the possible heritable aspects of the illness; and the patient takes her medication, which, at best, alleviates her symptoms only slightly, and has begun therapeutic work with a new and interested therapist.

THE CASE OF MRS. SMITH

Mrs. Smith is a 42-year-old, several times divorced mother of an 8-year-old son. The onset of her illness began at age 19, when she was hospitalized for depression during her sophomore year in college. In the hospital, she switched into a hypomanic episode; though her behavior was clearly documented in the medical chart, the patient was discharged with the diagnosis of a unipolar depression, unchanged. She was able to return to college and graduate. For the next 4 years, her history included numerous flights across the country and to the Caribbean, a sequence of marriages and divorces, and a progressively worsening series of jobs. She was again admitted to the hospital after coming to the attention of a mental hygiene clinic where she had been brought by friends who found her trying to jump from her apartment window "like supergirl." She thought that she was a misunderstood genius, "with an IQ of 187," who was certain to win a Pulitzer prize for her as yet unwritten novel. Mrs. Smith had a positive response to lithium, but after a year, decided she no longer needed the medication and was soon readmitted to the hospital once again in a manic state.

The patient was in seclusion for 4 weeks, during which time she was boldly psychotic, smearing feces and urine. Lithium was introduced again, with a good response, and family therapy sessions were begun. Her parents, through all of the turmoil surrounding her illness-related behaviors, had remained important in her life. They were a well-educated, upper-middle-class couple who expressed distress and humiliation over the change in the patient's behavior since her early years as an exemplary student and model daughter. By history, they tended to be overly controlling and intrusive, with high expectations of achievement for their only child. In the therapy, these issues were often addressed, and they lessened somewhat in the hospital to the extent that the patient was eventually able to leave the parental home.

The patient's dependence upon her parents, however, remains a current reality factor with qualitative differences. She remarried, but her husband deserted her after the birth of their child, again causing the patient to become financially dependent upon her parents. She was removed from lithium treatment during her pregnancy; during the postpartum period, she had a brief manic episode, which was managed out of the hospital, in the parent's home, by the therapists until lithium was reinstituted; subsequently, the patient returned with her child to her own apartment.

The vignette also may not seem a success story, but in the intervening years, Mrs. Smith has managed to work and raise her child with her parents' help and the support of her therapist. She has a better understanding of the relationship between her grandiosity and despair on the one hand, and the spoken and unspoken demands and expectations of others in her life on the other. She is seen for weekly psychotherapy and continues to take her lithium, and both parents feel able to call the therapist when they have concerns. The support that this family has received, and the fact that they have been willing to go beyond the family boundaries to seek it, enhances the possibility that Mrs. Smith's child will have the opportunity to be exposed to a larger community, to learn different ways of coping.

THE CASE OF MR. WHITE

Mr. White, a 42-year-old lawyer and separated father of three children, was admitted to the hospital in a hypomanic state. His wife's announcement that she intended to leave him for someone else had preceded a succession of disruptive hypomanic activities. At the time of admission, Mr. White was living with his parents. He was brought to the hospital by his father and brother after a night spent gardening by flashlight, followed by turning the hose into the home when attempts were made to restrain his activities. Although this was considered a first psychiatric admission, the history provided by the mother, who smiled continuously during the telling, suggested that Mr. White may have had an earlier hypomanic or manic episode while in college. That event involved Mr. White's driving over 90 miles per hour on a freeway before he crashed his car into a concrete abutment—a crash that he miraculously survived, though he did suffer numerous injuries and underwent a lengthy medical hospitalization. His history also included treatment for depression as an outpatient. Mr. White's father suffered from depressions, and during the course of our work with the family, he, too, was placed on lithium.

In addition to fearing the loss of his wife and children, Mr. White also feared the loss of his job in his law firm, although this latter information had not been shared by the patient with his family. The dual narcissistic injuries appeared to be more than he could bear. The patient's father, an obsessive man who had retired early from his government job and who still mourned its loss, was assisted in the sessions in becoming considerably more understanding and empathic.

Many of the interventions with this family seem, in retrospect, quite simple. The patient's wife decided to seek a divorce and gave custody of the children to her husband, who was ultimately able to reconcile himself to her loss and is now himself engaged to be married. He lives with their children in his parents' home and is functioning at a high level in a new law firm. He and his father both are now on medication, and the patient continues his psychotherapeutic treatment. His fiancée is also willingly participating in couples therapy. Again, the continuity of treatment and the availability of the therapist may have made a difference in the outcome.

THE CASE OF MS. GREEN

Ms. Green, a 21-year-old single college student, was admitted for her fifth psychiatric hospitalization in 2 years in a depressed state. The onset of her illness occurred in proximity to receiving unsatisfactory grades in her premed courses. At that time, her parents noted that the patient brooded and seemed upset, uncertain, and unlike her usual self. When she became quite lethargic, she was seen by the family doctor, who diagnosed "emotional exhaustion" and advised "rest." The patient then dropped out of school. Shortly afterward, she suddenly became hyperactive, made numerous telephone calls, rang doorbells after midnight to talk with neighbors, charged $1,500 in clothing to her parents, and seemed sexually preoccupied. An additional stress factor described by the parents appeared to be related to the patient's ambivalent feelings about her engagement and approaching marriage.

Ms. Green was first treated with Mellaril as an outpatient, but when she could not sleep and continued to be hyperactive, she was admitted to a hospital for 2 weeks. Her course over the next 2 years included treatment with neuroleptics and lithium carbonate, without noticeable success. Following her first hospital discharge, she immediately became depressed and had suicidal thoughts, necessitating rehospitalization after 4 days.

The parents, a warm and deeply concerned couple, were distraught as they described their grief and despair as well as their helplessness and inability to control the patient and set limits for her when her mood was elevated. They were sophisticated about the use of medication, understood the ramifications of her illness, and had hopes for a good prognosis. Initially, the couple denied there was affective disorder in the family. However, during the course of taking a systematic family history, the patient's mother referred to all of the women in her family as "high strung," and it was learned that her only sibling had had two postpartum depressions, that a maternal uncle had committed suicide, and that her mother had had periods of marked hyperactivity for many years, including cleaning the house at three or four in the morning. The parents felt that the patient's childhood and adolescent years had been quite normal. However, there were discrepancies in their recall, as it appeared that though not moody, "she easily became upset, even by little things." Described by the parents as "popular," the patient was also said to be "generally shy . . . always trying to get in," always "missing out on having girlfriends." It appeared that the patient, in order to maintain one steady relationship, had become engaged at an early age. The parents also described the patient's premorbid personality as "obsessive," as a "perfectionist," and as having a strong counterdependency phobia.

As the family therapy unfolded, a highly competitive family was revealed. Both parents were "self-made" and had achieved considerable wealth in a joint business endeavor. The patient's older brother and sister had been high achievers in college. The patient had never lacked for material things because of the family affluence which irritated the parents, who felt that wealth should be an asset for their daughter in the acquisition of friendships. Issues of oedipal and sibling rivalry and dependence–independence conflicts were addressed in the family therapy.

During this second hospitalization, lithium was again introduced and this time brought about positive results—the patient's episodes subsided. She remained in individual psychotherapy after discharge from the hospital and eventually returned to college.

TREATMENT ISSUES: DENIAL AND DEPENDENCY

Although the responsivity of the bipolar patient to medication supports the probability of biological abnormality, this may be only one determinant. Developmental arrests constitute a major part of the pathology these patients bring to the clinician, which are now accessible because of the combination of drug treatment and psychotherapy.

In a report in 1985 (Davenport & Adland), we expanded on denial and dependency as important issues in understanding and treating bipolar family psychopathology. Denial serves as a major avoidance mechanism against painful feelings and as an ego defense against processing distressing information. Attempts to cope with feelings of rage and helplessness are uncomfortable for patient and family because they provoke earlier feelings of helplessness, loss, and grief and reinforce the need for denial. In turn, this may precipitate even further withdrawal from those in the family and social environment, again representing further object loss and its consequences. Massive denial to avoid confrontation with conflict is a defensive maneuver observed over and over in the bipolar family and in the marital dyad. When a manic episode occurs, enormous anxiety is provoked; in the marital relationship, a primitive denial serves to protect patient and family against awareness of loss, reinforcing the desire for strict control of affects. Denial remains a consistent, pervasive, and persistent defense with which patient, family, and therapist must struggle.

In the marital relationship of the bipolar patient, the spouse is often viewed by the patient as the withholder or donor of gratifications. Provocativeness in their relationship is often the result of unresolved dependency issues and fears of object loss that predate the marriage. These are issues that serve to bring these couples together, perpetuating the unspoken pattern of need and mutual dependency and fears of loss from one generation to the next. In the bipolar marriages we have observed, there is always a need for one spouse to be in the dependent position; there is seldom parity at any given time. Needs must also be fulfilled in these marriages, even though the demand is never articulated. The patient bypasses the feelings of loss or sadness when needs are unmet, kindling an escalating rage. The rage then rebounds from one specific issue to encompass general condemnation of the depriving family member. When the infantile wish of the patient is unfulfilled and the demand warded off, anxiety rises and unbearable emotional pain explodes. Understanding this phenomenon, confronting and resolving dependency issues, and learning to reach reasonable resolutions constitute a major part of the therapeutic task in the treatment of the bipolar family.

CONCLUSION

We have attempted to address issues regarding therapeutic interventions in the treatment of bipolar patients and their families, and as is often true of the investigator in the laboratory, we cannot say with absolute assurance which strategies work. We can only provide a theoretical base for our treatment efforts, describe what happened, and report the outcome. This is a familial disorder. It occurs in families; its presence in one family member affects everyone else in the family. In the family therapy work, it is not just the identified patient who represents the problem. It is possible in the family sessions to address issues of loss, separation, and individuation, problems shared by bipolar families. The lives of these patients and their families have been impoverished by the presence of an illness, but in the family therapy setting, they can talk about the emptiness of their lives and the difficult aspects. Awareness of psychodynamic issues enables patient and family members to sort out together practical aspects of living with this recurrent disorder and enables them to engage further in preventative measures. Studies have begun as an outgrowth of our family work with children of bipolar patients, children at risk who were brought into a laboratory at NIMH 6 years ago. These studies may open new territories for further examination of family treatment of the bipolar patient (Zahn-Waxler *et al.*, 1988).

REFERENCES

Ablon, S. L., Davenport, Y. B., Gershon, E. S., & Adland, M. L. (1975). The married manic. *American Journal of Orthopsychiatry, 45*, 854–866.

Abraham, K. (1949). Notes on the psychoanalytical investigation and treatment of manic-depressive insanity and allied conditions. In D. Bryan and A. Strachey (Trans.), *Selected papers on psychoanalysis* (pp. 418–480). London: Hogarth Press. (Original work published 1924)

American Psychiatric Association (1987). *Diagnostic and statistical manual of mental disorders* (rev. 3rd ed.). Washington, DC: APA.

Carlson, G. A., & Goodwin, F. K. (1973). The stages of mania: A longitudinal analysis of the manic episode. *Archives of General Psychiatry, 28*, 221–228.

Cohen, M. B., Baker, G., Cohen, R. A., Fromm-Reichmann, F., & Weigert, E. V. (1954). An intensive study of 12 cases of manic–depressive psychosis. *Psychiatry, 17*, 103–137.

Connelly, C. E., Davenport, Y. B., & Nurnberger, J. L. (1982). Adherence to treatment regimen in a lithium carbonate clinic. *Archives of General Psychiatry, 30*, 585–588.

Davenport, Y. B., & Adland, M. L. (1985). Issues in the treatment of the married bipolar patient: Denial and dependency. In M. R. Lansky (Ed.), *Family approaches to major psychiatric disorders* (pp. 46–65). Washington, DC: American Psychiatric Press.

Davenport, Y. B., Adland, J. L., Gold, P. W., & Goodwin, F. K. (1979). Manic–depressive illness: Psychodynamic features of multigenerational families. *American Journal of Orthopsychiatry, 49*, 24–35.

Davenport, Y. B., Ebert, M. H., Adland, M. L., & Goodwin, F. K. (1977). Couples group therapy as an adjunct to lithium maintenance of the manic patient. *American Journal of Orthopsychiatry, 47*, 495–502.

Davenport, Y. B., Zahn-Wexler, C., Adland, M. L., & Mayfield, A. (1984). Early child-rearing practices in families with a manic–depressive parent. *American Journal of Psychiatry, 141*, 230–235.

Fitzgerald, R. (1972). Mania as a message: Treatment with family therapy and lithium carbonate. *American Journal of Psychiatry, 26*, 547–555.

Freud, S. (1950). Mourning and melancholia. In E. Jones (Ed.) and J. Riviere (Trans.), *Collected Papers* (Vol. 4, pp. 152–170). London: Hogarth Press. (Original work published in 1917)

Gibson, R. (1958). The family background and early life experience of the manic–depressive patient. *Psychiatry, 21*, 71–90.

Jacobson, E. (1956). Interaction between psychotic partners: I. Manic–depressive partners. In V. E. Eisenstein (Ed.), *Neurotic interaction in marriage* (pp. 125–134). New York: Wiley.

Janowsky, D. S., Leff, M., & Epstein, R. S. (1970). Playing the manic game: Interpersonal maneuvers of the acutely manic patient. *Archives of General Psychiatry, 22*, 252–261.

Kraepelin, E. (1921). Manic–depressive insanity and paranoia (M. Barclay, Trans.). Edinburgh: S. Livingstone Ltd. (Original work published in 1913)

Lansky, M. R. (1981). Introduction. In M. R. Lansky (Ed.), *Family therapy and major psychopathology* (pp. 3–17). New York: Grune & Stratton.

NIMH/NIH Consensus Development Conference Statement. (1985). Mood disorders: Pharmacologic prevention of recurrences. *American Journal of Psychiatry, 142,* 469–476.

Zahn-Waxler, C., Mayfield, A., Radke-Yarrow, M., Mcknew, D., Cytryn, L., & Davenport, Y. B. (1988). A follow-up investigation of offspring of bipolar parents. *American Journal of Psychiatry, 145,* 506–509.

9

Genetic Issues in Treatment

STEVEN D. TARGUM

Many individuals harbor fears that depressive disorders are "genetic" and may be transmitted from generation to generation in their families. These fears are not unfounded, given the consistency of research findings suggesting that genetic factors do contribute to the development of depressive disorders in some families (Gershon, Targum, Kessler, Mazure, & Bunney, 1977; Kay, 1979; Perris, Ericsson, & Knorring, 1982; Schlesser & Altshuler, 1983; Tsuang & Vandermey, 1980). The possibility that genetic determination may yield depression poses a psychological threat to many people because it affects their ability to consciously determine their mental life (Targum, 1981). In fact, the mere concept of "genetic" illness creates a powerful psychodynamic factor that can be sufficient to limit the progress of any course of therapy. Fears about genetic illness may yield overt anxiety or worry independent of the depressive disorder. Further, the affective components of depressive disorders may be compounded by these anxieties and misconceptions related to the spectre of "genetic" illness.

Consequently, the resolution of the emotional sequelae of a purported genetic illness may be necessary in order to facilitate the accomplishment of other goals in treatment. It is imperative that a therapist be open to examining genetic issues when they emerge in the course of treatment. Although many situations necessitate referrals to genetic counselors, it may be possible in some instances to incorporate the principles of genetic counseling into the ongoing therapy (Kay, 1979; Targum & Gershon, 1981; Targum & Schulz, 1982; Tsuang, 1978). Genetic counseling aims to provide scientifically valid information within the framework of a short-term, supportive therapeutic relationship (Kallmann, 1954; Targum & Schultz, 1982; Tsuang, 1978). It is the purpose of this chapter to consider the potential implications and clinical applications of psychiatric genetics in the treatment of depressive disorders. "Depression," as used in this chapter, refers to the description in the DSM III-R (American Psychiatric Association, 1987).

THE COMPONENTS OF
PSYCHIATRIC GENETIC COUNSELING

Several authors have described a systematic and rational approach to psychiatric genetic counseling that may be summarized as follows (Kay, 1979; Tsuang, 1978; Targum & Schultz, 1982; Kallmann, 1954; Targum & Gershon, 1981).

1. Establish a supportive, interactive relationship.
2. Assess the motive for the genetic consultation.
3. Assess the client's (the patient's) preconceptions and expectations about genetic counseling.
4. Assess the client's concepts about the illness and perceptions of the burden of the illness.
5. Assess the client's capacity to comprehend genetic information and statistical data.
6. Obtain accurate psychiatric diagnoses of all family members, and determine estimates of empirical risk for the occurrence of illness in unaffected family members.
7. Communicate the genetic information.
8. Help to alleviate anxiety and the emotional sequelae of a genetic diagnosis.
9. Assist but do not direct individuals in considering personal plans in light of the genetic information.
10. Monitor the client longitudinally through periodic follow-ups, in order to assess the outcome of counseling and the psychiatric status and course of illness in the family system.

It is important to consider the circumstances that lead up to the emergence of a genetic issue in the course of therapy. Often, it is important to examine where the individual or the family system is in the life cycle in order to ascertain the motive behind the genetic concerns. Frequently, psychiatric genetic counseling follows the emergence of psychiatric illness in a near relative and the resultant development of fears and/or curiosity about the risk of illness to other family members. Alternatively, genetic determination may become important when individuals are considering marriage, conception, abortion, or adoption. Depending upon the circumstances that have led up to the emergence of genetic issues, the therapeutic task will vary from alleviating anxiety and/or reactive depression, to clarifying misunderstanding through education, to assisting in decision making via a supportive therapeutic approach. The role of the therapist is complicated by the difficulties that exist in making specific psychiatric diagnoses in family members and by the lack of unequivocal genetic data relating to these psychiatric disorders. Given the poignancy inherent in a disorder that conveys both genetic and psychiatric implications and labels, it is critical that the therapist be open to his or her own feelings prior to examining the feelings, needs, and reactions of the patient. Genetic counseling requires a relationship based upon trust, respect, confidentiality, and receptivity between the patient and therapist (counselor). In some instances, a psychotherapist may believe that the supportive and interactive structure necessary for providing effective genetic counseling might inhibit the established structure of the therapeutic relationship. In these instances, it is better to refer the individual and/or the family to a genetic counselor, who can provide an independent assessment outside of the psychotherapeutic setting.

A depressive disorder may be viewed differently by family members based upon the effect that the illness has had on their own life experiences. The family may perceive the depressed patient's illness differently than the patient (Ablon, Davenport, & Gershon, 1975; Carlson, Kotin, & Davenport, 1974; Janowsky, Leff, & Epstein, 1970; Targum & Gershon, 1981). Janowsky and co-workers (Janowsky *et al.*, 1970) reported that the well spouse often felt that the manic phase of bipolar disorder was a willful, spiteful act, whereas the patient felt unfairly victimized and blamed for things beyond his or her control. Targum and Gershon (1981) documented the regrets about marriage and childbearing that the well spouse of bipolar patients expressed and the extensive denial by the patients themselves. In a sample of 19 couples, 53% of well spouses, in contrast to only 5% of bipolar patients, stated that they would not have married had they known more about the illness prior to marriage. Similarly, 47% of well spouses, compared to only 5% of bipolar patients, stated that they would not have had children had they known more about the illnes prior to making the decision about childbearing. Many of these families experienced the burden of bipolar disorder prior to the advent of lithium carbonate therapy, which has clearly improved the prognosis for a more functional life in affected individuals. In fact, some families may now discount the burdensome aspects of a depressive disorder in light of positive aspects they may attribute to the condition. Family members, including the patient, may emphasize the increased capacity and energy noted during the manic phase of bipolar disorder and may dismiss the possibility of personal failure, chronic illness, incapacity, or suicide in weighing the burden of the disorder for the family.

The communication of genetic information requires a description of statistical data. These figures are subject to personal interpretation. Some degree of mathematical sophistication is required in order to use numbers to reflect the perception of odds. Therefore it is helpful to examine the concept of mathematical risk as well as individual biases regarding genetic determination prior to providing empirical risk figures. Family members who deny the possibility of genetic determination of a depressive disorder may be shocked to hear the findings of genetic research data, whereas others who readily accept a concept of "genetic" depression may be entirely unaffected or relieved by a presentation of the same data.

An accurate diagnosis of all family members is critical in providing a useful psychogenetic assessment. The application of objective clinical criteria for psychiatric disorders is possible through the use of structured interviews, careful family history evaluations, and diagnostic criteria. Wherever possible, corroborative personal interviews with other family members may help to document the extent of illness in a particular family and to improve the meaning of the empirical risk figure. The inclusion of other family members, particularly more distant relatives, may become an issue in the course of treatment that could preclude these evaluations. The potential value of this information relative to its impact upon the existing therapeutic relationship must be weighed, and the alternative of a referral to a genetic counselor reconsidered, when family diagnoses through corroborative interviews are considered inadvisable. Ultimately, the assessment of the family psychiatric history will yield a pedigree that reveals the extent of psychiatric disorder in this family system. A family history that is loaded with homotypic (similar type) psychiatric disorder would indicate a greater genetic loading and higher risk for other family members than a family history that reveals little, if any, psychiatric disorder. There may be heterogeneity, such that all forms of psychiatric disorder in the family do not have the same presentation. A spectrum of depressive disorders, including dysthymia, cyclothymia, panic disorder, and alcoholism, may coexist with more specific major depressive disorders like bipolar and unipolar disorder (Gershon *et al.*, 1977; Targum & Gershon, 1981; Gershon *et al.*, 1982). The information gathered from the pedigree is incorporated with published pooled data relating empirical risk figures developed from accumulated studies in order to consider the possibility of genetic factors in the development of depressive disorder in a particular family. A summary of empirical risk figures for depressive disorders is provided later in this chapter.

A description of the risk for developing a depressive disorder is not given until all of the preceding information is gathered. At this point, the counselor or therapist ought to be prepared to facilitate the client's comprehension of the genetic information and to deal with his or her emotional response to it. In genetic counseling, it is generally preferable to use a nondirective approach in which decisions regarding the genetic information are left to the client. In psychotherapy, the response to the information may yield new material that can be explored as part of the treatment.

Genetic counseling for psychiatric disorders is a longitudinal process in which there is a need for periodic follow-up in the family system. Depressive disorders are not constant, and the need for clinical management and new interventions may change over time. Other family members may become ill, and this will influence the perception of burden within the entire family system.

THE GENETICS OF DEPRESSIVE DISORDERS

Numerous studies have suggested that genetic factors do contribute to the development of depressive disorders (Gershon *et al.*, 1977; Gershon *et al.*, 1982; Kay, 1979; Perris *et al*, 1982; Schlesser & Altshuler, 1983; Tsuang & Vandermey, 1980). Though purists may forever argue the validity of these studies, the data supporting genetic hypotheses are overwhelming and compelling. Studies of twins, families, and adopted children have consistently shown a significantly higher risk rate for the development of depressive disorder in the first-degree relatives (parents, siblings, offspring) of depressed patients as compared to the general population.

Studies of twins compare concordance rates between monozygotic (MZ) and dizygotic (DZ) twins. The actual concordance rates determined vary among investigators because of methodological differences in their studies. However, all studies have revealed high concordance rates for MZ twins—rates that are substantially greater than those for DZ twins (Gershon *et al.*, 1977; Kay, 1979; Perris *et al.*, 1982; Schlesser & Altshuler, 1983; Tsuang & Vandermey, 1980). Pooled data from nine studies reviewed by Schlesser and Altshuler (1983) revealed an MZ concordance rate for depressive disorders, (both bipolar and unipolar) of 74.7%, in contrast to a 19.8% rate among DZ twins. The data might be criticized because MZ twins are unique in their similarity, which sets them apart from the general population, and their unique relationship could conceivably exacerbate problems if they were reared together. However, Price (1968) reviewed the outcome of 12 MZ twin pairs who were reared apart and found in that group a concordance rate of 67% for the development of depressive disorders, implying that the MZ concordance rate is not due to a shared environment.

Family studies of depressive disorders include, as part of the methodology, both the indirect accumulation of family history and direct personal interviews with family members. These studies invariably demonstrate a greater rate of depressive disorder in the first-degree relatives of depressed individuals than the rate found in such relatives in the general population (Gershon *et al.*, 1977; Gershon *et al.*, 1982; Kay, 1979; Perris *et al.*, 1982; Schlesser & Altshuler, 1983; Tsuang & Vandermey, 1980). Pooled data from 12 family studies of bipolar patients revealed an overall rate of depressive disorder of 23% in first-degree relatives (11.5% bipolar and 11.5% unipolar). Pooled data from seven family studies of unipolar patients revealed an overall rate of 14.9% in first-degree relatives (1% bipolar disorder and 13.9% unipolar disorder). Most studies have found the rate of bipolar disorder in the general population to be less than 1%, and the rate of unipolar disorder, 2–3% (Gershon *et al.*, 1977; Gershon, *et al.*, 1982; Targum & Schulz, 1982; Tsuang & Vandermey, 1980). Thus the rate of depressive disorder in the first-degree relatives of depressed individuals is 10 to 20 times greater than that found in the general population (Gershon *et al.*, 1977; Gershon *et al.*,

1982; Kay, 1979; Perris *et al.*, 1982; Schlesser & Altshuler, 1983; Tsuang & Vandermey, 1980). It is of interest that the rate of illness found in second-degree relatives is not significantly greater than that found in the general population. These studies found a rate of schizophrenia among first-degree relatives that was no greater than that found in the general population (less than 1%), supporting the belief that depressive disorders and schizophrenia are distinct entities (Gershon *et al.*, 1982; Schlesser & Altshuler, 1983).

Gershon and co-workers (Gershon *et al.*, 1982) completed a comprehensive study of depressive disorders in families of patients admitted for treatment to the National Institute of Mental Health as well as in families of a comparison group of nonpsychiatric patients who were admitted to the medical units of the National Institutes of Health. Psychiatric patients had diagnoses of schizoaffective disorder, bipolar I (manic–depressive) disorder, bipolar II (hypomanic–depressive) disorder, and unipolar disorder. The investigators directly interviewed 1,254 adult relatives of patients and controls and found a lifetime prevalence of depressive disorders of 20%–37% in the relatives of the psychiatric patients in contrast to only 7% in the relatives of patients in the medical comparison group. This study also examined the consequences of illness upon offspring. Whereas 74% of the offspring of two depressive parents developed illness, only 27% of the offspring of one depressive parent did. The rate of depressive disorders in grandparents, uncles, and aunts (second-degree relatives) was considerably lower than that found in first-degree relatives and not higher than the prevalence in the general population (Gershon *et al.*, 1982).

Several studies have drawn attention to the high rate of depressive disorders that develop in the offspring of depressed patients (Beardslee, Bemporad, Keller, & Klerman, 1983; Cytryn, McKnew, & Bartko, 1982; Gershon *et al.*, 1982; Orvaschel, Weissman, & Kidd, 1980). They have noted considerable social and psychological difficulties and a range of psychiatric symptoms developing in these children. The overt manifestation of a major psychiatric disorder may be only a small part of a broader range of psychopathology from which these offspring may suffer, perhaps as a consequence of living in the home of a depressed parent.

Studies of adopted children have sought to distinguish the genetic component from the environmental component in the development of a depressive disorder. One strategy for adoption studies is to examine retrospectively the biological and adoptive parents of individuals who have developed a psychiatric disorder. In one study, Mendlewicz and Rainer (1977) examined the biological and adoptive parents of individuals who had been adopted away as infants and later went on to develop bipolar disorder. They found depressive disorder in 31% of the biological parents in contrast to 12% of the adoptive parents. In a control population, depressive disorder was found in only 2% of the biological parents but in 10% of the adoptive parents of individuals who were adopted away as infants and who did not go on to develop depressive disorder. In another study, using a different strategy, Cadoret (1978) studied the offspring who were given up for adoption by normal and by depressed biological parents. These individuals were raised in homes in which the adoptive parents were determined to be normal (without psychiatric disorder). In this study, 38% of the children of biologically depressed parents developed depressive disorders (unipolar or bipolar) in contrast to only 7% of the offspring of normal biological parents. The data from these two adoption studies offer compelling evidence of a genetic factor in the development of depressive disorders. On the other hand, some recent studies have failed to find a significant correlation between adoptee depression and depressive disorder in the biological parents and have noted that some environmental factors (alcoholism, early death of an adoptive parent) were significantly correlated.

Table 9.1 offers a summary of empirical risk figures for the development of major depressive disorder that take into account the results of the numerous genetic studies that have been reported. These data must be used with circumspection, given the diverse methodologies and differing enthno-

Table 9.1. Empirical Risk Figures for the Development of Major Depressive Disorder (MDD)

Relationship to patient	Empirical risk for MDD*
Patient with bipolar (manic–depressive) illness	
MZ twin	75%
DZ twin	15%–25%
Offspring of one ill parent	15%–25%
Offspring of two ill parents	50%–75%
Sibling	15%–25%
Parent	10%–15%
Aunt, uncle, grandparent	2%–3%
Cousin	1%–2%
General population	1%
Patient with unipolar illness	
MZ twin	40%–50%
DZ twin	15%
Offspring	15%–20%
Sibling	10%–15%
Parent	10%–15%
Aunt, uncle, grandparent	2%–5%
Cousin	2%–3%
General population	2%–3%

*Relatives of bipolar patients develop both bipolar and unipolar illness, reflecting the heterogeneity of the expression of illness, whereas relatives of unipolar patients develop primarily unipolar illness.

graphic and geographic distributions of the population studied. Overall, it appears that a first-degree relative of a bipolar patient has a 15%–25% risk of developing a major depressive disorder, and that a first-degree relative of a unipolar patient has a 10%–20% risk. Whereas MZ twins have a 40%–75% risk of developing concordant depressive disorder, DZ twins have a risk similar to that of any other siblings. The offspring of two depressed patients have an extremely high risk for developing depressive disorder (greater than 50%) and represent a high-risk group. On the other hand, the second-degree relatives of bipolar or unipolar patients have a rather low risk for the development of depressive disorder, a risk that is only slightly greater than that found in the general population.

CLINICAL ISSUES IN PSYCHIATRIC GENETICS

Psychiatric Genetics and Suicide

Suicidal behavior as part of an acute depressive disorder may cause shock waves in a family, particularly when it is preceded by a lack of awareness or denial of illness. Completed suicide may be the most dramatic example of an acute psychiatric condition, leading to substantial unrest in the remainder of the family. Although it is not well documented, some studies suggest that genetic factors may contribute to overt suicidal behavior.

In a recent family study, Egeland and Sussex (1985) reported on suicide among the old-order Amish located in southeastern Pennsylvania. They counted 26 persons who had committed suicide between 1880 and 1980, the majority of whom were diagnosed as having major depressive disorder and as being situated within four multigenerational pedigrees with heavy loading for bipolar, unipolar, and other affective illnesses. These data are consistent with data from other studies that suggest that the risk of suicide in the relatives of patients with a depressive disorder is considerably greater than that in the normal population. Alec Roy (1983) found attempted suicide in 48.6% of psychiatric inpatients who had a family history of suicide in contrast to only 21.8% of inpatients with no family history of suicide. In a Danish adoption study, 57 adoptees without previously diagnosed psychiatric disorder who had committed suicide were found to have substantially more biological relatives with a history of suicide than were 57 nonsuicidal adoptee controls (Schulsinger, Kety, Rosenthal, & Wender, 1979). Given these data, Schulsinger and co-workers suggested the possibility of a genetically determined transmission of suicidal behavior independent of depressive disorder.

Genetic concerns about suicide may emerge during the course of treatment. In some instances the potential for suicide can become a treatment issue with a "genetic" twist. For example, a 28-year-old woman came to her psychiatrist in a state of acute alarm on the day following the completed suicide of her cousin. While she had been in and out of psychotherapy for several years because of lingering depression, she had not been aware that other members of her family had been in treatment as well. The suicide of her cousin had forced an opening of honesty that had been precluded by the family's embarrassment over, and avoidance of, the stigma of psychiatric disorder. Given her own difficulties, this woman was realistically concerned about her personal risk for suicide. Further exploration revealed additional family members who had been in treatment for depression and another relative who had completed suicide. The therapist had diagnosed this particular woman as having dysthymia and had not previously considered the risk of suicide, the use of pharmacotherapeutic drugs, or the possibility of genetic determination in the etiology of her difficulties. The shock of the suicide had made it possible for the family to reveal the extent of depressive disorder within the system and opened up new possibilities in the course of treatment.

In this example, the mere description of an empirical risk figure for suicide for the client would have been largely irrelevant. It was more important to note the heavy loading for major depressive disorder with suicide in the pedigree and, consequently, to consider pharmacotherapy for this patient with dysthymia.

Family Planning and Psychiatric Genetics

Family-planning decisions may be difficult for individuals who have had a major psychiatric disorder or who believe that their offspring may be at risk for a serious psychiatric disorder. For some patients, pregnancy exacerbates the risk for the development or recurrence of an acute depressive disorder (particularly in the postpartum period) and places constraints upon the use of some psychotropic medications (i.e., lithium; Targum, 1981). Single individuals may wonder about issues of inheritance when they are considering marriage, whereas already married individuals may seek genetic information to weigh the desirability of conceiving children, aborting unintentional pregancies, adopting children, or getting divorced.

In all cases, the description of genetic data requires delicate and cautious handling because of the psychological importance it holds for these individuals. The motivation for seeking genetic information is particularly relevant in these circumstances. Although most situations involve only mild to moderate risk for illness, there are conditions that involve particularly high risks to the offspring. Clearly, elective childbearing in patients with chronic schizophrenia, rapidly cycling bipolar disorder, or intractable severe depression with suicidal behavior reflects poor judgment and consequently increases the burden of illness for the putative parent (Targum, 1981). As noted earlier, the offspring of parents who both have a major depressive disorder may have a greater than 50% risk for developing a similar depressive disorder during their lifetimes. One may also presume that the home environment of these children may be strained by the burden of illness, which will increase the likelihood of adjustment problems and psychopathology for them. However, most patients with a major depressive disorder can lead functional lives and can often manage the course of the illness. Environmental factors may be the ultimate determinants of which predisposed individuals will actually develop a depressive disorder in their lifetimes (Cadoret, O'Gorman, Heywood, & Troughton, 1985; Knorring, Cloninger, Bohmon, & Sigvardsson, 1983; Wynne, Cromwell, & Matthysse, 1978). Wynne and colleagues maintain that the offspring of one ill parent can grow to be quite healthy if the impact of the ill parent is counterbalanced by an active, presumably well spouse and support system. Unlike schizophrenia, the outcome of most patients with a major depressive disorder is favorable.

Because marriage and family-planning decisions are personal options for individuals, therapists are usually noncommittal regarding these issues. With the exception of couples where both individuals have had unstable psychiatric courses, most individuals can make their own decisions about their lives without the interference of mental health professionals.

Often, the perception of genetic risk (given as a percent risk figure) is overestimated by the client. Frequently, clients presume a 50%–100% risk for the development of illness in their offspring if either parent is ill. Naturally, individuals who underestimate the risk or deny any risk at all are unlikely to inquire about genetic concerns. Couples may have widely divergent views about genetic determinations of depression, and exploring these differences may become a paramount issue in working with them.

Genetics, Depression, and Adoption

There are occasions when a biological parent may consider giving a child up for adoption because of genetic concerns. There are also some instances when genetic issues encumber the adoption process. For instance, a schizophrenic parent may elect to give a child up for adoption because of genetic concerns and a desire to provide for the child's welfare, but the adoption agency may find it difficult to present this child to potential adoptive parents because of the stigma and confusion surrounding the biological parent's schizophrenic illness. Although it is the responsibility of the adoption agency to address the possibility of an increased risk for psychiatric disorder in the child, the difficulties inherent in making both an accurate psychiatric diagnosis of the parent and an accurate determination of risk for the child can obfuscate the discussion.

Genetic issues constitute only a part of the complex set of factors that potential adoptive parents must consider in the process of adoption. Sometimes the infants of psychiatrically ill parents are underweight and psychologically undernourished at the time they are placed for adoption, particularly when they have lived in the parental home for some time. On the other hand, the majority of these children will not go on to develop a major psychiatric disorder. As noted earlier, Wynne and colleagues (Wynne *et al.*, 1978) have emphasized the positive role that clear communication in the family home can provide for any child and the possibility that a healthy psychosocial environment can counterbalance any genetic predisposition to psychiatric disorder that these children may have inherited. It is important that the adoption counselor provide as much descriptive information as possible to the prospective parents and assist them in objectively exploring the risks and potentials that these children have. The sharing of information with prospective parents not only will protect the agency against the liability of withholding the information but also will allow adoptive parents to digest these issues before the child is ready to ask about his or her biological background.

The Influence of the Environment

Adoption studies have documented behavioral similarities shared by adoptees and their biological relatives in contrast to their adoptive parents. Numerous studies have shown evidence for a genetic factor in psychiatric disorders as diverse as schizophrenia, bipolar disorder, antisocial personality, alcoholism, and panic disorder. Although a genetic factor appears to contribute to the overt development of these disorders, it has been suggested that a continuum of genetic expression may exist, which could range from normality to the most severe expression of the genetic diathesis. Further, several studies have demonstrated the modifying effect that the environment can have upon the expression of any genetic disease, particularly one that expresses itself as psychiatric disorder (Cadoret, 1978; Cadoret, Cain, & Crowe, 1983; Cloninger, Bohman, & Sigvardsson, 1981; Knorring *et al.*, 1983; Wynne *et al.*, 1978). For instance, Cadoret and colleagues have demonstrated that the incidence of adolescent antisocial behavior in adoptees increases when a biological background of alcoholism and/or antisocial behavior is combined with the presence of adversity in the adoptive home (Cadoret *et al.*, 1983). In another study, involving 48 adoptees who had developed depressive disorders, it was found that alcoholism and the early death of an adoptive parent significantly correlated with the development of depression (Cadoret, O'Gorman, Heywood, & Troughton, 1985). Since depressive disorder tends to be a recurrent condition, the environment will continually influence the course of the disorder through the lifetime of the individual. Thus a supportive, secure environment may minimize the severity of expression of a depressive disorder, whereas a more stressful, less structured milieu may exacerbate the expression and yield more severe disruption and more frequent recurrence. The following example of a bipolar MZ twin pair exemplifies the effect of the psychosocial environment upon the longitudinal course of the disorder.

An MZ twin pair was followed for 10 years subsequent to the development of concordant bipolar disorder in the latter twin (B) 1 year after the emergence of mania in her sister (A). The longitudinal course was markedly different in these identical twins and was clearly related to the life experience of each. Twin A became manic coincidental with the engagement of her sister (B) to a man they had both dated. She went on to have numerous hospitalizations for both mania and depression with suicide attempts over the next 10 years, whereas Twin B had only two distinct episodes (one manic, one depressive) requiring hospitalization and otherwise appeared relatively stable throughout the same period. Twin A was married twice during the 10 years, first to a man 35 years her senior, and later to a man she had met while she was manic. Twin B was married prior to the onset of manic episodes and remained married to the same man throughout the 10-year period. Psychological evaluations, including projective testing, revealed marked similarities between these two women, with the exception that Twin A was considerably more aggressive than her co-twin. Further, Twin A revealed a profound sense of inadequacy and inferiority relative to her co-twin and acknowledged that she always wanted to be as good as her co-twin. Twin A suffered frequent and protracted depressive episodes interspersed with mania, which reflected her internal pressure to succeed and the external social failures that she experienced. Twin A developed manias characterized by promiscuity, acting-out behaviors, and impulsive activities, whereas Twin B became grandiose and religious, without any acting-out behavior. Over the course of 10 years, the significance of the genetic predisposition to bipolar disorder seemed less important than the psychosocial consequences of their behaviors, which continually affected how they viewed themselves and how they were viewed by others. Thus, although they shared an identical genetic predisposition to bipolar disorder, their clinical courses were largely determined by their environmental experiences.

Psychiatric Genetics and Treatment

Some studies have demonstrated a relationship between a family history of depressive disorder and better response to psychopharmacological treatment. The demonstration that genetic factors contribute to the development of depressive disorders in some families kindles the possibility that intrafamilial diagnoses and selection of pharmacotherapeutic agents will be enhanced when these families can be identified. This concept led Winokur and his colleagues to develop a diagnostic classification system based upon a family history of depressive disorder (Winokur, 1979). In this system of diagnostic differentiation of subtypes of depression, patients with a family history of depression among first-degree relatives are considered to have "pure depressive disease," whereas patients with no family history of depression, alcoholism, or antisocial personality are said to have "sporadic depressive disease." Depressed patients with a family history of alcoholism or antisocial personality in first-degree relatives fall into a third category, that of "depressive spectrum disease." Several studies have attempted to demonstrate differential responses to treatment among the three familial subtypes of depressive disorder, as well as differences in course of illness, suicidal behavior, and biological markers (Van Valkenberg & Winokur, 1977).

Currently, this system of diagnostic classification does not offer any specific clinical utility to the practicing therapist. On the other hand, some investigators have demonstrated that pharmacotherapy can be facilitated by a carefully conducted psychopharmacological family history. For instance, patients who present with atypical symptom patterns or insufficient symptoms to meet criteria for major depression may still be candidates for pharmacotherapy when family histories demonstrate heavy loading for depressive disorder. In these cases, a subthreshold affective problem may be a minor variant of the genetic diathesis for major depressive disorder within the family system. These patients might respond to the same antidepressant medications that helped other family members with more severe depressive disorders. Pare (1970) compared pharmacological treatment of ill patients to that of their ill relatives and found a tendency for family members to respond to the same antidepressant medications. In another study, Angst (1961) compared the treatment effectiveness of imipramine in nine biologically related pairs of depressed patients and noted concordant responses to the drug in eight of the nine pairs (five pairs improved, three did not improve, and one pair had a mixed response). Although the similarity of drug responsiveness noted in these studies may or may not be related to genetic factors, the findings support the suggestion that a psychopharmacological family history may be helpful in determining appropriate pharmacotherapy.

Mendlewicz and co-workers have reviewed the effect of lithium carbonate in depressed patients with and without family histories of bipolar disorder (Mendlewicz, Fieve, & Stallone, 1973). These investigators found that lithium carbonate was more effective prophylactically in bipolar patients who had first-degree relatives with bipolar disorder than in bipolar patients who had no family history of bipolar disorder. Furthermore, a family history of bipolar illness was correlated with greater lithium efficacy in the treatment of unipolar patients as well. Thus the clinical response to lithium carbonate may be related to an underlying genetic predisposition for the development of bipolar disorder in specific families.

Metabolic factors such as the rate of acetylation of antidepressant drugs (particularly monoamine oxidase inhibitors) or the rate of achieving a steady-state plasma level of antidepressant drugs have been shown to be under genetic control independent of the psychiatric disorder for which the drug might be given (Targum & Schultz, 1982). The clinical efficacy of antidepressant drugs can depend upon the metabolism of these drugs related to factors under genetic control. For instance, Johnstone and Marsh (1973) found that the efficacy of tranylcypromine (a monoamine oxidase inhibitor) was related to acetylator status in 72 depressed patients in their study. Patients who were considered to be slow acetylators had a much greater clinical response to tranylcypromine than patients who were fast acetylators or those who received a placebo drug.

Clinicians may hesitate to use antidepressant medications in patients who are diagnosed as having acute schizophreniform disorder (acute psychotic episodes with a duration of less than 6 months). However, some, but not all, of these patients will go on to develop well-defined major depressive disorder (Gershon *et al.*, 1977; Hirschowitz, Casper, Garrer, & Chang, 1980; Targum & Schultz, 1982). The early introduction of antidepressant medications and/or lithium carbonate therapy may facilitate more effective clinical management in those cases (Hirshowitz *et al.*, 1980). A family history of depressive disorder is one variable to consider when selecting the treatment plan, and schizophreniform patients with heavy loading for depressive disorder might be good candidates for antidepressant or lithium carbonate trials.

FUTURE PROSPECTS FOR CLINICAL PSYCHIATRIC GENETICS

The future promises that specific genetic markers of physiological or biological vulnerability to developing depressive disorder will be identified, which will, in turn, facilitate treatment decisions. Currently there are no specific markers that have reliable clinical value. Psychogeneticists have attempted to identify specific genes as well as specific psychobiological or psychophysiological deficits that would be invariably linked to depressive disorders (Gershon *et al.*, 1977; Targum & Schultz, 1982). Although numerous associations have been reported, linkage has not yet been demonstrated in a replicable fashion (Goldin, Gershon, Targum, Sparkes, & McGinnis, 1983). One promising approach examined the human leukocyte antigen (HLA) system, which is located on the sixth chromosome and has been associated with some medical and neurological diseases (i.e., ankylosing spondylitis; Weitkamp, Stancer, Persad, Flood & Guttormen, 1981). However, HLA studies of major depressive disorder have been contradictory, and most linkage studies have failed to demonstrate segregation of specific HLA alleles with depressive disorder in selected families (Goldin, Clerget-Darpoux, & Gershon, 1982; Targum,

Gershon, VanEerdewegh, & Rogentine, 1979). In another promising approach, Nadi and co-workers reported a higher density of muscarinic cholinergic binding sites on cultured human skin fibroblasts in patients and relatives who had histories of major or minor depressive disorder than in normal relatives or normal controls (Nadi, Nurnberger, & Gershon, 1984). The possibility exists that this marker might identify family members who are at risk for the development of depressive disorder but who have not yet manifested symptoms. Unfortunately, methodological problems and nonreplication by the same investigators have limited the development of this concept. Other investigators have considered specific sleep markers (REM latency or density) or neuroendocrine deficits (blunted thyrotropin responses to thyrotropin-releasing hormone stimulation), but studies published thus far have not provided a consistent framework to support a genetic relationship between these markers and depressive disorder. It is likely that the peripheral markers that have been studied to date do not have a direct etiological relationship to the underlying genetic diathesis, although they may coexist with the expression of major depressive disorder. In summary, the empirical risk figures developed from the numerous twin, family, and adoption studies published thus far are still the best data available for an approximate determination of risk for the development of depressive disorder within families.

The future treatment of major depressive disorder may include diagnostic sybtyping along biological–genetic lines rather than the more commonly used descriptive–phenomenological methods. The demonstration of genetic determination of depressive disorder does not preclude the importance of examining the interpersonal and intrapsychic difficulties that patients also manifest. The therapist must remain open and informed about the possibility that genetic factors may contribute to depression in a particular patient and must also be aware that the fear of genetic illness may obstruct the course of treatment unless fully explored. This chapter has considered genetic issues that may emerge during the course of treatment for a depressive disorder and has described some clinical applications that might be relevant to the practicing clinician. It must be emphasized, however, that genetic illnesses constitute a specific medical discipline and that genetic counseling forms only a part of the whole. Therefore referrals to genetic counseling programs may be appropriate adjuncts to utilize in conjunction with ongoing treatment in many situations.

REFERENCES

Ablon, S. L., Davenport, Y. B., & Gershon, E. S. (1975). The married manic. *American Journal of Orthopsychiatry, 45*, 854–866.
American Psychiatric Association (1987). *Diagnostic and statistical manual of mental disorders* (rev. 3rd ed.). Washington, DC: APA.

Angst, J. (1961). A clinical analysis of the effects of Tofranil in depression. *Psychopharmacology, 2*, 381-407.

Beardslee, W. R., Bemporad, J., Keller, M. B., & Klerman, G. L. (1983). Children of parents with major affective disorder: A review. *American Journal of Psychiatry, 140*, 825-832.

Cadoret, R. (1978). Evidence for genetic inheritance of primary affective disorder in adoptees. *American Journal of Psychiatry, 134*, 463-466.

Cadoret, R., Cain, C. A., & Crowe, R. R. (1983). Evidence for gene-environment in the development of adolescent antisocial behavior. *Behavior Genetics, 13*, 301-310.

Cadoret, R., O'Gorman, T. W., Heywood, E., & Troughton, E. (1985). Genetic and environmental factors in major depression. *Journal of Affective Disorders, 9*, 155-164.

Carlson, G. A., Kotin, J., & Davenport, J. B., (1974). Follow-up of 53 bipolar manic–depressive patients. *British Journal of Psychiatry, 124*, 134-139.

Cloninger, C. R., Bohman, M., & Sigvardsson, S. (1981). Inheritance of alcohol abuse: Cross-fostering analysis of adopted men. *Archives of General Psychiatry, 38*, 861-868.

Cytryn, L., McKnew, D. H., & Bartko, J. J. (1982). Offspring of patients with affective disorders: II. *Journal of the American Academy of Child Psychiatry, 21*, 389-391.

Egeland, J. A., & Sussex, J. N. (1985). Suicide and family loading for affective disorders. *Journal of the American Medical Association, 254*, 915-918.

Gershon, E. S., Hamovit, J., Guroff, J. J., Dibble, E., Leckman, J. F., Sceery, W., Targum, D. D., Nurnberger, J. I., Goldin, L. R., & Bunney, W.E., Jr. (1982). A family study of schizoaffective, bipolar I, bipolar II, unipolar, and normal control probands. *Archives of General Psychiatry, 39*, 1157-1167.

Gershon, E. S., Targum, S. D., Kessler, L. R., Mazure, C. M., & Bunney, W. E., Jr. (1977). Genetic studies and biologic strategies in the affective disorders. *Progress in Medical Genetics, 2*, 101-164.

Goldin, L. R., Clerget-Darpoux, F., & Gershon, E. S. (1982). Relationship of HLA to major affective disorder not supported. *Psychiatry Research, 7*, 29-45.

Goldin, L. R., Gershon, E. S., Targum, S. D., Sparkes, R. S., & McGinnis, M. (1983). Segregation and linkage analyses in families of patients with bipolar, unipolar, and schizoaffective mood disorders. *American Journal of Human Genetics, 35*, 274-287.

Hirschowitz, J., Casper, R., Garver, D. S., & Chang, S. (1980). Lithium response in good prognosis schizophrenia. *American Journal of Psychiatry, 137*, 916-920.

Janowsky, D. S., Leff, M., & Epstein, R. S. (1970). Playing the manic game. *Archives of General Psychiatry, 22*, 252-261.

Johnstone, E., & Marsh, W. (1973). Acetylator status and response to phenelzine in depressed patients. *Lancet, 1*, 567-570.

Kallmann, F. J., (1954). Genetic principles in manic–depressive psychosis. In P. Hoch & J. Zubin (Eds.), *Depression*. New York: Grune & Stratton.

Kay, D. W. K. (1979). Assessment of familial risks in the functional psychoses and their application. *British Journal of Psychiatry, 33*, 385-403.

Knorring, A. L. von, Cloninger, R., Bohman, M., Sigvardsson, S. (1983). An adoption study of depressive disorders and substance abuse. *Archives of General Psychiatry, 40*, 943-950.

Mendlewicz, J., Fieve, R., & Stallone, F. (1973). Relationship between the effectiveness of lithium therapy and family history. *American Journal of Psychiatry, 130*, 1011-1013.

Mendlewicz, J., & Rainer, J. (1977). Adoption study supporting genetic transmission in manic–depressive illness. *Nature, 268*, 327-329.

Nadi, N. S., Nurnberger, J. I., & Gershon, E. S. (1984). Muscarinic cholinergic receptors on skin fibroblasts in familial affective disorder. *New England Journal of Medicine, 311*, 225-255.

Orvaschel, H., Weissman, M. M., & Kidd, K. K. (1980). The children of depressed parents; the childhood of depressed patients; depression in children. *Journal of Affective Disorders, 2*, 1-16.

Pare, C. (1970). Differentiation of two genetically specific types of depression by the response to antidepressant drugs. *Humangentik, 9,* 199–201.

Perris, C., Perris, H., Ericsson, U., & Knorring, L. von (1982). The genetics of depression. *Archiv fuer Psychiatrie und Nervenkrankheiten, 232,* 137–155.

Price, J. (1968). The genetics of depressive behavior. In A. Coppen & A. Walk (Eds.), *Recent developments in affective disorders* [Special issue]. *British Journal of Psychiatry, 2,* 37–54.

Roy, A. (1983). Family history of suicide. *Archives of General Psychiatry, 40,* 971–974.

Schlesser, M. A., & Altshuler, K. Z. (1983). The genetics of affective disorder: Data, theory and clinical applications. *Hospital and Community Psychiatry, 5,* 415–422.

Schulsinger, F., Kety, S., Rosenthal, D., & Wender, P. H. (1979). A family study of suicide. In M. Schou & E. Stromgren (Eds.), *Origin, prevention and treatment of affective disorders* (pp. 277–287). New York: Academic Press.

Targum, S. D. (1981). Psychotherapeutic considerations in genetic counseling. *American Journal of Medical Genetics, 8,* 281–289.

Targum, S. D., Dibble, E. D., Davenport, Y. B., & Gershon, E. S. (1981). Family attitudes questionnaire: Patients and spouses view bipolar illness. *Archives of General Psychiatry, 38,* 562–568.

Targum, S. D., & Gershon, E. (1980). Genetic counseling for affective illness. In R. Belmaker & H. Van Praag (Eds.), *Mania: An evolving concept* (pp. 119–126). Holliswood, NY: Spectrum Publications.

Targum, S. D., & Gershon, E. (1981). Pregnancy, genetic counseling, and the major psychiatric disorders. In J. Schulman & J. Simpson (Eds.), *Genetic counseling in pregnancy* (pp. 413–438). New York: Academic Press.

Targum, S. D., Gershon, E., VanEerdewegh, & Rogentine, N. (1979). Human leukocyte antigen (HLA) system not closely linked to or associated with bipolar manic–depressive illness. *Biological Psychiatry, 14,* 615–636.

Targum, S. D., & Schulz, S. C. (1982). Clinical applications of psychiatric genetics. *American Journal of Orthopsychiatry, 52,* 45–57.

Tsuang, M. T. (1978). Genetic counseling for psychiatric patients and their families. *American Journal of Psychiatry, 12,* 1465–1475.

Tsuang, M. T., & Vandermey, R. (1980). *Genes and the mind: Inheritance of mental illness.* London: Oxford University Press.

Van Valkenberg, C., & Winokur, G. (1979). Depressive spectrum disease. *Psychiatric Clinics of North America, 2,* 469–482.

Weitkamp, L. R., Stancer, H. L., Persad, E., Flood, C., & Guttormen, S. (1981). Depressive disorders and HLA: A gene on chromosome 6 that can affect behavior. *New England Journal of Medicine, 305,* 1301–1306.

Winokur, G. (1979). Unipolar depression: Is it divisible into autonomous subtypes? *Archives of General Psychiatry, 36,* 447–452.

Wynne, L., Cromwell, R., & Matthysse, S. (1978). *The nature of schizophrenia: New approaches to research and treatment.* New York: Wiley.

10

Common Clinical Predicaments

MELVIN R. LANSKY

In discussing affective disturbance and the family, I will deal with four clinical predicaments that are often characterized by overwhelming affect: mania, recurrent depression, the overlap between affective disorder and personality disorder, and the problem of suicide. The problem of conceptualizing affective disorders is greater than our terminology suggests. We have no basis for classifying "affective" disorders other than phenomenologically, that is, as situations that present clinically with overwhelming affect at the forefront of the clinical picture. Whether the affective disorders actually have a common basis other than one based on surface phenomenology that warrants their classification together is still far from clear. The question is, in principle, undecidable without our being able to apply Koch's postulate, that is, to know with reproducible certainty that diseases can be classified on the basis of what causes them, rather than on their striking surface features.

The nomenclature of DSM-III-R (American Psychiatric Association, 1987) is still held captive—more than is commonly realized—by a psychology (usually implicit) that assumes that there really *are* specific disorders of mental faculties: of thinking (schizophrenia), of feeling (affective disorders), of conduct or will (personality disorders), and of body (organic disorders). Such a "faculty" psychology lends an apparent credibility to the reification of the concept of "disorders of mood" with the implicit assumption that such a classification has a basis in some central and essential feature rather than in similarities of surface phenomena. The DSM-III-R is, at its best, a phenomenological document, a classification that is not based in any meaningful way on thought, mood, will, and body, but that is a first approximation for systematic study correlations of relatively clear-cut symptom clusters associated with a general course of illness and response to treatment. If DSM-III-R is denuded of faculty psychological presuppositions, that is, of assumptions that there are, in anything other than a descriptive sense, disorders of mood, thought, conduct, and body, it is a useful classification, but by its very phenomenological (presuppositionless) nature, not one that helps us gain a useful method of classifying mood disorders. "Affective

213

disorder" should have the same tentative classificatory status as "febrile disorder" might have had in a diagnostic manual a century ago.

At first blush, one might be tempted to argue that medication response supports the idea that affective disorders are separable from other disorders on the basis of treatment response. Neuroleptic medication modifies some features of schizophrenic disorders, but not depression; antidepressants do not help schizophrenics and may worsen their illness; and lithium has been thought to be a mood-regulating drug somewhat specific for bipolar disorders. This relative specificity of major classes of medication may lend an apparent credibility to faculty psychology by buttressing the notion that we medicate somewhat distinctly schizophrenia, depression, and bipolar illness. But to revive and reify a faculty psychology overgeneralized from this rough-hewn and approximate clinical phenomenology is as unacceptable a rationale for classification as would be a classification of infectious diseases by antibiotic response. We do not know what affective disorders are. The basis, then, for separating a class of affective disorders from others remains poorly grounded.*

In this discussion, I make no attempt to put forward a classification that is either exhaustive or based on some principle of classification other than striking surface features. The "entities" I describe are familiar to anyone who treats severely disturbed psychiatric patients. The clinical phenomenology is at least as likely to remain significant than is the rationale for classifying these situations as affective disorders.

The treatment attitude, then, is agnostic. No etiological presuppositions are made. It should always be presumed that constitutional difficulties (deficits) and turbulence in close attachments (conflict) are both potentially relevant in any one case. Any contrast of organic with dynamic posits a false antithesis for these disorders, as it does for any serious psychiatric disorder. That severe depressions may be unresponsive to interventions other than medication or electronconvulsive therapy (ECT) does not mean that they are thereby "biological" and therefore without significant dynamics. Likewise, amelioration of disorders by psychosocial means does not imply that the disorder is unrelated to biology or constitution.

I am taking a decidedly integrative view and stressing that the different clinical pictures mentioned here require different treatment strategies. In discussing family strategies and approaches for these disorders, it should be

*In contrast, psychoanalysis conceptualizes virtually all symptoms as compromises between expression and defense that are formed to keep the psyche from being flooded with unmanageable affect. Behind the acting out of the personality disorder (Vaillant, 1975), the fabricated reality of the psychotic, and the symptoms of the neurotic, are defensive distortions—methods of handling affect that would otherwise be overwhelming. Viewed psychoanalytically, each of these types of disorder at bottom derives from a response to overwhelming mood and is, in some sense, an affective disorder.

borne in mind that family therapy is virtually never the only modality used. Hospitals, medications, groups, ECT, milieu therapy, individual psychotherapy, management sessions, and self-help groups, among others, are always potential ingredients in the treatment package. Any attempt to treat these disorders by psychotherapy or medication alone is insufficient. Therapy depends on an intimate knowledge of psychopathology and its impact on the interpersonal environments. Models derived from one method—for example, models based on learned helplessness, biological models, or psychoanalytic models—have been put forward in ways that have held their own adherents captive. But the adoption of such one-sided models works against the integration required to deal optimally with these disorders. They are, for the most part, chronic disorders and do not remit without residual deficits. Preconceptions of these disorders that do not acknowledge chronicity, incomplete treatment results, and residual illness, even in the best-treated cases, are evasions on the part of the therapist.

The four clinical situations I will address are mania (bipolar illness), recurrent unipolar depression (with no implication that this category is a uniform one), personality disorder with strong affective accompaniment (including the overlap between the problematically conceptualized "borderline personality disorder," with anger, empty depression, and massive anxiety in the picture, and the equally problematic "bipolar II disorder"), and the role of the family in the evaluation of suicide. Unmanageable affect is in each type of case the dominant clinical feature. The discussions fall short of providing detailed programs for family intervention. Rather, attitudes toward family intervention in major illness are put forward, with an attempt to highlight interpersonal features typical of the clinical situation.

Family intervention is not the same as family therapy. A 30-second phone call to persons close to a suicidal patient is often a major family intervention, but it is not family therapy. Nor is a simple collaborative conference involving relatives, patients, and hospital staff concerning details of the currrent episode for which the patient is hospitalized and assessment of support systems available after the patient leaves the hospital. It should never be supposed that family therapy refers to one type of intervention or that family therapy appropriate to any one of these four entities is at all similar to that of any of the others. "Family therapy," like "surgery," is a feature of the treatment of many types of illness. Like the surgeon, the family therapist must have definite skills, training, discipline, and knowledge of specific procedures. But the surgery for a peptic ulcer is not the same as that for an inguinal hernia, nor is the family therapy for mania the same as that for depression or for risk of suicide.

In each case, the procedure employed derives from a knowledge both of the disorder and of the specific patient or family in treatment. My clinical illustrations are provided so as to highlight commonly found interpersonal aspects of the psychopathology in question insofar as it is an often neglected target for therapeutic strategy. Technique evolves from an understanding of the pathology encountered. The therapeutic approaches portrayed are of secondary importance.

MANIA

Mania may be diagnosed by any of a variety of criteria (World Psychiatric Association, 1983). Those from DSM-III-R (American Psychiatric Association, 1987) stress psychotic episodes with elevated expansive or irritable moods, with or without a clinically significant depression. Manic "episodes" are so dominant and so striking a feature of the illness that manic–depressive psychosis may be oversimplified and seen as a series of manic episodes only—recurrent, self-limited, "biological" states in patients with a high family incidence of this same disorder and often responsive to neuroleptics, ECT, or lithium carbonate. Mania may remit with either depressive episodes of euthymic periods during which the patient is not manic.

The high prevalence of the disorder in the families of manic patients, the unique flavor of high periods of mania, and the response of manic episodes to biological interventions have given some clinicians the impression that bipolar illness is biological, without significant dynamics, an illness treatable by biological methods alone. Close scrutiny of cases regularly shows this view to be disastrously oversimplified (Davenport, 1981). Manic–depressive illness is chronic and recurring. Manic states may remit, but many patients in their "euthymic" states, if they have them, are not normal (Carlson, Kotin, Davenport, & Adland, 1974). During mania, patients usually have a marked inability to acknowledge inner reality. The interpersonal difficulties of such patients are enormous. No other difficulty, not even homicide in the family, has such a high degree of enduring familial chaos nor such a high likelihood that family will be unable to tolerate the patient and give up on him or her. This volatility takes place with a sensitivity within the patient to rejection and narcissistic wounding, such that abandonment or rejection may precipitate depressive dips, which, in turn, precipitate full-blown manic episodes. Manic–depressive patients are often left destitute of close relationships because people, even family, do not tolerate them. Alternatively, such patients may form collusive relationships, usually clingy marriages, organized around denial and dependency that provide security at a fearful price (Davenport & Adland, 1985).

Family therapy is indicated in every case of manic–depressive illness. This prescription does not presume that such family work alters or works through the essential difficulty, the vulnerability to become manic, nor does family therapy by itself modify manic attacks themselves. The presumption that family therapy is indicated for every case of bipolar illness derives from these considerations:

1. *Interpersonal precipitants* of manic attacks are quite commonly found when a proper history is taken. Often, such a history reveals narcissistic wounding followed by depression, followed by mild hypomania, denial of dependency, drug discontinuance, and then a full-blown manic attack.

2. *Management*, especially rapid management, is a crucial component in the treatment of the majority of manic patients. This is because of the nature of the illness and because mania is so poorly understood by the legal system that legal detention procedures are too cumbersome to aid the clinician. Denial is so much a part of the picture of early mania that collaboration often cannot be made in the early phases of exacerbation unless family members are strongly involved and supported in their involvement.

3. *Empathic contact and education* about the illness are important for family members, both for their own and for the patient's well-being, and for the purpose of keeping them from being overwhelmed and ultimately abandoning the patient.

4. *The pattern and the actual deficits and residual problems* in the manic–depressive are almost never so simple as conveyed in the notion of "recurrent manic bouts," with the implication that intervals between such bouts are normal. The treatment team, the patient, and the family are needed in a collaborative coalition formed to understand what actually has transpired in order to appreciate the full significance of what is wrong with the patient and to respond to it appropriately.

Initial family sessions with an acute manic patient may take place, for the most part, without the patient present, until the mania is at least in a partial state of remission. Nonetheless, it is usually worthwhile to include the acutely psychotic patient for a short time at first, even if that meeting is very disruptive and results in the exclusion of the patient after a few minutes. The disruption itself provides an invaluable opportunity for the therapist to make empathic contact with the family members right at the point where their terrified efforts to reason with the patient have failed to contain the patient's chaos or to exert some sort of control. By conveying understanding of and empathy for their experiences at these points where their ability to contain chaos has failed, the therapist is best able to cement an alliance that leaves family members feeling understood and good about themselves when they had hitherto felt overwhelmed, ashamed, and inadequate to the task before them.

Family contacts should then proceed to an educative phase. The family should be told that the patient appears interpersonally strongest when he or she is becoming manically ill, and that if, at such times, the patient presses for special exemptions from limits, professional help should be obtained immediately. Compromise and reasoning—usually appropriate negotiating strategies for most human predicaments—should be eschewed when a patient is in the early phases of mania or at any time while the patient is still manic. The patient must be managed, and managed rapidly.

Family education should proceed *pari passu* with a workup that looks for family history of the illness, the circumstances that precipitated the illness, and the effect both of interpersonal events on the illness and of the illness on interpersonal events. Manic patients are exquisitely sensitive to rejection and to separations and respond to these with an exuberance and expansiveness that is likely to compound and amplify the original rejection.

The illness affects both work and close relationships, and the patient's actual failures in these areas powerfully affect his or her self-esteem. The bipolar individual who cannot be an adequate provider, caretaker, spouse, or parent is exquisitely sensitive to the (real, not fantasied) humiliation that accompanies such chronically defective functioning, even when the patient is not clinically manic. Such patients in close relationships show both excessive dependency and a gross (and often irritating) denial of that dependency. Chronic humiliation is usually a key feature in the narcissistic wounding that is often seen to be closely related to the beginning of a manic attack.

Details of past manic episodes should be explored with the family and understood fully. Do they have a typical course? Do they involve drinking as an attempt to soothe the mood? Do they involve spending, job losses, reckless driving, promiscuity, querulousness? The patient's past patterns often hold true and thus provide some guidelines for management in manic attacks in the future.

Constant pressing of limits, together with loud, expansive, insensitive behavior, makes patients in a manic episode difficult for both family and therapist to deal with. The therapist is at high risk of employing distancing maneuvers that remove him or her from the patient when that patient is most in need. As a group, individuals in manic states are likely to be unattractive to therapists: They are loud, insensitive, and overwhelmingly extroverted, with seemingly little curiosity about, or access to, their inner workings. For therapeutically oriented professionals, they don't "feel" like good therapy patients. Sadly, many such patients suffer from less than optimal treatment because of therapists' unwarranted aversion to them. This aversion detracts from the treatment's taking an optimal course. Although family therapy and individual psychotherapy often do not proceed in ways that give the therapist emotional satisfaction, they frequently combine with pharmacological and hospital treatments to decisively alter the course of the illness and to lower the overall morbidity significantly beyond that which would occur with the provision of hospital treatments and medications alone (Davenport & Adland, 1985). Therapists giving up on family work with manic patients are often, unbeknownst to themselves, responding to countertransference problems of serious proportions that compromise the overall treatment results immensely.

CASE EXAMPLE

A 38-year-old first-break manic patient was brought in to the hospital with expansive mood, flight of ideas, delusions, overactivity, and querulousness. He had not slept for nights, had made many phone calls over the preceding weeks, had proposed extravagant business deals, was overactive and on the move, and had been sexually promiscuous for some weeks prior to admission. He was brought in by his family after admitting that he needed help after he was arrested for speeding in a school zone. His marriage had been in difficulty for some years and appeared to be headed imminently toward separation. Nonetheless, his wife appeared, as did his parents and teen-age son. The patient pressed to leave and was placed on involuntary detention. A family session was called immediately, and was held on the day after he was admitted.

The family was seated in the therapist's office when the patient entered, greeted the therapist, and immediately requested a half-day pass to take care of business matters. The therapist noted that he was new to the hospital and asked if anybody in the family could help with those details. The patient pressed, and the family at first looked at the therapist, inclined to go along with the patient's request. But the therapist said, "He has just been admitted as dangerous to himself and perhaps others. Aren't you trying to reason when it's not possible to do so because of the way his illness is?"

The patient became angry and more demanding, saying he was in better shape than many of the patients on the ward already, and defied the therapist to produce evidence that he could not handle a pass. He said, "Look, you've spent only an hour with me. How do you know I can't handle it? There are other people here in much worse shape than I am who get passes." The therapist turned to the patient's upset wife and crying mother, saying, "Perhaps this is what you've had to deal with over these last weeks." They cried, then looked greatly relieved, and the therapist continued, "With this illness, you have to see him as sicker the more he presses for things like this, and to be firm about saying no."

The patient became angry and boisterous to the point where he had to be escorted out of the room, but the session continued, with the therapist saying, "So this is what you've put up with over the last few weeks." All agreed. The therapist continued, "We have a whole experienced hospital staff that is used to dealing with these things, and knows something about them. What has it been like for all of you?" The wife cried for some time and told about the marriage, which was near the breaking point, and became overwhelming when he became demanding, unrealistic, and expansive. After a few minutes, the therapist turned to the parents, who told of their tribulations in trying to be reasonable with the patient, and of their regrets at their own failures to protect him early in his life. The son acknowledged his upset and talked about his deteriorating grades in school over the last month.

The therapist then said, "This is an illness that you must know something about. The first thing to stress is that when he is like this, he has to be in a hospital as soon as possible." The session continued, with the therapist giving information about manic–depressive illness and its treatment, interspersed with empathetic comments and questions about the family's experience of the patient's psychosis and their fears of what this meant, the shame over their failures, and public embarrassment and guilt because they felt they should have done more and had begun to resent the patient and wanted to be rid of him. They left greatly relieved and eager to return for the next session.

RECURRENT UNIPOLAR DEPRESSION

A major depressive episode is one characterized more by neurovegetative signs—disturbances of sleep, appetite, libido, and concentration—than by mood *per se*. Evidence that severe depressive disorders are not in immediate steady state with the interpersonal environment is overwhelming: The obviously somatic nature of neurovegetative signs, the imperviousness of such states to psychotherapy and their responsiveness to medication or ECT, and the likelihood that there are biological markers either for depressive states themselves or for persons liable to experience recurrent depressive episodes all attest to the biological contribution to depressive states.

But it is an entirely false antithesis to posit a biological "lesion" as opposed to a dynamic one. We do not know what the basic disorder in depression is. There are biological approaches to understanding depressive phenomena, but we are far from an understanding of specific biological factors—not just correlates—in their connection to the defects in self-esteem regulation, the dependence of "will," and the difficulty with direct expression of anger that are so much a part of the attachment behavior and emotional makeup of depressive persons. Constitutional factors powerfully affect interpersonal (attachment and expressive) behaviors, which, in turn, affect mood. At present, we lack good integrative models to conceptualize the central defect in depression.

The curious and unbiased clinician is always perplexed by the depressive patient, sensing the biology behind the dynamics, and the dynamics behind the biology. Behind the "dynamics" of a middle-aged man whose wife has found out about his having an affair is the depression, providing both the need to prove himself with another woman and the need to be caught. So, perhaps the depression was primary and the circumstances were "downstream" from the affective disorder. But behind the depression lurks a hopelessness about a failure of promotion, or a job loss—a failure to experience his will as sufficiently powerful to accomplish his aspirations: a dynamic frame of reference again. Perhaps he fears competition, suffers guilt over successes, depends too much on approval from superiors to be a leader, has an endopsychic perception of these weaknesses, and is depressed about them. But behind those dynamics are the basics of his personality— the combination of his constitutional givens and his life experience. This perplexity in the relation of mood to circumstances would still be with us even if we had clear markers—biological correlates—for either depressive states or persons vulnerable to them. Biology and dynamics are inseparable with the depressed patient. There are no depressive disorders, no matter how responsive to medications, without major characterological features that should be considered in overall treatment approaches. Its origins and etiology notwithstanding, severe depression of mood always has accompaniments in difficulties in close, especially familial, relationships. The family should be in focus if the therapist is to understand the history of the patient's difficulties and pave the way for dealing with the interpersonal aspects of them.

No one pattern of interpersonal relationships typifies all depression, though typical patterns, and ones with common themes, are found. Slipp (1984), using an object relations perspective to characterize one type of depressive dynamics, has described a familial constellation in which one parent uses both spouse and child for regulation of that parent's narcissistic equilibrium. That parent's bad parts are projected onto the spouse, and the good ones onto the child, who is driven to succeed but who is simultaneously filled with guilt and unable either to enjoy success or to separate from the parent in question.

Certainly, attachments that are intense and extremely limiting are found in the families of origin of depressive patients (Bemporad, 1970). Often, the future depressive is keenly sensitive to the depression of a parent and is both limited by that depression and burdened with a need to take care of that parent. Such a predicament saddles the future depressive with deficits from parenting that come from a depressed or preoccupied parent; poor models of interpersonal effectiveness provided by that parent, which the child can use in the course of development; and the burden of responsibility for that parent's emotional state, which forces the future depressive, as a child, into a parental role vis-à-vis his or her depressed parent. All of these factors combine powerfully to retard separation from the family of origin, to make for a powerful but constrictive parent–child bond that generates in the future depressive an intense resentment that often cannot be expressed or resolved for fear of damaging the parent. The parent–child bond and the subsequent constrictions and unresolved anger that arise are usually recreated in the family of procreation (often with the overattachment to the family of origin persisting and creating conflict in the family of procreation). In both the family of origin and the family of procreation, the depressive feels a sense of overwhelming obligation, no sense of choice, and a fear of deep anger that is seen as destructive when expressed.

There are many variations on this basic pattern. Some depressives get lost in a maze of dutiful performances on the job or for the family of procreation, with obsessional "false selves" existing only for people with whom they work or only for family members with whom they are close and—despite protestations from those in the family—never having an independent time or independent projects of their own (Winnicott, 1955). Others express anger in unmodulated, explosive ways; compensate by guilty atonements; and oscillate between outbursts and exaggerated atonements, neither of which emanate from a sense of self-worth and self-respect. Yet others may take an overtly regressed posture toward their own families: They are quarrelsome, combative, blaming, substance abusing, whining, self-pitying, or negativistic (Rosenthal & Gudeman, 1967). Alternatively, an unconscious struggle—a desperate one—may exist against an identification with a depressed parent of the same sex who showed these traits in a manner felt to be contemptible in the family of origin (Greenson, 1954; Lansky, 1985).

The family therapy of such persons must proceed with awareness of these patterns, and especially of the resonances between family of origin and family of procreation. The therapist not mindful of major dynamic features is at high risk of oversimplifying or of aiming treatment at superficial or irrelevant issues, or of neglecting central matters altogether. A feeling of responsibility for a depressed parent or spouse is not the same issue as a struggle against an unconscious identification with a contemptible parent that is handled by projection onto a spouse. Fear of autonomous gratification is almost never as simply handled as it might appear to be. The overly encumbered depressed patient engages in self-sabotaging maneuvers, picks fights, provokes "realistic" circumstances that preclude independence, or simply fails to let the issue of autonomy stay in focus. Some depressives will "parent" the therapist, either by helping with the session arrangement or fees or by quietly regulating the therapist's self-esteem, or keeping his or her mood "up." Alliances so formed are, in my experience, always costly to the overall result. The therapist should question any alliance with the depressed person that becomes too convenient, that is, where hours are easily changed, where the depressive person is the only one approachable about fees, where the depressive person placates or soothes upset members of the family, and so forth.

Another strong indication for family involvement, and a commonly neglected one, is the need for assessing and monitoring the effects of medication (Lansky, 1981b). Not all the effects of antidepressant medication can be assessed by reports of the patient's subjective responses, that is, by improvement in self-reported mood, or by change in neurovegetative signs. A spouse is often able to note very definite changes in abrasiveness with even minute changes in antidepressant medications. It is essential that such abrasiveness come into focus in the treatment, because the depressed patient is often unaware of his or her own abrasiveness or tension but notices, instead, the anger, quarrelsomeness, or lack of soothing support coming from close persons—responses that always frustrate the patient. Medication effects provide the basis for a method of assessment of inner tension states in persons who all too frequently never see themselves as tense, on edge, and quarrelsome until they experience some other baseline feeling. Antidepressants have a good effect on patients who are quarrelsome, belligerent, touchy, and blaming and who only in retrospect can see that they have carried a low-key, chronic depression into close relationships and have provoked unkind reactions to themselves by their style of relating. A common finding with such patients is that they feel exposed and humiliated by having to be on medication in the first place, and that they are likely to discontinue that medication, no matter how good the effects, after some unempathic or outright wounding remark is made by a family member.

CASE EXAMPLE

A 37-year-old mother of two came in with her husband for marital therapy complaining of so many of his shortcomings that it was difficult to keep track of them. She worked in his medical office as a manager, receptionist, and general office assistant and complained that he had pushed her around, exploited her constantly, and was unappreciative, unaffectionate, and unloving. He, in turn, complained that she argued; was nervous, sleepless, and uninterested in sex; and avoided closeness. She was unremittingly critical of him and of the two children. These transactions had been a typical pattern over the years but had increased dramatically over the last 2 months. The therapist commented on how intertwined their lives were. They both explained that she did work equivalent to a professional position at least and that to replace her would cost many times her salary. The therapist noted that the family had adequate funds to forgo the financial advantages of her working in the office. They came to work together and went home together. When they came home, she made dinner but ate almost nothing, criticized the children constantly, and berated her husband. He retreated, reading magazines most evenings in his room. She spent the evening taking long baths and just resting in a state of exhaustion. She had sunk into a state of clear-cut depression, with early morning awakening, complete loss of libido, pronounced weight loss, and some difficulty concentrating, but she was also querulent, blaming, critical, and fault finding of those closest to her. The latter behaviors were not observed at the office. The therapist suggested antidepressants and began a moderate dose of this medication.

At the next session a week later, the wife reported that there was no change, but her husband disagreed: "No, she's much less prickly, and she's calmer, and there's no problem sleeping now." She agreed about the sleep problem. He said that she attacked the children less. She wondered why she had to take medication and he didn't. He was the cause of her unhappiness, and he was much more disturbed than she. He said that she was considerably better. The dose was increased.

A week later, she did notice that she was calmer and somewhat less attacking, and very definitely slept better. She had even started to feel some libido. He said she had missed some of her medication one day, and he could tell from the tension that she was taking less than a full dose. She went back on the medication and, after a few weeks, started to feel better. The question arose again why she was so intertwined with her husband that she had no autonomous life, and why she didn't work elsewhere if life was as intolerable as she claimed. The husband said that she did the work of several staff persons and that in her absence it would have been necessary to hire several professionals and administrative staff to replace her. They agreed that the office required her to continue to work that way. The issue of her overinvolvement at home and in the office surfaced repeatedly, with her guilt and sense of overresponsibility brought more sharply into focus.

She was the eldest daughter in a family where the parents quarreled and threatened divorce within deliberate earshot of the children, making the patient, in particular, fear that they were imminently about to leave the house, arguing over which of them was to leave, and ultimately deciding that both would leave. She recalled a feeling of panic, constant pleading with them to stay together, and running alternatively after one and then the other, thinking they were really both going to leave. Only later in life did she realize the durability of her parents' marriage, despite the perpetual instability that drew her in.

When her inability to free herself from servitude to her husband's office and to her family came up again, she went a day and a half without medication and became quarrelsome. In the midst of an argument, the husband told her abruptly, "Stop yelling and take your pills," and she refused to take medications thereafter. The same depressive stalemate reasserted itself.

BORDERLINE PERSONALITY DISORDERS

Before discussing the family treatment of patients carrying the unhappily chosen label "borderline," I will attempt to disentangle that term from its many pejorative associations and linkages to theoretical assumptions that are untenable.

The word derives from two sources. Early in its usage, it was linked to thinking about psychosis, or even schizophrenia. In its early (and inaccurate) usage, it denoted preschizophrenic, ambulatory schizophrenia, latent schizophrenia, or not-quite-manifest schizophrenia. This usage carried with it an implication that the adjective "borderline" somehow modified the noun "schizophrenia." This line of thinking gained apparent support from the observations of Robert Knight (1953) that deeply disturbed, presumably neurotic patients in psychoanalysis were vulnerable to short-lived psychotic episodes, that is, "borderline states." The tendency to cluster borderline states and borderline patients has found no support in systematic research (Grinker, Werble, & Drye, 1968). The natural history of the two disorders, schizophrenia and the borderline disorder, have been discontinuous: Borderline condition does not develop into schizophrenia, and schizophrenia does not remit into a borderline state.

The 1980 DSM-III (American Psychiatric Association, 1980), and subsequently DSM-III-R (American Psychiatric Association, 1987), considered "borderline" as a personality disorder distinct from other personality disorders and as having no connection with schizophrenia. The virtue of this approach is that it has worked from specific discriminating criteria for the identification and study of such patients. These criteria carry us as far as a purely phenomenological method can. There are, however, problems with the DSM-III-R classification of "borderline" as one among many disorders of personality. First, it has been argued (Bursten, 1982) that the classification, based as it is on the phenomenology and not on personality organization or basic deficit, is too reified and lacks a central concept of disturbance in personality. Hence it constructs a typology entirely wedded to appearance—a typology that is not refined by feedback from relatively clear-cut treatment response as is the case with the psychoses. Second, the classification is tainted by the faculty psychology inherent in the term "personality disorder," which has nothing really to do with the methodology of DSM-III-R. That methodology is Kraepelinian and phenomenological, deriving its strength from the linkage of observable traits with the natural history of illness and treatment response, and not at all from the postulation of any fundamental reason to classify any particular illness as a disorder of thought, mood, personality, or brain.

I belabor these points because currently, the literature reflects a growing awareness of the prevalence of affective disorder among patients with presumed personality disorders (Gunderson & Elliott, 1985; Akiskal, Chen, & Davis, 1985). Certainly, the following evidence can be garnered to support the notion that patients with these disorders:

1. The phenomenology of the disorder is dominated by overwhelming disturbances of mood, intense and often explosive rage, affective instability, intolerance of both separation and closeness (and affective storms precipitated by either of these), empty depression and mood-related quarrelsomeness, social withdrawal, preoccupation, or impulsive action.

2. When patterns of impulsive actions, including substance abuse, are interrupted, overwhelming disturbances of mood often result (Vaillant, 1975).

3. Psychotherapeutic intervention of any kind has as one of its final achievements the integration of personality to the point where the patient can tolerate previously unbearable affects (guilt, mourning, anxiety, etc.; Klein, 1946; Paul, 1973) without engaging in a rageful and controlling action that inevitably destroys close relationships.

4. Pharmacological intervention for disorders of this type is never complete, but major gains are often made with antidepressant medications or lithium carbonate. These medications also prove highly effective in treating symptoms far different from those thought to be classical—that is, neurovegetative signs (for depressions) and demonstrative cyclic moods or manic episodes. Neither neuroleptics nor minor tranquilizers have as central a role in the treatment of borderline conditions.

These considerations are at least as supportive of classifying these disorders under the reification "affective disorder" as under the reification "personality disorder," even though deep disturbances of both mood and conduct are prominent in each case. If it is borne in mind that the personalities of such patients are usually vulnerable to disorganization, and that reactions to this disorganization are (in part) attempts to control people who provide cohesion, it can be asserted that in thoroughly treated cases at least, the major efforts, pharmacological, and psychotherapeutic, are aimed at controlling overwhelming disturbances of mood.

The family of the borderline patient is important to treatment in a number of ways, not just in terms of participation in conjoint psychotherapy sessions. Because of the high prevalence of lability of relationships both in this type of patient and in family members, it is important to maintain the focus on the family, even if the patient and family insist that there is no current contact between them. Serious mistakes are made in not focusing on absences of family contact (Lansky, Bley, Simenstad, West, McVey, 1983). It is important to consider the family in the following areas when treating borderline patients:

1. *The workup.* An intergenerational perspective on such patients is essential. Histories of the borderline patient almost invariably reveal easily ascertainable massive trauma prior to the age of 10 (Lansky, 1981a). Such trauma can take the form of absence of, or instability in, close intimate persons; actual separations or emotional absences due to serious depression, substance abuse, or chronic preoccupation; continually threatened separations in a volatile marriage; the patient's involvement in an immature and difficult marriage and in an attempt to control it by his or her being scapegoated, parentified, or blamed; or sustained sexual or physical abuse,

continuing with the knowledge of at least one parent. It is the rule that borderline patients come from unsatisfying or strife-ridden marriages in the family of origin, often those where the same-sex parent was held in contempt within the family circle (Lansky, 1985). Mate choice in such patients, as Bowen (1966) has noted, is powerfully affected by the family of origin and current level of the patient's functioning. Many of the difficulties that arise in the family of procreation or that are related to an absence of family can be usefully seen as being derived from unfinished business in the family of origin. The workup is not an idle historical preamble to treatment of these patients. The overreactivity and proneness to humiliation of these patients makes an intergenerational stance the beginning of an ongoing therapeutic process and a method of pointing out to the patient his or her characterological vulnerabilities in close relationships, without flooding him or her with shame.

2. *The assessment and management of overt conflict.* I have previously described blaming relationships, stably unstable, conflictual marriages that despite their surface discomfort, typically endure for decades (Lansky, 1980, 1981c). These relationships, despite their seeming volatility and chaos, are tightly regulated, enduring structures, providing for both security and thematic repetition of infantile trauma. Such marriages, organized as they are around transgressions and rage, cannot be treated in the same ways as are relatively normal or neurotic marriages organized around inhibition. The therapist may too soon see the central purpose of the couple's treatment as the management and diminution of overwhelming affect, but such an assumption should never be the basis for therapeutic goals without a total appreciation of the protective and expressive functions of such collusive transactions for the couple, however unpleasant they may seem to the therapist. Often, couples do not see such episodes as something they want treated, or, because of the extreme sensitivity to humiliation in the partners, they are not able to go forward with treatment and the risk of exposure that goes along with it. Treatment of a marriage characterized by blaming is always a complex issue, involving the following modalities: (a) conjoint treatment for the spouses or treatment in a couples group, often with the aim of minimizing malignant effects of the couples (collusive defensive operations); (b) involvement of children of the marriage, for the purpose of providing perspective for them and enabling them to free up emotionally from the debilitating effects of the family process; (c) antidepressant medication, in moderate dosage, for the habitual blamer, no matter what other indications for medication are present; and (d) some enduring methods of support, provided by either long-term psychotherapy or open-ended couples groups. Conjoint treatment should be aimed at overreactivity, and couples encouraged to speak through the therapist, as Bowen (1966) has advocated; this strategy is employed because the therapist does not react and because the couples overreact to each other to the point that they cannot learn from

experience by talking to each other. Intergenerational reconstructions are crucial in providing patients with a sense of unfinished business in their families of origin. This business is triggered by conflict in their current familial situation and is repeated at great cost and without the likelihood of resolution. The use of intergenerational reconstructions should be thought of as a technique for dealing with affect in two main ways: It relocates anger to the original objects, and it allows spouses to appreciate vulnerabilities without being flooded with shame and without covering the shame with an omnipotent, infantile rage directed at the other. Such crippling emotional forces that affect children in the family can be recognized and acknowledged in the countertransference by experienced therapists. I cannot emphasize too strongly the importance of getting children in sessions, to free them up from false hopefulness about changing the family process or from the responsibility for refereeing continued marital disputes. Antidepressant medication for the blamer produces effects that are almost always dramatic both to the spouse and (often, later) to the blamer, who comes to appreciate that the edgy, depressive state that is transiently abetted by blaming transactions and the constriction and anhedonia that become personified and are attributed to the shortcoming of the blamed spouse are variants of depression. Finally, establishing long-term psychotherapy for the patient or having both spouses participate in open-ended couples groups will help maintain improvement and provide support into the future.

3. *The management of crises.* Borderline patients react to the interpersonal environment by inducting in others strong affect, guilt, anxiety, terror, and futility. The intrapsychic accompaniment of such transpersonal maneuvers is projective identification (Klein, 1946; Lansky, 1980), or the fantasy that part of the self is split off and resides in others whom the patient controls. Such affective force, detectable in the countertransference feelings of the therapist, puts strong pressure on others to collude with the unconscious fantasy that they carry the responsibility for somehow regulating the patient or to leave the emotional field. In treating patients who are undergoing borderline crises, not only the issues but the method of communication and the emotional climate must be scrutinized and interpreted. Absence of family members almost always becomes more understandable when these issues have been explored: Although excess demands for support or intimidations may control people at first, they eventually wear out the support systems—employers, friends, therapists, and finally even spouse, parents, and children. It is crucial that these emotional forces be understood, lest repetitive self-sabotaging actions arising from them be continued.

4. *The management of symptoms.* Symptoms, especially if they are impulsive acts (Lansky, in press), slashing, binge drinking, communication of suicidal impulses, violence, or intimidation, are found to have a complex structure and a regulatory function among intimates of the patient. A precipitant, usually a narcissistic wound or an emotional absence, detonates

a personality disorganization in a person vulnerable to such fragmentation. This experience of disorganization may have conscious elements, or it will be superseded almost entirely by the more visible parts of the process. There may be a conscious prodromal experience, a fleeting paranoia, cravings to complete a compulsive act, or eerie, edgy moods and experiences of disintegration. The impulsive act itself may be followed by either shame or guilt; these sequelae tend to hide the earlier experiences of disorganization that so flood the patient with shame. The act often restores optimal distance to supportive persons who have become either too close or too far away. The distance-regulating effect of borderline symptoms must be appreciated if the symptoms, the family, or the individual are to be treated appropriately. Such treatment often includes antidepressant medication or lithium carbonate. Use of these mood-regulating drugs may prospectively (but usually not retrospectively) seem to be based on arbitrary indications. I shall elaborate on the problem of impulsive action in the section on suicide that follows.

CASE EXAMPLE

A 43-year-old married man was admitted for excessive drinking, job loss, depression, and legal difficulties that were the results of his exhibiting his penis in public. In the hospital, he stopped drinking, with help from Alcoholics Anonymous, and discussed his sexual difficulties with his resident physician. In the course of family evaluation, his marriage was felt to be an unusually difficult one. The resident physician felt that the case was too tumultuous and too difficult to deal with and referred the patient and his wife to an experienced co-therapy team for evaluation and treatment.

In an early session, when the wife was 10 minutes late for an appointment, the husband flew into a rage, berating his wife for her lateness and hurling vile epithets at her for letting him down and being unreliable. The accusatory episode took place in an atmosphere of intense rage on his part and a child-like neediness on hers that seemed helpless in the face of the angry blast coming from him. The therapists, acting on a sense of helplessness, inquired about the couple's mutual understanding of their arrangements about arrival place and time and attempted to negotiate a compromise solution to the conflict. Looking back on their reaction, the therapists agreed that they had felt responsible for stopping the chaos, helpless to do so, and repelled by the aggressive outbursts. More rage attacks continued from the husband every time his wife would be late, let him down, or even exclude him from a conversation. Once, when she locked the bathroom door while bathing, he flew into a rage and broke down the door, furiously proclaiming that he would not be locked out.

Asked about the marriage, the couple agreed that such interchanges were typical of a marriage that had endured for two decades without talk of divorce. They had three adolescent children. The husband had had a number of jobs and worked somewhat below his intellectual capacity. The wife had been in charge of an auditing department in a large retail store for many years.

He had been born in wartime Europe to a woman widowed when she was still pregnant with the patient. He had been passed back and forth early in life from one resentful female caretaker to another. His wife was the youngest of three daughters born to alcoholic parents. The parental marriage collapsed, and the two elder sisters went with the father. She went with her mother for a few years until the mother was institutionalized. Then she was taken in by her father, but resented by the sisters. She developed a *modus operandi* that consisted of enduring indignities from these two sisters as a method of securing herself in the family, in a degraded but somewhat secure position.

As the therapy continued, the couple began to appreciate their collusive defenses from an intergenerational perspective. His rage and humiliation at being dependent on women was compounded by a fragility—not unrelated to his tenuous and unwelcome status early in life—that manifested itself in actual disorganized states precipitated by lateness, rejection, and even exclusion from conversations by his wife. This vulnerability was compensated for in the intense relatedness accompanying his self-righteous blaming attacks. The wife endured, and even encouraged, indignities as she had in her family of origin, to feel secure by being needed, however degraded the relationship made her feel. She encouraged blaming attacks in her marriage by repeated maneuvers, such as the lateness and her ineffectual protestations when he began to attack her. This was her method of inflicting punishment on, and exerting control over, her husband. As his rage attacks became less upsetting to the therapists, the depressive element in the husband's attacks could be sensed and confirmed in the actual content of the blaming transaction, that is in his protestations that she had deserted him, let him down, not been there for him, and been unreliable for him. The blaming transaction, together with the provocation to blame, was found to serve complex distance-regulating functions for both, locking the couple into a secure relatedness, and at the same time warding off the intimacy that both also feared.

A course of moderate-dose antidepressant medication modulated both the rageful blaming attacks and the vulnerability to disorganization and intense fear behind them.

THE PROBLEM OF SUICIDE

The problem of suicide is so often felt by therapists to be parallel to the problem of depression that unwarranted assumptions are made that increasing depression is the reason for suicide. Though in many cases there are indeed strong connections between depression and suicide, the assumption that people kill themselves simply because of overwhelming depression is unwarranted and potentially disastrous. Depression is one of many pathways to suicide and is usually not a sufficient explanation of the death of depressed persons who commit suicide. "Depression" is too constricted a concept for the turmoil that leads people to self-destruction. "Suicide" or "suicidal," also has an ambiguity of usage that has a broader connotation than completed self-destruction. "Suicidal" may refer to acute or chronic gestures, threats, or communications of intent to kill oneself that terrify persons who feel responsible for the patient. These communications may either organize supportive persons in attempts to be helpful to the patient or cause them to become exhausted and abandon the patient (Lansky, 1982). Alternatively, "suicidal" may refer to any of a variety of self-harming, impulsive acts, such as wrist slashing or overdosing, that have a structure of typical impulsive action, that is, a disorganizing experience, together with a distance-regulating effect. People employing such pathological distance regulation are most likely to kill themselves not during impulsive acts that serve to organize people but rather when the restitutive or distance-regulating function of such acts fails, that is, when support systems give out (Straker, 1958).

Suicidal intent is often communicated either indirectly or in such a manner that a useful alliance cannot be formed with the assurance that the patient, too, is worried about being suicidal. Faced with a patient who communicates that he or she does not want to live, the therapist may feel that all of the responsibility is his or hers, and none the patient's. Such a feeling of responsibility without the assurance of a treatment alliance, especially if the lack of alliance is not addressed by the therapist directly, inevitably produces turmoil or panic in the therapist and the push either to overregulate the patient or to desert him, physically or emotionally. These responses of the therapist are far from harmless. Such overregulation and desertion often reiterate the very kind of object relations in the patient's life history that has contributed to his or her despair, shame, and hopelessness about the kind of attachments that make life worth living. An overregulatory or too distanced response, then, may push the patient closer to despair and self-harm than a methodical, communicative approach that is mindful of the patient's history of relationships with supportive persons and that is attentive to the nature of the therapeutic alliance and the communications within it.

The family is crucial to the assessment of the following factors.

1. *Developmental history* is often crucial in determining if the patient's presumed suicidal intent refers to self-destructive impulsive actions typical of patients with borderline personality organizations. This sort of history was discussed in the previous section. Impulse-ridden patients often cope with their defects in personal cohesion by excessive demandingness, provocation, and a sense of entitlement that provokes current supportive persons,

often in the family of procreation, to overregulate, distance, or finally desert.

2. *The current status of support systems* can often be evaluated quickly by the simple suggestion of a family meeting or by a phone call to family members. Overeager family can be mobilized, but there is risk, in the short run, of their impinging on the patient and amplifying regression and envy, or in the long run, of exhausting the support system. Frightened or overwhelmed family must be responded to in a way that is mindful of their fears of being blamed for the patient's difficulties or their feeling that impossible demands are being placed on them. Faint or absent interest indicates that the support system is chronically rejecting or unempathic, or, more likely, that the disinterest results from repetitive communications of suicidal intent from the patient that have worn out his or her welcome and have exhausted the support system. Absent family participation (Lansky *et al.*, 1983) is often a strong indication that the patient's characterological maneuvers have worn out support systems and resulted in rejection. Such absence is a crucial issue for therapy and should never be overlooked. Often, patients' depression, despair, and completed suicide are related to the shame and hopelessness they feel upon realizing that they are repeatedly destructive in close relationships and repeatedly drive off the very people they require for a sense of well-being. The realization that one inevitably does this in close relationships may be more lethal than the actual loss of a particular person, which may be overemphasized.

3. *Multisystem containment interpretation* is the most perspicacious method of dealing with the patient's current problems. Disruptions in relations with persons on whom the patient depends, especially if they occur in more than one social system, may point to areas of potential caution and potential change in the treatment collaboration; for example, if similar themes are found in the family of origin, the family of procreation, the job, previous marriages, and even the treatment setting, the therapist is in a better position to focus on these areas for emphasis and to beware of them in the helping relationship as well. Special care should be taken by the therapist to observe feelings or actions on his or her part that reveal inappropriate reactions to the patient's pathology—that is, countertransference reactions. The therapist may notice helplessness or panic at the patient's communications, especially indirect or disowned communications of suicidality, and may deal with these emotions by being oversolicitous—that is, too involved, which is likely to produce regression and envy and to wear out the therapist—or overtly indifferent or overly contractual—that is, too emotionally indifferent to the patient. Certain behaviors in the treatment team usually indicate that unresolved hostility has been evoked in the therapist or treatment team. These include joking about the patient, any sort of self-righteousness, and overattention to manipulative aspects of the patient's behavior, as well as overt hostility or dislike. The therapist with a

perspective on other systems that provoke this response in the helper will be more likely to be able to communicate the feeling, and the maneuvers that elicit such a feeling, to the patient and the family. Once the therapist's curiosity is drawn to difficulties with the treatment alliance and to their perpetration by overt or covert communications, he or she, aided by an intergenerational perspective, may look for pathological features behind these communicative modes that shed light on the suicidality as well as on the disturbed treatment alliance.

A common pattern includes indirect communication of suicidal intent and disowning of intent. This snares intimates into caretaking situations and fills them with panic when the patient does not ally with the protectors or profess any acknowledgment of suicidal intent or interest in helping himself or herself. The therapist's metacommunication, that is, communication about communication, often leads to a realization that the very panic stirred up in others was felt by the patient in crucial relationships early in life. The patient's communication may *split* helpers, with one party being too solicitous, and the other too critical, of the patient. Usually, such a pattern resonates with significant events in the family of origin and is likely to appear in the treatment situation also, with helpers split into rescuers and persecutors. Again, inter-generational interpretation is a powerful method of freeing up malignant aspects of the communicative process that work against an alliance. Knowing *secrets* in the family of the suicidal patient, whether these be the patient's suicidal plans or, for example, the knowledge of a spouse's affair or intent to divorce, puts the therapist in a disastrous and thoroughly impossible bind. The therapeutic team should refuse to be bound to secrecy on issues that may affect the treatment alliance or the ability to communicate.

Removal of these difficulties in the alliance is not tantamount to removing the problem of suicide, but in a surprising number of cases of suicidal patients, the reasons for poor alliance are so intimately linked with the reasons—found in early and repeated pathological object relations—for suicidal feelings in the first place that metacommunication with an intergen-erational perspective addresses the alliance only to end up at the center of the patient's basic difficulties.

In the presence of a reliable working alliance, in direct communication, the patient, therapist, and family can collaborate to do what is possible to best provide for the patient's needs.

CASE EXAMPLE

A man in his late 50s was admitted to the hospital after a communication of suicidal intent to his first wife. That woman, who had divorced him 20 years previously, became concerned and, finally, terrified and brought him to the hospital where he was admitted, not only for safekeeping but also for evaluation of his general difficulties, which included a turbulent relationship with his second wife and stepson. He also had depression, which was accompanied by neurovegetative signs; sleep, appetite, and libido disturbance; and decreased ability to concentrate.

He described a childhood replete with deprivations. He was raised in orphanages and never knew his father. His mother, a woman with many characterological difficulties, could not provide stable nurturance and finally gave him up for adoption. His first marriage had ended 20 years previously. He explained the failure of that marriage in the way he explained so many other things, in a vague manner that suggested either offhandedness on his part or shortcomings in persons other than himself. His evasiveness consistently failed to provide the listener with a clear view of his difficulties in either marriage, or of life in general. He had remarried soon after the first marriage ended and represented himself as a stable and steadily employed man, providing for his wife and her son from a previous marriage. Two years prior to his admission to the hospital, he had had spinal surgery, which incapacitated him and rendered him unable to work. His wife began to work and support the family. The stepson, now 20 years old, had utterly failed, in the patient's words, to show him any respect and provoked quarrels. His wife sided with her son. The patient became sullen and angry and began drinking heavily. He attempted to convince his wife to leave the area and leave the stepson behind. He described the stepson in vehement terms that suggested projected self-reproaches: The lad was lazy, parasitic, manipulative, and underhanded, provoking people to get undeserved caretaking and special status. In the hospital, he made much of his sufferings, but demanded grounds privileges, missed meetings, and in general proved to be elusive and very difficult to engage in treatment.

An intergenerational perspective on his hatred of caretakers and his fear of abandonment and on the passivity in his family of origin allowed the staff, and later, the patient, to appreciate his fears of dependent relationships. These were previously compensated for by a relatively stable work history that provided a source of self-esteem. This source of self-esteem had become undone, and he did poorly in the regressive status left him after the spinal surgery. The feelings of deviousness and worthlessness that he had felt in trying to get caretaking early in life resonated throughout his current circumstances with his wife and son and in his relationships at the hospital. Evening staff, in particular, disliked his evasiveness, suspected that he was drinking, and thought him to be generally elusive. These circumstances in the hospital gave the therapists a good deal of insight into his conduct in both marriages and into the context of his precarious sense of self-worth that was compensated for by the control he exerted with his threats of intent to commit suicide. His previous somewhat stable compensation had become undone when the combination of physical illness (loss of status as breadwinner) and competition with his stepson flooded him with a sense of neediness, shame, and depression that precipitated the hospitalization.

CONCLUSION

I have provided an overview of treatment approaches for four prominent clinical predicaments involving affective disorders. My treatment approaches and attitudes have been put forward more definitively in this chapter than might have been the case in a longer and less clinically oriented presentation, where a review of the evidence and justification of my specific line of thinking would have been set forth in comparison with other approaches.

Those familiar with the current literature will notice that my approach fails to comment at all on shorter, more cognitive approaches to depression, especially Beck's (Beck & Shaw, 1977), or on behavioral approaches, for example, those emphasizing learned helplessness. I have placed no emphasis on the use of biological markers, and in particular, on the dexamethasone suppression test. Fully explaining these omissions would carry me into lines of reasoning that go beyond space constraints and beyond the immediate clinical purpose of this discussion. That purpose is to highlight aspects of the family treatment of severe affective disorders from an integrative point of view, emphasizing the importance of treatment strategy, including family involvement, arising in response to the specific psychopathology in question.

The four predicaments pose different treatment problems, and for that reason, the flavor of each set of family interventions is different. Despite the differences in particular approach, there are certain commonalities, which taken together, constitute a treatment attitude toward these disorders with major pathology present. This treatment attitude involves the following elements:

1. *No etiological presuppositions are made*; hence there is no reason to assume that a psychotherapeutic approach presumes a dynamic etiology as opposed to one deriving from constitutional deficit, or that a pharmacological intervention implies an organic as opposed to a conflictual origin of the difficulties.

2. *Treatment of major psychopathology is integrative*, in three complex ways, when treating the affective disorders. First, it is usually multimodal. Insistence on one method alone, for example, psychotherapy or pharmacotherapy is never a virtue and is confined in its usefulness to simpler cases and less sick patients. Second, integration is required between considerations dealing with dynamics or conflict and those concerning deficit or constitution; both are present, in almost every instance, in patients with severe affective disorders. This requires complex integration for the therapist, who must see himself or herself as responsible for every aspect of competent treatment and yet must avoid overregulating or overorchestrating the patient's movements to the point where the patient loses responsibility for elements of conflict and for his or her own life. Practical decisions

about who is responsible for what remain extremely difficult in the treatment of the affective disorders and require extreme skill and patience on the part of the therapist. Third, the same kind of integration is necessary for keeping in focus the upset, turmoil, and affective storms undergone by a patient (how he or she feels) and what he or she does (including what he or she does not do, omissions in responsibility). This is most difficult with characterologically impaired patients. The therapist must keep an eye on those demands for special status based on how damaged and upset the patient feels and on evasion of responsibility for what the patient actually does.

3. *The family can be usefully conceptualized using a container model* (Lansky, 1981a). The family provides a support system when the personality system fails to contain the chaos imposed by the patient's disorder. This model provides a conceptualization for hospitalization that is very useful. The hospital is a temporary container when the personality and family systems do not contain the chaos posed by the disorder. The indications for family intervention can be conceptualized quite simply: Family therapy is indicated any time containment fails, certainly in any hospitalized case or major psychotic disorder involving uncontrolled impulsivity or a threat to self or others. The patient's right to reasonably refuse family involvement is justified by his or her ability to contain self, no matter how much duress is undergone by the illness. The focus of family work should begin with the experience of failed containment for the disorder, and empathic contact should be made with both patient and family. An intergenerational perspective begins with a focus on the family of origin as container and proceeds to a comparison of containment in the current family of procreation, absent family, job, or treatment team. Family involvement, so conceptualized, is far more inclusive than is the notion of family therapy as usually conceived for outpatients when only minor disorders are present.

4. *Treatment strategies arise in response to psychopathology.* The therapist adapts general skills in psychotherapy and family systems to particular pathological predicaments as a surgeon would adapt general surgical principles to the particular kind of operation being done. In the case of mania, heavy emphasis is placed on rapid management of a psychosis characterized by denial and requiring tight regulation for the entire time that the patient is manic. For the kind of depressive states discussed here, family intervention includes the use of family members to assess medications and to focus on the patient's constricted, anhedonic, and overly involved depressive dynamics, which are usually evident in the family of origin and in the patient's current environment, including the current family. Borderline conditions require a sharp intergenerational perspective and a sensitivity to the following: countertransference reactions as indications that the patient may be evoking unmanageable affect in others, the patient's overfocusing on disturbed feelings in the service of evading personal responsibilities for actions, evi-

dence of collusive defensive patterns and pathological distance regulation to avoid personality disorganization and the use of symptomatic impulsive action as a method of keeping intimates at a comfortable distance, one that is neither too close nor too far away. The suicidal patient is best approached with a careful eye on difficulties in the treatment alliance and on indirect communication as a key to the same type of disturbed object relations that are so often intimately tied to the basic suicidal problem; only then can an appropriate response be made to the patient, a response that is neither overregulatory nor emotionally distanced.

REFERENCES

Akiskal, H. A., Chen, S. E., & Davis, G. C. (1985). Borderline, an adjective in search of a noun. *Journal of Clinical Psychiatry, 46*, 41–48.

American Psychiatric Association. (1980). *Diagnostic and statistical manual of mental disorders* (3rd ed.). Washington, DC: APA.

American Psychiatric Association. (1987). *Diagnostic and statistical manual of mental disorders* (rev. 3rd ed.). Washington, DC: APA.

Beck, A. T., & Shaw, B. F. (1977). Cognitive approaches to depression. In A. Ellis & R. Gruger (Eds.), *Handbook of rational emotion theory & practice*. New York: Springer.

Bemporad, J. V. (1970). New views on the dynamics of the depressive character. In S. Avieti (Ed.), *World biennial of psychiatry and psychotherapy* (Vol. 1, pp. 219–243). New York: Basic Books.

Bowen, M. (1966). The use of family theory in clinical practice. *Comprehensive Psychiatry, 7*, 345–374.

Bursten, B. (1982). Narcissistic personalities in DSM-III. *Comprehensive Psychiatry, 23*, 409–420.

Carlson, G. A., Kotin, J., Davenport, Y. B., & Adland, M. (1974). Followup of 53 bipolar manic-depressive patients. *International Journal of Psychiatry, 124*, 134–139.

Davenport, Y. (1981). Treatment of the married bipolar patient in conjoint couples psychotherapy group. In M. R. Lansky (Ed.), *Family therapy and major psychopathology* (pp. 123–144). New York: Grune & Stratton.

Davenport, Y., & Adland, M. (1985). Issues in the treatment of the married bipolar patient: Dependency and demand. In M. R. Lansky (Ed.), *Family approaches to major psychiatric disorders* (pp. 45–65). Washington, DC: American Psychiatric Press.

Greenson, R. (1954). The struggle against identification. *Journal of the American Psychoanalytic Association, 2*, 200–217.

Grinker, R. R., Werble, B., & Drye, R. (1968). *The borderline syndrome: A behavioral study of ego functions*. New York: Basic Books.

Gunderson, J. G., & Elliott, G. R. (1985). The interface between borderline personality disorder and affective disorder. *American Journal of Psychiatry, 142*, 277–288.

Klein, M. (1946). Notes on some schizoid mechanisms. *International Journal of Psychoanalysis, 27*.

Knight, R. P. (1953). Borderline states. *Bulletin of the Menninger Clinic, 17*, 1–12.

Lansky, M. (1980). On blame. *International Journal of Psychoanalytic Psychotherapy, 8*, 429–456.

Lansky, M. (1981a). Family psychotherapy in the hospital. In M. R. Lansky (Ed.), *Family therapy and major psychopathology* (pp. 395–414). New York: Grune & Stratton.

Lansky, M. (1981b). Medication and family process. In M. R. Lansky (Ed.), *Family therapy and major psychopathology* (pp. 375–393). New York: Grune & Stratton.

Lansky, M. (1981c). Treatment of the narcissistically vulnerable marriage. In M. Lansky (Ed.), *Family therapy and major psychopathology* (pp. 163–182). New York: Grune & Stratton.

Lansky, M. R. (1982). The role of the family in the evaluation of suicidality. *International Journal of Family Psychiatry, 3,* 105–118.

Lansky, M. R. (1984). Violence, shame, and the family. *International Journal of Family Psychiatry, 5,* 21–40.

Lansky, M. R. (1985). Preoccupation and pathologic distance regulation. *International Journal of Family Psychoanalysis and Psychotherapy, 11,* 409–425.

Lansky, M. R. (in-press). The explanation of impulsive action. *International Journal of Psychoanalysis and Psychotherapy.*

Lansky, M., Bley, C. R., Simenstad, E., West, K. L., & McVey, G. G. (1983). The "absent" family of the hospitalized borderline patient. *International Journal of Family Psychiatry, 4,* 155–171.

Paul, N. (1973). The need to mourn. In E. J. Anthony (Ed.), *The child in his family* (pp. 219–224). New York: Wiley.

Rosenthal, S. N., & Gudeman, J. E. (1967). The self-pitying constellation in depression. *British Journal of Psychiatry, 113,* 485–489.

Slipp, S. (1984). *Object relations: A dynamic bridge between individual and family treatment.* New York: Jason Aronson.

Straker, M. (1958). Clinical observations on suicide. *Canadian Medical Association Journal, 19,* 473.

Vaillant, G. (1975). Sociopathy as a human process: A viewpoint. *Archives of General Psychiatry, 32,* 178–183.

Winnicott, D. W. (1955). Metapsychological and clinical aspects of regression within the psychoanalytic setup. *International Journal of Psychoanalysis, 36.*

World Psychiatric Association. (1983). *Diagnostic criteria for schizophrenic and affective psychosis.* Washington, DC: American Psychiatric Press.

PART FOUR

ISSUES IN RESEARCH

The final section—and chapter—of this volume comes full circle to the advances we have made in the field and the questions that are now clearer but that remain unanswered. The authors, Haas and Docherty, review trends of the past decade in research on family/marital treatments for the affective disorders. They are optimistic regarding the prospects for the development and implementation of well-designed programs of clinical research on family/marital treatments for the affective disorders.

11

Family Intervention in Affective Illness: A Review of Research

GRETCHEN L. HAAS
JOHN DOCHERTY

CURRENT STATUS OF RESEARCH IN THE FIELD

If one were to ask us, What is the status of research in family/marital treatments for affective disorders?, we would respond by offering a comparison utilizing examples from the larger field of clinical psychopharmacology and individual psychotherapy research. Among the clinical treatments for affective disorders, family therapies are among the most recent and the least researched in the field. At a recent meeting of the Society for Psychotherapy Research, John Rush, MD, noted that the research on pharmacological agents for affective disorders closely approximates a traditional model of systematic treatment research, including a stepwise sequence of investigations, from laboratory (e.g., analogue animal) research, to preliminary clinical trials on human subjects, to controlled clinical trials on select patient samples, and finally, to cross-validation studies on larger samples. Research on individual psychotherapies for affective disorders (utilizing, for example, cognitive and interpersonal therapeutic interventions) has graduated from single case reports and controlled clinical trials and has now achieved the stage of cross-validation studies on large samples (a primary example being the recently completed National Institute of Mental Health Collaborative Study on Psychotherapy for Depression).

By comparison, research on family treatments for affective disorders is at an earlier stage of development—that of the transition from clinical observation and preliminary single case reports to more systematic empirical investigations using large samples and random assignment to comparison (e.g., Chapter 6, this volume) and control (e.g., Chapter 3, this volume) treatments. Drawing on the knowledge gained from basic studies of normal and pathological family functioning, we are beginning to understand more about the instrumental role of interpersonal variables and the interpersonal context in the etiology and course of affective disorders (e.g., Chapters 1 and 3, this volume). Moreover, research on interpersonal (specifically, marital/family) functioning has radically influenced our theoretical models of affective disorder and has informed the design and implementation of some of our most advanced assessment (Chapter 2, this volume) and treatment (Chapters 3, 4, and 6, this volume) strategies and technologies.

As the field of family therapy research matures and begins to integrate many core features of systematic clinical research into its methodologies and procedures, family therapy researchers are drawing criticism from family clinicians who promote the "new epistemologies," or cybernetic models of causality, that is, models that describe *systems* rather than *elements* and that are circular rather than linear models of causality. These models assume an interdependence of events rather than a simple linear relationship between events. For example, a cybernetic model of depression might describe an individual's depressive symptoms as both a stimulus for, and a response to, critical communications from a spouse. Several models of family treatment based on principles of general systems theory (von Bertalanffy) or cybernetics (Bateson) gave birth to a new "breed" of family therapists during the 1970s (e.g., Watzlawick, Haley, Weakland). The debate among clinicians regarding theoretical/epistemological models of family therapy has been heated. Gurman, Kniskern, and Pinsof (1986) have observed that one unexpected outcome of this debate has been a growing split between contemporary family therapists who adhere to the "systems" models, and family researchers, for whom the linear models are more readily adapted to empirical research (Wynne, 1983; Gurman *et al.*, 1986).

The biggest challenge for family treatment researchers today is to find a means of utilizing important insights generated by systems theory and other nonlinear models while simultaneously incorporating the most useful tools of empirical research technology. Systems theorists warn against a too restrictive research methodology—one based solely on linear models of causality and methods of analysis that attempt to isolate components of behavioral processes independent of a surrounding behavioral "system."

On the other hand, family researchers note that systematic research on family intervention has been lacking; the family therapy field is currently dominated by clinical reports on the efficacy of a particular approach with a particular patient/family presenting a particular symptom constellation. This kind of clinical report is essentially equivalent to the inductive stage of research. Graduation to controlled comparative study designs has been handicapped by a lack of clarity in hypothetical models of therapeutic action and goals of treatment and by a lack of operational descriptions of our treatment techniques. Progress in the field has also been encumbered by a lack of sophisticated assessment tools and methods for systematically measuring and documenting clinical change.

Nonetheless, the field has, in recent years, made important progress. Certain indicators of this progress are reflected in the foregoing chapters. In reviewing the work presented in this volume, we can begin to highlight important milestones in the development of an empirical approach to family and marital treatments for the affective disorders.

1. *The work of skilled family clinicians adds to the theoretical and clinical base for empirical study.* Dr. Lansky's clinical observations (Chapter 10) offer significant clinical data on family assessment and treatment of some of the more intractable correlates of depression (e.g., personality disorder and suicidal behavior). This is the kind of creative clinical data base from which systematic, programmatic research on family therapy outcome must be generated.

2. *Knowledge gained from basic studies of normal and pathological family functioning is being used in the design of treatment for depression* (Chapters 1, 2, and 3). Evidence of the important influence of psychosocial variables on the course of the affective disorders has promoted development of psychosocial treatments for these disorders. For example, the wealth of empirical data on the social and interpersonal factors that contribute to depression (Ilfeld 1977; Klerman, 1982; Paykel, 1982; Weiss & Paykel, 1974) has inspired the investigation of family and marital treatments for depression. Psychosocial and epidemiological research has also contributed to a more comprehensive conceptualization of the affective disorders—a conceptual model of depression that takes into account the psychosocial context and the interpersonal problems commonly associated with the disorder.

3. *Interpersonal and behavioral models of depression have encouraged both clinicians and researchers to experiment with the use of family/marital-based treatments for the affective disorders.* Hence we observe an outcropping of treatments that capitalize on the inclusion of significant persons from the patient's interpersonal environment. These interventions share an emphasis on identifying and inviting into the treatment domain these members of the patient's interpersonal world. These family/marital treatments tend to vary, however, in terms of their rationale for engaging significant others in the treatment process. We can identify at least three major reasons for using family and marital constellations in treatment: (a) evidence that the family or marital spouse can be instrumental in promoting change; (b) a need to focus on maladaptive patterns of interaction that may contribute to or reinforce the illness; and (c) a need to reduce the "psychological fallout" of depressive symptoms in the family. Davenport and Adland (Chapter 8) utilize an approach based on the rationale of a spouse's helping to promote change—a marital couples group format that emphasizes the social support functions of the spouse and the group. Such treatment may be particularly effective in enhancing adherence to a prescribed treatment regimen. The work of Coyne and colleagues (Chapter 4) focuses on the second rationale, emphasizing the need to modify important elements of the interpersonal context in order to alter the depressive condition. Addressing the third rationale is the inpatient family intervention for treatment of depression (Chapter 6).

4. *The development of theoretical models of treatment that can be systematically enriched by controlled observation has moved the field toward the development of more empirically based family treatments.* Until recently, the lack of any coherent theoretical models that consider psychosocial factors in the pathogenesis and treatment of depression has handicapped empirical investigation of family/marital treatments for depression. Systematic studies of marital treatment outcome (represented by the work of Jacobson and colleagues, Coyne, Weiss, Hops and Patterson, Baucom, and others) have evolved out of a research ethic informed by theoretical and technical innovations such as Stuart's (1969) social exchange theory, Lewinsohn's (1974) social reinforcement theory, Beck's (1967) cognitive theory, and Coyne's (1976) interpersonal interaction theory, among others. These theoretical formulations begin to offer a more sound empirical foundation than that which previously existed for the study of family and marital treatments with affective disorders. Falloon, Hole, Mulroy, Norris and Pembleton (Chapter 5) present the theoretical basis for use of behavioral family therapy with mood disorders. Although no controlled study of this treatment approach has yet been conducted, the authors present an excellent example of a theory-based treatment model with procedures for family assessment and intervention linking directly to the model.

5. *With the formulation of explicit models of depression and therapeutic change processes, we have begun to develop manuals that define these treatments and describe, in operational terms, the methods for implementing them* (Chapters 3 and 6). "Manualization" of a treatment represents an important breakthrough in the development of an empirical approach to assessment of its therapeutic efficacy. The use of treatment manuals allows for standardization in the teaching and tracking of progress with student therapists. A detailed manual includes specific descriptions of therapeutic strategies and techniques and thus provides a means of developing and maintaining quality control in the delivery of a particular treatment. It also serves as an index for assessment of therapist skill and for study of therapist variables and patient–therapist interaction variables that can influence patient/family outcome.

6. *The development of structured family assessment tools is also necessary for translating clinical observation into the domain of controlled research on family therapy for affective disorders.* Here, there is a need for reliable and valid measures of major dimensions of family behavior, attitude, and affect. The Family Assessment Device (FAD) developed by Epstein and colleagues (Chapter 7) represents an important step in this direction. The development and more extensive use of similar assessment tools is necessary in order to identify major dimensions of family functioning that are related to the therapeutic outcomes for the affectively ill patient being treated with a family intervention (Chapter 2).

7. *"Dismantling strategies" designed to compare different components of therapeutic intervention programs have contributed to our understanding of therapeutic processes and the relative efficacy of specific techniques (e.g., cognitive vs. behavioral).* The work of the behavioral and cognitive–behavioral therapists (Baucom, 1984; Beck, 1967; Jacobson, 1977; Lewinsohn, 1974; Stuart, 1969) is most notable in this respect. Dobson, Jacobson, and Victor's review (Chapter 3) of the empirical literature in the field of cognitive, behavioral, and cognitive–behavioral treatments reveals an uncommon degree of sophistication in the design and implementation of programmatic work on marital treatments for depression. Of course, these studies can be classified as a form of "analogue" research (i.e., studies that are conducted in a semicontrolled, nonnaturalistic setting with experimental interventions that may depart from the type used in the naturalistic, clinical setting), and as such, they offer both advantages and disadvantages. The investigator who opts for the stronger experimental controls of more laboratory-like research is usually restricted to working with nonclinical populations. Thus the "power" to be gained by well-controlled experimental manipulations or comparative strategies that involve a dismantling of the therapy (e.g., focusing on a comparison of single components of a therapy) may ultimately be diminished by limited generalizability or clear inapplicability to some (e.g., the more severely disturbed) clinical populations. Nonetheless, this type of analogue research is quite necessary in the development of an empirically based family/marital intervention in the clinical setting.

8. *The need for treatment techniques that address the full range of affective disorders calls for the use of pharmacological treatment strategies. Many pharmacological treatment regimens are enhanced by inclusion of family members in the presentation and implementation of the pharamacological treatment program.* Epstein, Keitner, Bishop, and Miller, (Chapter 7) and Falloon, Hole, Mulroy, Norris and Pemberton (Chapter 5) discuss useful combinations of family/marital treatments and medication for affective disorders. Some of the more innovative treatments include the use of genetic counseling, prophylactic medication strategies, and interventions designed to modify environmental conditions that might predispose a genetically vulnerable individual to the onset of an affective illness. As both Targum (Chapter 9) and Falloon *et al.* (Chapter 5) have discussed, the family can be an important participant in preventive strategies, particularly those that utilize information on family history of affective illness or other psychiatric disorder. This work is revolutionary in that it utilizes treatment strategies that draw on *both* state-of-the-art biological *and* psychosocial diagnostic tools and treatment technologies.

9. *The next stage in research on family/marital treatments for affectively disordered patients calls for controlled clinical trials of family/marital therapies alone and in combination with pharmacotherapy.* In an era in

which the efficacy of pharmacological treatments for affective disorders has been reliably demonstrated, there is a need for controlled studies of the incremental benefits of adding family and marital treatments to outpatient maintenance and continuation treatments for affective disorders. Epstein and colleagues (Chapter 7) have reported their clinical observations regarding the benefits of adding family intervention to the pharmacological treatment of affective disorders. Similarly, Davenport and her colleagues at the National Institute of Mental Health (Chapter 8) have reported data bearing on the question of the relative benefit of including the spouse in the continuation phase of pharmacotherapy for bipolar patients. Their creative use of treatments that involve members of the family or marital dyad in the implementation of long-term medication regimens now needs further study under controlled conditions.

10. *We have developed the capacity to conduct full-scale controlled clinical trials of family interventions for affective disorders.* This "next step" in the evolution of a scientific family therapeutics is comparable to the clinical pharmacologist's shift from a controlled laboratory trial to controlled field trials of a specific drug. The work of Epstein and colleagues (Epstein, Miller, Keitner, Bishop, & Kabacoff, 1985) on the inpatient family treatment of bipolar disorders and that of Glick, Haas, and colleagues (Glick *et al.*, 1985; Haas *et al.*, 1986) on the inpatient family treatment of affective disorders represent a much needed *preliminary effort* in this direction. These clinical trials of family treatment are notable for their application of controlled or semicontrolled experimental designs to the study of family treatments with the more severely disturbed affectively disordered patients. However, inpatient studies (e.g., Glick *et al.*, 1985) of this nature often suffer from the complex problems involved in integrating controlled research into the daily activities of a clinical treatment/teaching setting. Hence we see the difficulty in instituting study designs that permit sensitive tests of the incremental benefits of adding a family treatment to an already complex and highly "active" multimodal treatment regimen. Equally problematic in the existing research on inpatient family treatments has been the lack of dismantling designs that permit the investigation of the specific components of a multicomponent family intervention (e.g., an intervention program that includes *both* psychoeducation and cognitive–behavioral problem-solving strategies.) The inherent practical problems of implementing studies of this nature are many. Nevertheless, a next step in the stage of clinical investigations of family therapeutics would involve the use of a controlled comparison design or dismantling strategy to identify the relative efficacy of various types of family interventions, such as psychoeducation and cognitive–behavioral problem-solving approaches, each of which may be beneficial but will exert its effects by different means, on perhaps different dimensions of the affective disorder, and with varying degrees of success.

11. *With the evolution of family-based therapeutic strategies, there has*

been a growing recognition of the need for diagnostic and assessment procedures relevant to the marital dyad or family. The advantages of family-based assessment strategies are well enumerated by Clarkin and Haas (Chapter 2). Their discussion speaks to the value of using family assessment procedures in differential treatment planning, regardless of the ultimate choice of treatment format (be it individual or family based). For example, one of the more effective applications of family assessment strategies has been in the assessment of medication adherence and clinical treatment response. Melvin Lansky (Chapter 10) presents a strong argument for the use of a standard clinical interview and/or self-report assessment procedure with the spouse or family members of the affectively ill patient. He notes that one advantage of gathering information from the family is that it may yield a more reliable and accurate assessment of a patient's clinical status and response to pharmacological or other therapeutic interventions. A family diagnostic assessment can also provide essential information regarding the social support system, environmental stressors, and role demands that may be intrinsically linked to affective symptomatology within the identified patient. Work in the realm of *psychosocial diagnostics* represents a major challenge for psychosocial researchers and psychometricians in the 1990s. The potential value of systematically assessing major dimensions of the patient's interpersonal environment is well illustrated in the observations of Davenport and Adland (Chapter 8) in their work with bipolar disorder patients. Coyne's clinical interventions with depressed patients and their spouses (Chapter 4) are well-articulated examples of how a marital-based assessment strategy can very effectively inform the clinician's understanding of the ecological constraints on the change process and thereby influence the choice of particular interventions and techniques in treating a depressed patient and his or her spouse. Syndrome diagnosis has dominated psychiatric practice. This system of categorizing has clear limitations for psychosocial interventions. The field of individual psychotherapy has begun to develop specific treatments for specific subcategories of individual disorder that vary in terms of psychosocial context and psychosocial factors that influence change. For example, in interpersonal psychotherapy for depression, four subcategories of depressive disturbance (grief, transition, interpersonal dispute, and interpersonal deficit disorder) call for specific therapeutic strategies (Klerman, Weissman, Rounsaville, & Chevron, 1984). Nonetheless, progress in the field of family/marital interventions is still limited by a lack of clarity regarding the relevant *unit* (family or individual) of study and a simultaneous lack of well-controlled empirical investigations of the relationship between individual psychopathology and the interpersonal (family and other) environment. The need for reliable and valid diagnostic tools and procedures for assessing the patient *in* his or her psychosocial context is obvious, and this area constitutes one of the new frontiers open to young investigators in the behavioral sciences.

CONCLUSION

Recent advances in the field of family interventions for affective disorders include (1) the development of theoretical models of family therapy with greater emphasis on explication of the specific mechanism of therapeutic action, (2) the development of family interventions enriched by research on interpersonal variables related to affective disorders, (3) well-operationalized manuals of family therapy that outline specific therapeutic strategies and techniques, (4) methods for assessment of key therapeutic processes, (5) methods for assessment of family and individual outcome, and (6) a growing awareness of the need for a psychosocial diagnostics that takes into account the psychosocial context of a clinical psychiatric syndrome. These achievements suggest that the field has developed the capacity to conduct full-scale controlled clinical trials of specific family treatments. Thus the time is ripe for controlled clinical investigation of the efficacy of family interventions for affective disorders.

REFERENCES

Baucom, D. H. (1984). The active ingredients of behavioral marital therapy: The effectiveness of problem-solving/communication training, contingency contracting and their combination. In K. Hahlweg & N. S. Jacobson (Eds.), *Marital interaction: Analyses and modification* (pp. 73–88). New York: Guilford Press.

Beck, A. T. (1967). *Depression: Clinical, experimental and theoretical aspects.* New York: Harper & Row.

Coyne, J. C. (1976). Depression and the response of others. *Journal of Abnormal Psychology, 85,* 186–193.

Epstein, N. B., Miller, C. W., Keitner, G. I., Bishop, D. S., & Kabacoff, R. I. (1985, May). *Family dysfunction in bipolar disorder: Description and pilot treatment study.* Paper presented at the meeting of the American Psychiatric Association, Dallas.

Glick, I. D., Clarkin, J. F., Spencer, J. H., Haas, G. L., Lewis, A. B., Peyser, J., DeMane, N., Good-Ellis, M., Harris, E., & Lestelle, V. (1985). A controlled evaluation of Inpatient Family Intervention: I. Preliminary results of the six-month follow-up. *Archives of General Psychiatry, 42,* 882–886.

Gurman, A. S., Kniskern, D. P., & Pinsof, W. M. (1986). Research on the process and outcome of marital and family therapy. In S. L. Garfield & A. E. Bergin (Eds.), *Handbook of psychotherapy and behavior change* (pp. 565–624). New York: Wiley.

Haas, G. L., Glick, I. D., Spencer, J. H., Clarkin, J. F., Lewis, A. B., Good-Ellis, M., Peyser, J., DeMane, N., Harris, E., & Lestelle, V. (1986). The patient, the family, and compliance with posthospital treatment for affective disorders. *Psychopharmacology Bulletin, 22,* 999–1006.

Ilfeld, F. W. (1977). Current social stressors and symptoms of depression. *American Journal of Psychiatry, 134,* 161–166.

Jacobson, N. S. (1977). Marital therapy and the cognitive–behavioral treatment of depression. *the Behavior Therapist, 7,* 143–147.

Klerman, G. L. (1982). Testing analytic hypotheses: Do personality attributes predispose to depression? In A. Jacobson & D. Parmelee (Eds.), *Psychoanalysis: A contemporary appraisal* (pp. 56–73). New York: Brunner/Mazel.

Klerman, G. L., Weissman, M. M., Rounsaville, B. J., & Chevron, E. S. (1984). *Interpersonal psychotherapy of depression.* New York: Basic Books.

Lewinsohn, P. M. (1974). A behavioral approach to depression. In R. J. Friedman & M. M. Katz (Eds.), *The psychology of depression: Contemporary theory and research* (pp. 157–185). New York: Wiley.

Paykel, E. S. (1982). Life events and early environment. In E. S. Paykel (Ed.), *Handbook of affective disorders* (pp. 146–161). New York: Guilford Press.

Stuart, R. B. (1969). Operant–interpersonal treatment of marital discord. *Journal of Consulting and Clinical Psychology, 33,* 675–682.

Weissman, M. M., & Paykel, E. S. (1974). *The depressed woman: A study of social relationships.* Chicago: University of Chicago Press.

Wynne, L. C. (1983). Family research and family therapy: A reunion? *Journal of Marital and Family Therapy, 9,* 113–118.

Index

Abraham, Karl, 180
Adjustment disorder
  assessment, 32
  combined pharmacologic and
    inpatient family therapy, 155
Adoption and genetic issues in
    depression, 201, 202, 205, 206
Affect, inappropriate, unstable, or
    restricted, DSM-III-R Axis II
    criteria, 37
Affective involvement/responsiveness,
    problem-centered systems
    therapy of family, 160
Affiliation, dysfunctional, DSM-III-R
    Axis II criteria, 37
Age of patient
  family/interpersonal context, 4
  assessment, 29
  inpatient family intervention, 148
Agitated, restless behavior, 127, 128
Alcohol abuse, 12, 144, 145, 155, 165,
    229, 234
Alcoholism
  manic episodes, management, 176
  parental, 144, 168, 230
  psychiatric genetics, 199, 202, 206,
    208
Amish, suicide among, 203
Amitriptyline, 158
Amoxapine, 158
Analogue research, 245
Anger, marital, 77, 78, 80, 81
  strategic therapy in depression, 107
Antidepressants, 124, 127, 129, 144, 214
  borderline personality disorder, 226,
    228, 230

depressive disorders, classification,
    91
  genetic considerations, 208, 209
  and inpatient family therapy, 156,
    159, 169
  MAO inhibitors, 187
    genetic considerations, 209
    with inpatient family therapy, 159
  poor prognosis with marital distress,
    91, 92
  tricyclic
    with inpatient family therapy, 156,
      159, 169
    manic episodes, management, 187
  unipolar depression, recurrent, 223, 224
Antisocial personality, psychiatric
    genetics, 206, 208
Anxiety, social, DSM-III-R Axis II
    criteria, 37
Areas-of-Change Questionnaire, 44, 45,
    68
Assertive behavior, inappropriate,
    DSM-III-R Axis II criteria, 37
Assessment
  family- or couple-relevant, research
    issues, 246, 247
  inpatient family intervention in
    affective disorders, 139, 140
  problem-centered systems therapy of
    family, 161
  as therapeutic role induction,
    affective disorders, 46, 47
  tool development, research issues, 244
  see also Family/interpersonal
    context, affective disorders,
    assessment

Assortative mating and marital
    support, 16, 17
Attitude of family toward affective
    disorder, 45, 46
Attribution
    cognitive–behavioral marital therapy,
        71, 72, 74, 75
    depression, 55, 59–61
Attributional Style Questionnaire, 39
Automatic thoughts, 65
Automatic Thoughts Questionnaire, 39
Aversiveness, interpersonal, DSM-III-
    R Axis II criteria, 37
Avoidance, DSM-III-R Axis II
    criteria, 37
Axis I disorders, 35, 36
Axis II disorders, 35–37, 151

B

Basic tasks, problem-centered systems
    therapy of family, 159
Beck, Aaron, 65, 66
Beck Depression Inventory, 33, 38, 81,
    82
Beck Hopelessness Scale, 41
Behavioral family therapy, 115, 117–132
    behavioral analysis, 121–123
        information about family
            members, 121, 122
        therapeutic alliance with family
            members, 121
    bipolar manic–depressive disorders,
        119, 125, 126, 129, 130, 131
    depression, 117, 118, 124
    family-based stress management, 120
    functional analysis, 123–125
        case example, 124, 125, 129
    intervention during acute episodes,
        125–129
    intervention therapies, 120
        case example, 127, 128
        education about episodes, 125–129
        family stress management, 126
        hospitalization, 125, 127
        symptom management, 126–128

prevention of episodes, 129–132
    case, 130
    communication skills, 131
    problem-solving behavior, 119, 126,
        129, 131
    six-step approach, 126, 131
    schizophrenia, 129
    stress, vulnerability, and family
        coping behavior, 118, 119
Behavioral marital therapy, 67–72, 75–
    77, 82; *see also* Cognitive-
    behavioral marital therapy
Behavior control, problem-centered
    systems therapy of family, 160
Behavior exchange, cognitive and
    marital interventions in
    depression, 68–70, 80
Bipolar disorders, 10, 92
    I cf. II, 215
    behavioral family therapy, 119, 125,
        126, 129, 130, 131
    family/interpersonal context,
        assessment, 31
    inpatient family intervention, 135,
        137, 140–146, 149, 150
    pharmacologic and inpatient family
        therapy, combined, 153–155, 167
    psychiatric genetics, 199–204, 206,
        207, 208, 209
    symptomatology, 175–180
        cf. unipolar, 176
    see also Manic episodes,
        management
Bipolar families, 174, 183–187
Borderline personality disorder
    DSM-III-R, 225
        Axis II criteria, 37
    lithium in, 226
Borderline personality disorder, family
    intervention, 116, 213, 215, 224–
        230, 236
    antidepressants, 226, 228, 230
    case example, 229, 230
    characterization, 225, 226
    conflict, overt, assessment and
        management, 227, 228
    crisis management, 228

intergenerational perspective, 226,
227, 236
cf. schizophrenia, 224, 225
symptom management, 228, 229
Buckingham Mental Health Service
Project, 119

C

Camberwell Family Interview, 6, 19, 46
Carbamazepine, 187, 188
Carroll Rating Scale for Depression,
33, 38
Change, beliefs about, cognitive-
behavioral marital therapy, 70,
71, 74
Character spectrum disorder, 12
Children
bipolar families, 187
death of, 78, 79, 80, 82, 124
family stress and, 118
Chlorpromazine, 143
Chromosome, 6, 209
Clinical data, importance, research
issues, 243
Clinical trials with and without
pharmacotherapy, need for, 245,
246
Closure, problem-centered systems
therapy of family, 162
Cognitive and marital interventions in
depression, 65-72
behavioral marital therapy, 67-72,
75-77, 82
behavior exchange, 68-70, 80
communication/problem-solving
training, 68, 69, 81
problem-solving, 67, 73, 81
cognitive therapies, 65-67
communication training (homework),
66
Cognitive aspects
depression, 54, 55
family/interpersonal context,
assessment, 39, 40, 47
and intervention, 23

Cognitive–behavioral marital therapy,
51, 53, 54, 61, 64, 69, 82
attribution, 71, 72, 74, 75
case example, 77-82
change, beliefs about, 70, 71, 74
classic couples, 76
denial couples, 76, 77
expectancies, self and spouse, 70, 73
planning of week, 80
problem definition, 70, 72, 73
social support couples, 77
Socratic questioning of nondepressed
spouse, 75
systemic couples, 77
Cognitive Bias Questionnaire, 39
Cognitive style, self-enhancing illusory, 66
Communications, indirect, suicidal
intent, 233
Communications skills
bipolar families, 187
cognitive and marital interventions
in depression, 68, 69, 81
maladaptive, assessment, 47
manic episodes
management, 187
prevention, 131
problem-centered systems therapy of
family, 160
Communication training (homework),
cognitive and marital
interventions in depression, 66
Compliance, 141
problems, manic episode
management, 174
Computers, family/interpersonal
context assessment, 30
Conflict
marital/family, 13-15
overt, borderline personality
disorder, family intervention,
227, 228
Container model, family, 236
Contingency
contracting, decline of, 71
on individual actions, family/
interpersonal context, affective
disorders, 14

Contracting, problem-centered systems
    therapy of family, 161, 162
Control/power issues, family/
    interpersonal context, affective
    disorders, 19, 20
Coping, 12, 13
    and intervention, 23
    style, family/interpersonal context,
        affective disorders, 16
    tasks, strategic marital therapy in
        depression, 101, 102
Costs, assessment, 30
Couples. *See* Marital *entries*
Crisis management, borderline
    personality disorder, family
    intervention, 228
Criticism, constructive, from spouse,
    cf. hostility, 15
Cybernetics, 242
Cyclothymia, 31
    psychiatric genetics, 199

D

Death
    of child, 78, 79, 80, 82, 124
    of mother, 118
    see also Suicide *entries*
Demographics, affective disorders, 10
Denial
    couples, cognitive–behavioral marital
        therapy, 76, 77
    and dependency, manic episodes,
        management, 192, 193
Dependence, DSM-III-R Axis II
    criteria, 37
Depressed parents, children of, 18, 20
Depressed women. *See under* Women
Depression/depressive disorder, 53–64
    behavioral family therapy in affective
        disorders, 124
    helplessness in, 117, 118
    cognitive aspects, 54, 55
        attribution, 55
        distortion, 54, 55
    differential treatment planning, 42

endogenous vs. reactive, 92
family/interpersonal context, 3–5, 9,
    10, 21, 22
    assessment, 29, 31, 32
    behavioral aspects, 55–64
    current research, 9, 10
    future research, 243
    insularity, 4
    feedback loops, 62
    inpatient family intervention. *See*
        Inpatient family intervention in
        affective disorders
    interactive model, 62–64
    intrapsychic causes, 63
        attributions, 59–61
        marital consequences, 56–62
        observational studies, 57
        problem-solving deficits, 62
        skill deficits, 56
    major, combined pharmacologic and
        inpatient family therapy, 153,
        155, 156
    prevalence, U.S., 3, 10
    pure, 11, 12, 208
    sporadic, 208
    see also Cognitive and marital
        interventions in depression;
        Genetic issues in treatment of
        depression; Strategic marital
        therapy in depression; Suicide,
        depression and, family
        intervention; Unipolar
        depression, recurrent
Depressive spectrum disease, 11, 208
Desipramine, 158
Developmental history, suicide and
    depression, family intervention,
    231, 232
Deviation amplifying process,
    depression, 56
Dexamethasone suppression test,
    classification of depressive
    disorders, 91
Diagnostic and assessment procedures,
    family- or couple-relevant,
    research issues, 246, 247
Diagnostics, psychosocial, 247

Diagnostic systems, individual, 8
Dimensional assessment, affective
    disorders, 36, 38–41
Dismantling strategies, research issues,
    245
Distortion and depression, 54, 55
Divorce, 110, 111
Dominance/submission, DSM-III-R
    Axis II criteria, 37
Double-bind communication,
    schizophrenia, 5
Drug abuse, 144, 165
Drug metabolism, genetic
    considerations, 209
DSM-III, 136, 151, 163, 225
    Axis I, 35, 36
    Axis II, 35–37, 151
DSM-III-R, 196, 216
    affective disorder vs. schizophrenia,
        213, 214
    bipolar illness, 176
    borderline, 225
    faculty psychology, 213, 214
    and family/interpersonal context,
        affective disorder assessment,
        31, 32, 35, 36
Dyadic Adjustment Scale, 33, 43
Dysfunctional affiliation, DSM-III-R
    Axis II criteria, 37
Dysfunctional Attitude Scale, 33, 39,
    40, 45
Dysthymia, 170
    psychiatric genetics, 199, 204

E

Education
    and empathy, mania, 217, 218
    about episodes, and behavioral
        family therapy, 125–129
    and inpatient family intervention,
        137–139, 148
        with pharmacologic therapy, 159,
        167
Electroconvulsive therapy, 127, 147,
    214, 215, 220

England, 7
Environmental influence and genetic
    issues in treatment of
    depression, 206, 207
Environmental mastery/coping,
    affective disorders, 12, 13
Environmental resources, affective
    disorders, 16–20
Etiological presuppositions, avoiding,
    235
Expectancies, self and spouse,
    cognitive–behavioral marital
    therapy, 70, 73
Expressed emotion (EE)
    depression, 59
    inpatient family intervention in
        affective disorders, 135
    schizophrenia, 6, 19
Extratherapy task assignments,
    strategic marital therapy in
    depression, 97, 99–101, 105, 109,
    110

F

Faculty psychology, DSM-III-R, 213,
    214
Family Adaptability and Cohesion
    Evaluation Scales, 33, 46
Family Assessment Device, 33, 45, 155,
    156, 244
Family Attitude Scale, 139, 144, 145,
    148
Family-based stress management, 120
Family, container model, 236
Family Evaluation Form, 46
Family history, mania, 217, 218
Family/interpersonal context, affective
    disorders, 3–24
    current research, 7–10
        individual diagnostic systems, 8
    depression, 3–5, 9, 10
        current research, 9, 10
        insularity, 4
        linkage with interpersonal context,
        21, 22

Family/interpersonal context, affective
    disorders (*continued*)
  environmental resources, 16–20
  cf. individual focus, 3, 4
  intervention, indications for, 22–24
  manic episodes, management, 182,
      183
    interactional patterns, 182
  marital therapists, 4, 8
  personal resources, 10–13
  schizophrenia and family therapy, 5–
      7
  stressful life circumstances, 13–16, 21
  type of illness and interpersonal
      context, 20, 21
Family/interpersonal context, affective
    disorders, assessment, 29–47
  age of patient, 29
  assessment as therapeutic role
      induction, 46, 47
  communication, maladaptive, 47
  depression, differential treatment
      planning, 42
  DSM-III-R classifications, 31, 32,
      35, 36
  family/interpersonal context, 41–47
  goals of assessment, 32, 33
  instruments, 30, 31, 33, 35, 36
  interviews, 34
  problem-solving, maladaptive, 47
  Research Diagnostic Criteria, 35
  symptomatology, 29, 32, 38, 39, 47
    cognitions, 39, 40, 47
    dimensional assessment, 36, 38–41
    social skills, 40
    suicide potential, 40, 41
  see also Assessment
Family pathology
  broader, 167, 168
  minimal, 166, 167
Family planning and genetic issues in
    treatment of depression, 204, 205
Family roles, problem-centered systems
    therapy of family, 160
Family stress management, behavioral
    family therapy in affective
    disorders, 126

Family support, family/interpersonal
    context, affective disorders, 17
Family therapy. *See* Behavioral family
    therapy; Pharmacologic and
    inpatient family therapy,
    combined
Feedback loops, depression, 62
Fitzgerald, R., 187
Fluphenazine decanoate, 130, 131
Freud, Sigmund, 180
Frustration, spouse, and strategic
    marital therapy in depression,
    107
Future research issues, 150–152

G

Genetic counseling, psychiatric, 196–
    199
Genetic issues in treatment of
    depression, 116, 173, 196–210
  adoption and, 205, 206
  depressive disorders, genetics, 200–
      204, 207
    risk figures, 202–204
  environmental influence, 206, 207
  family planning, 204, 205
  genetic counseling, psychiatric, 196–
      199
  HLA-markers, 209
  muscarinic cholinergic binding sites,
      210
  REM markers, 210
  suicide, 203, 204, 207
  treatment considerations, 207–209
Global Assessment Scale, inpatient
    family intervention, 140, 143,
    145, 147
  with pharmacologic therapy, 157
Goals
  defining, strategic marital therapy in
      depression, 101
  mediating cf. final, inpatient family
      intervention, 135–136, 140, 141,
      149
    compliance, posthospitalization, 141

Grandiosity, manic episode
  management, 177, 178
Great Britain, 7

H

Hamilton Rating Scale for Depression,
  33, 38
Helplessness in depression, 117, 118
Heterogeneity
  of clinical problems, combined
    pharmacologic and inpatient
    family therapy, 115, 163–165
  patient sample, inpatient family
    intervention, 151
Histrionic behavior, DSM-III-R Axis
  II criteria, 37
Homework, strategic marital therapy,
  97, 99–101, 105, 109, 110
Hospitalization
  behavioral family therapy in affective
    disorders, 125, 127
  bipolar families, 185, 186
  manic episodes, management, 185, 186
  see also Inpatient family intervention
    in affective disorders;
    Pharmacologic and inpatient
    family therapy, combined
Hostility
  avoiding, strategic marital therapy in
    depression, 107, 108
  cf. constructive criticism, from
    spouse, 15
  and intervention, 23
Housecleaning/household
  management, 79, 80, 127, 128,
    130, 131
Human leukocyte antigens (HLA)
  markers, 209
Hypomania cf. mania, 173, 175, 177,
  179, 185, 187–190

I

Illusory glow, depression, 61
Imipramine, 208

Individual focus cf. family/
  interpersonal context, affective
  disorders, 3, 4
Infantile narcissism, 180
Inpatient family intervention in
  affective disorders, 23, 115, 134–
    152, 243
  affective disorders, working model,
    138
  age, 148
  assessment, 139, 140
    Family Attitude Scale, 139, 144,
      145, 148
    Global Assessment Scale, 140, 143,
      145, 147
    Psychiatric Evaluation Form, 140,
      143, 145, 147
    Role Performance and Treatment
      Scale, 139, 140
  brief intervention vs. therapy, 137, 148
  cases, 142–148
    bipolar, 142–146
    unipolar, 146, 148
  depression, 135
    bipolar, 135, 137, 140–146, 149, 150
    unipolar, 135, 137, 140–142, 146,
      148–151
  education, 137–139, 148
  expressed emotion, 135
  future research, 150–152
  goals, mediating and final, 135, 136,
    140, 141, 149
    compliance, posthospitalization,
      141
  impact on family, 151
  long-standing family conflicts, 138,
    151
  monitoring intervention, 150
  outpatient treatment and, 151, 152
  patient sample, 136, 137
    heterogeneity, 151
  schizophrenia, 134, 135, 150
  timing of intervention, 150, 151
  treatment goals and therapeutic
    strategies, 138, 139, 141, 142
  see also Pharmacologic and inpatient
    family therapy, combined

Integrativeness of treatment, 235, 236
Interactive model, depression, 62–64
Intergenerational perspective,
    borderline personality disorder,
    226, 227, 236
Interpersonal aversiveness, DSM-III-R
    Axis II criteria, 37
Interpersonal Behavior Role-Playing
    Test, 40
Interpersonal context. *See* Family/
    interpersonal context *entries*;
    Marital *entries*
Interpersonal Events Schedule, 43
Interpersonal precipitants of manic
    attacks, 217
Interpersonal relationships, behavioral
    aspects of depression, 55–64
Intervention, 120
    during acute episodes, 125–129
    assessment, 45
    indications for, 22–24
    strategic marital therapy for
        depression
        focused, 100–110
        initial, 99, 100
    see also Cognitive and marital
        interventions in depression;
        Inpatient family intervention in
        affective disorders
Interview(s)
    assessment, 34
    initial, strategic marital therapy in
        depression, 97–99
    time-limitations, 98
Intrapsychic causes, depression, 63
Irrational Beliefs Test, 39
Irritable bowel syndrome, 78, 79

J

Janowsky, D. S., 181

K

Kraepelin, E., 175

L

Lansky, M. R., 183, 184
Lithium carbonate, 92, 129–131, 143, 214
    borderlines, 226
    manic episodes, 173, 174, 180, 181,
        187–189, 191
Locke-Wallace Marital Adjustment
    Test, 43, 44, 45
LSD abuse, 144

M

Mania, assessment, 29, 43
Mania, family intervention, 213, 215–
    220
    case example, 219, 220
    education and empathy, 217, 218
    family history, 217, 218
    interpersonal precipitants of attacks,
        217
    rapid management, 217
Manic episodes, management, 116,
    173–194
    alcoholism, 176
    antidepressants, tricyclic, 187
    bipolar families, 174, 183–187
    bipolar illness, symptomatology,
        175–180
        children of, 187
    communications skills, 187
    hospitalization, 185, 186
    multigenerational, 174, '188, 192
    cf. unipolar, 176
    cases, 178, 179, 187–192
    compliance problems, 174
    denial and dependency, treatment
        issues, 192, 193
    cf. depressive phase, 179, 180
    early phase of episodes, 177
    family issues in treatment, 182, 183
        interactional patterns, 182
    historical perspective, 174, 175, 180–
        182, 184
        infantile narcissism, 180
    psychoanalytic view, 174, 180, 184

cf. hypomania, 173, 175, 177, 179,
185, 187–190
lithium carbonate, 173, 174, 180,
181, 187–189, 191
mini-episodes, 177
stages, 177, 178
grandiosity, 177, 178
paranoia, 177, 178
see also Bipolar disorders
Manic-State Rating Scale, 33, 39
"Manualization" of treatment, 244
Maprotiline, 158
Marijuana abuse, 144
Marital Activities Inventory, 45
Marital anger, 77, 78, 80, 81
Marital assessment packages, 44, 45
Marital interaction, assessment, 43, 44
Marital Interaction Coding System, 43
Marital intervention. *See* Cognitive
and marital interventions in
depression
Marital intimacy, lack of, and
intervention, 23
Marital Precounseling Inventory, 44
Marital satisfaction/commitment,
assessment, 43
Marital Satisfaction Inventory, 33, 43,
45
Marital support and assortative
mating, 16, 17
Marital therapists, affective disorders,
4, 8
Marital therapy, behavioral, 67–72, 75–
77, 82; *see also* Cognitive-
behavioral marital therapy;
Strategic marital therapy in
depression
McMaster model, 159, 160
Melancholic cf. nonmelancholic
patients, 11
Mellaril, 191
Menopause, 124
Men, pharmacologic and inpatient
family therapy, combined,
154
Millon Clinical Multiaxial Inventory,
36

Minnesota Multiphasic Personality
Inventory, Depression Scale, 38,
39
Monoamine oxidase inhibitors, 187
genetic considerations, 209
with inpatient family therapy, 159
Mother, death of, 118
Multisystem containment
interpretation, suicide and
depression, 232
Muscarinic cholinergic binding sites,
210

N

Narcissism
DSM-III-R Axis II criteria, 37
infantile, 180
Narcissistic disequilibrium disturbance,
221
National Institute of Mental Health,
180, 182–184, 194, 201, 246
Collaborative Study on
Psychotherapy for Depression,
241
/NIH Consensus Development
Conference on Mood Disorders,
173
National Institutes of Health, 173, 201
Negative self-statements, 128
Neuroleptics, 191, 214, 216
Noxious behavior negotiation, strategic
marital therapy in depression,
108, 109

O

Observational studies, 18–20
depression, 57
research issues, 244
Obsessive–compulsive, DSM-III-R
Axis II criteria, 37
Outpatient treatment and inpatient
family intervention in affective
disorders, 151, 152

P

Panic disorder, psychiatric genetics,
    199, 206
Paranoia, manic episode management,
    177, 178
Parent(s)
    alcoholic, 144, 168, 230
    death of, 118
    depressed, children of, 18, 20
"Parenting" of therapist by depressive,
    222
Parenting skills and intervention, 23–24
Passive–aggressive, DSM-III-R Axis II
    criteria, 37
Patient Rejection Scale, 46
Patient sample, inpatient family
    intervention, 136, 137
    heterogeneity, 151
Personality disorders, family/
    interpersonal context, 10–12; *see
    also* Borderline personality
    disorder *entries*
Personal resources, 10–13
Pharmacologic and inpatient family
    therapy, combined, 115, 153–
    171
    adjustment disorder, 155
    alcohol dependence, 155
    bipolar disorder, 153–155, 167
    case examples, 165–170
        broader family pathology, 167,
        168
        freeing family of severely
        depressed patients, 168–170
        minimal family pathology, 166,
        167
        rapid response to treatment, 165,
        166
    depression, major, 153, 155, 156
    education, 159, 167
    Family Assessment Device, 155,
    156
    Global Assessment Scale, 157
    heterogeneity of clinical problems,
    115, 163–165
    men, 154

pharmacologic approach, 157, 158, 167
    monoamine oxidase inhibitors, 159
    tricyclic antidepressants, 156, 159, 169
    problem-centered systems therapy of
    family, 159–163
    schizophrenia, 155, 156
    women, 154, 156
    see also specific drugs
Pharmacologic treatment, research
    issues, 245, 246
Phenothiazines, 178
Planning of week, cognitive–behavioral
    marital therapy, 80
"Playing the Manic Game" (Janowsky
    et al.), 181
Pleasant Events Schedule, 43
Prevention, affective disorders, 129–132
    case, 130
    communication skills, 131
Primary affective disorders, 10
Problem-centered systems therapy of
    family, 159–163
Problem definition
    cognitive–behavioral marital therapy,
    70, 72, 73
    strategic marital therapy in
    depression, 101
Problem-solving
    behavioral family therapy, 119, 126,
    129, 131
        six-step approach, 126, 131
    cognitive and marital interventions
    in depression, 67, 73, 81
    deficits, depression, 62
    maladaptive, assessment, 47
    problem-centered systems therapy of
    family, 160
Psychiatric Evaluation Form, 140, 143,
    145, 147
Psychoanalysis, 214n, 225
    on mania, 174, 180, 184
Psychosocial diagnostics, 247

Q

Quaalude abuse, 141, 144

R

Rapid management, mania, 217
Rapid response to treatment,
    pharmacologic and inpatient
    family therapy, combined, 165,
    166
Reasons for Living Inventory, 41
Recurrent depression. *See* Unipolar
    depression, recurrent
Reframing, strategic marital therapy in
    depression, 90, 103, 106, 107,
    109, 110
REM markers, depression, 210
Renegotiation, relationship, strategic
    marital therapy in depression,
    94, 95, 104
Research Diagnostic Criteria, 35
Research issues, 239, 241–248
    assessment tool development, 244
    clinical data, importance, 243
    clinical trials with and without
        pharmacotherapy, need for, 245, 246
    depression, interpersonal and
        behavior models, 243
    diagnostic and assessment
        procedures, family- or couple-
        relevant, 246, 247
    dismantling strategies, 245
    observation, controlled, 244
    pharmacologic treatment, 245, 246
    systems vs. elements, 242
    treatment design, 243
    treatment, "manualization" of, 244
Responsiveness, affective, problem-
    centered systems therapy of
    family, 160
Restless, agitated behavior,
    intervention, 127, 128
Restraining maneuvers, strategic
    marital therapy in depression,
    102, 103
Role Performance and Treatment
    Scale, 139, 140
Roles, family, problem-centered
    systems therapy of family, 160
Rush, John, 241

S

Schedule for Affective Disorders, 33,
    35
Schematic thinking, 65
Schizoaffective disorder, 201
    assessment, 32
    psychiatric genetics, 201
Schizophrenia, 115, 183, 184
    cf. affective disorder, DSM-III-R,
        213, 214
    behavioral family therapy in affective
        disorders, 129
    cf. bipolar illness, 175, 176
    cf. borderline personality disorder,
        family intervention, 224, 225
    double-bind communication, 5
    and family therapy, 5–7
        expressed emotion, 6, 19
        systems theories, 5, 6
    inpatient family intervention in
        affective disorders, 134, 135, 150
    pharmacologic and inpatient family
        therapy, combined, 155, 156
    psychiatric genetics, 201, 204–206
Self-Control Questionnaire, 39
Self-enhancing illusory cognitive style, 66
Self-statements, negative, intervention,
    128
Sexual Interaction Inventory, 44, 45
Skill deficits, depression, 56
Sleep, REM markers, 210
Social Adjustment Scale–Self-Report,
    33, 40, 45
Social anxiety, DSM-III-R Axis II
    criteria, 37
Social skills, 12
    assessment, 40
    poor, intervention, 23
Social support, 15
    couples, cognitive–behavioral marital
        therapy, 77
Socratic questioning of nondepressed
    spouse, 75
Spouse
    demands/criticism, strategic marital
        therapy in depression, 103, 104

Spouse (*continued*)
  family/interpersonal context,
    affective disorders, 19
  nondepressed, Socratic questioning
    of, 75
Spouse Observation Checklist, 44
  Pleasing and Displeasing, 45
Strategic marital therapy in depression,
    51, 72*n*, 89–111
  classification of affective disorders,
    biology and, 90–93
  conceptualizing depression in marital
    context, 93–95
  daily stress, 93
  divorce as solution, 110, 111
  extratherapy task assignments, 97,
    99–101, 105, 109, 110
  intervention, focused, and specific
    agenda, 100–110
    anger, spouse, 107
    coping tasks, 101, 102
    frustration, spouse, 107
    goal definitions, 101
    hostile reaction, avoiding, 107, 108
    noxious behavior negotiation, 108,
      109
    problem definitions, 101
    renegotiation, relationship, 94, 95,
      104
    restraining maneuvers, 102, 103
    spouse demands/criticism, 103,
      104
    time-limitations, 98
    working with couple, 108–110
    working with depressed person,
      100–105
    working with spouse, 105–108
  interview, initial, 97–100
  rationale for working with each
    partner separately, 95–97
    vs. conjoint, 95
  reframing, 90, 103, 106, 107, 109, 110
  women, depressed, 92, 94, 95, 101,
    103
Stress
  daily, and strategic marital therapy,
    93

and depression, 92
  spouse's, intervention, 128
  vulnerability, and family coping
    behavior, 118, 119
Stressful life circumstances, 13–16, 21
Structural Analysis of Social Behavior,
    36
Structured Clinical Interview for
    DSM-III-R, 33, 35, 36
Suicide
  attempt, 102, 165, 167–170
  genetic issues in treatment of
    depression, 203, 204, 207
  potential, assessment, 40, 41
Suicide, depression and, family
    intervention, 116, 213, 215, 229–
    234
  case example, 233, 234
  developmental history, 231, 232
  multisystem containment
    interpretation, 232
  suicidal intent, 231
    indirect communication, 233
  support system, current status, 232
Suicide Intent Scale, 33, 40
Support system, current status, suicide
    and depression, family
    intervention, 232
Symptom management
  behavioral family therapy in affective
    disorders, 126–128
  borderline personality disorder,
    family intervention, 228, 229
Systemic couples, cognitive–behavioral
    marital therapy, 77
Systems vs. elements, research issues, 242

T

Therapeutic alliance with family
    members, behavioral family
    therapy, 121
Thinking, schematic, 65
Thioridazine, 128
Thoughts, automatic, 65
  questionnaire, 39

Time
  and cost considerations, family/
    interpersonal context,
    assessment, 30
  limitations, and initial interview, 98
Tranylcypromine, 209
Trazodone, 158
Treatment design/planning
  depression, differential, 42
  genetic issues, depression, 207–209
  inpatient family intervention, 138,
    139, 141, 142
  integrativeness of, 235, 236
  "manualization" of, research issues,
    244
  and psychopathology, 236, 237
  research issues, 243
Tricyclic antidepressants. *See under*
  Antidepressants
Twin studies, depressive disorders, 200,
  202, 203, 207

U

Unemployment, 118, 166
Unipolar depression, recurrent, 213,
  215, 220–224
  antidepressants, 223, 224
  case example, 223, 224
  inpatient family intervention, 135,
    137, 140–142, 146, 148–151

narcissistic disequilibrium
    disturbance, 221
  parenting of therapist by depressive,
    222
  psychiatric genetics, 199–203
United States, 6
  depression prevalence, 3, 10
Unpleasant Events Schedule, 43

V

Verbal Problem Checklist, 43
Videotape, 167
Vietnam War, 142

W

Winokur, G., 208
Women
  combined pharmacologic and
      inpatient family therapy, 154,
      156
  depressed, 17, 18
    attention from spouse, 80, 81
    strategic marital therapy, 92, 94,
      95, 101, 103
  urban, in relationship with male,
      stressful life circumstances,
      15

DATE DUE

NOV 2 9 2006			
GAYLORD			PRINTED IN U.S.A.